Imaging of Diffuse Lung Disease

Editor

STEPHEN HOBBS

RADIOLOGIC CLINICS OF NORTH AMERICA

www.radiologic.theclinics.com

Consulting Editor
FRANK H. MILLER

November 2022 • Volume 60 • Number 6

ELSEVIER

1600 John F. Kennedy Boulevard • Suite 1800 • Philadelphia, Pennsylvania, 19103-2899

http://www.theclinics.com

RADIOLOGIC CLINICS OF NORTH AMERICA Volume 60, Number 6
November 2022 ISSN 0033-8389, ISBN 13: 978-0-323-98729-5

Editor: John Vassallo (j.vassallo@elsevier.com)
Developmental Editor: Karen Solomon

Radiologic Clinics of North America (ISSN 0033-8389) is published bimonthly by Elsevier Inc., 360 Park Avenue South, New York, NY 10010-1710. Months of issue are January, March, May, July, September, and November. Periodicals postage paid at New York, NY and additional mailing offices. Subscription prices are USD 529 per year for US individuals, USD 1335 per year for US institutions, USD 100 per year for US students and residents, USD 624 per year for Canadian individuals, USD 1362 per year for Canadian institutions, USD 717 per year for international individuals, USD 1362 per year for international institutions, USD 100 per year for Canadian students/residents, and USD 315 per year for international students/residents. To receive student and resident rate, orders must be accompanied by name of affiliated institution, date of term and the signature of program/residency coordinatior on institution letterhead. Orders will be billed at individual rate until proof of status is received. Foreign air speed delivery is included in all *Clinics* subscription prices. All prices are subject to change without notice. **POSTMASTER:** Send address changes to *Radiologic Clinics of North America*, Elsevier Health Sciences Division, Subscription Customer Service, 3251 Riverport Lane, Maryland Heights, MO63043. **Customer Service: Telephone: 1-800-654-2452** (U.S. and Canada); **1-314-447-8871** (outside U.S. and Canada). **Fax: 1-314-447-8029. E-mail: journalscustomerservice-usa@elsevier.com (for print support); journalsonlinesupport-usa@elsevier.com (for online support)**.

Reprints. For copies of 100 or more of articles in this publication, please contact the Commercial Reprints Department, Elsevier Inc., 360 Park Avenue South, New York, New York 10010-1710. Tel.: +1-212-633-3874; Fax: +1-212-633-3820; E-mail: reprints@elsevier.com.

Radiologic Clinics of North America also published in Greek Paschalidis Medical Publications, Athens, Greece.

Radiologic Clinics of North America is covered in *MEDLINE/PubMed (Index Medicus), EMBASE/Excerpta Medica, Current Contents/Life Sciences, Current Contents/Clinical Medicine, RSNA Index to Imaging Literature, BIOSIS, Science Citation Index,* and *ISI/BIOMED.*

Contributors

CONSULTING EDITOR

FRANK H. MILLER, MD, FACR, FSAR, FSABI
Lee F. Rogers, MD, Professor of Medical
Education, Chief, Body Imaging Section and
Fellowship, Medical Director, MRI, Professor,
Department of Radiology, Northwestern
Memorial Hospital, Northwestern University
Feinberg School of Medicine, Chicago, Illinois

EDITOR

STEPHEN HOBBS, MD, FSCCT
Associate Professor of Radiology and
Medicine, Vice-Chair, Radiology Informatics
and Integrated Clinical Operations, Chief,
Division of Cardiovascular and Thoracic
Radiology, Medical Director, UK HealthCare
Imaging Informatics, University of Kentucky,
Lexington, Kentucky

AUTHORS

AYODEJI ADEGUNSOYE, MD
Assistant Professor, Section of Pulmonary and
Critical Care, Department of Medicine,
University of Chicago, Chicago, Illinois

WILLIAM F. AUFFERMANN, MD, PhD
Associate Professor of Radiology, Interim
Section Chief of Cardiothoracic Imaging,
Department of Radiology and Imaging
Sciences, University of Utah School of
Medicine, University of Utah Health, Salt Lake
City, Utah

MELISSA B. CARROLL, MD
Department of Radiology, University of Kansas
Medical Center, Kansas City, Kansas

CATO CHAN, MD
Resident, Cedars Sinai Imaging, Cedars Sinai
Medical Center, Los Angeles, California

JESSICA CHAN, MD
University of Utah Health, Salt Lake City, Utah

APEKSHA CHATURVEDI, MD
Department of Imaging Sciences, University of
Rochester Medical Center, Rochester, New
York

LYDIA CHELALA, MD
Assistant Professor, Department of Thoracic
Imaging, University of Chicago Medicine,
Chicago, Illinois

KATHERINE A. CHENG, MD
Department of Radiology, Duke University,
Duke University Medical Center, Durham,
North Carolina

CHRISTOPHER LEE, MD
Attending Physician, Cedars Sinai Imaging,
Cedars Sinai Medical Center, Los Angeles,
California

JONATHAN H. CHUNG, MD
Professor, Department of Thoracic Imaging,
University of Chicago Medicine, Chicago,
Illinois

BRITTANY A. CODY, MD
Fellow, Department of Pathology, University of Chicago Medicine, Chicago, Illinois

OLIVIA DIPRETE, MD
Department of Radiology, Beth Israel Deaconess Medical Center, Boston, Massachusetts

BASTIAAN DRIEHUYS, PhD
Professor, Department of Radiology, Duke University Medical Center, Durham, North Carolina

FLORIAN J. FINTELMANN, MD
Department of Radiology, Division of Thoracic Imaging and Intervention, Massachusetts General Hospital, Boston, Massachusetts

DANE A. FISHER, MD
Department of Radiology, Division of Thoracic Imaging and Intervention, Massachusetts General Hospital, Boston, Massachusetts

JEFFREY R. GALVIN, MD
Department of Diagnostic Radiology and Nuclear Medicine, University of Maryland, Baltimore, Maryland

FRANCIS G. GIRVIN, MD
Department of Radiology, NewYork-Presbyterian/Weill Cornel Medical Center, New York, New York

DANIEL B. GREEN, MD
Department of Radiology, NewYork-Presbyterian/Weill Cornel Medical Center, New York, New York

JAMES F. GRUDEN, MD, FCCP
Clinical Professor of Radiology, UNC School of Medicine, Department of Radiology, The University of North Carolina at Chapel Hill, Chapel Hill, North Carolina

ROBERT W. HALLOWELL, MD
Division of Pulmonology and Critical Care Medicine, Massachusetts General Hospital, Boston, Massachusetts

LIDA P. HARIRI, MD, PhD
Department of Pathology, Massachusetts General Hospital, Boston, Massachusetts

TRAVIS S. HENRY, MD
Department of Radiology, Duke University, Duke University Medical Center, Durham, North Carolina

ALIYA N. HUSAIN, MD
Professor, Department of Pathology, University of Chicago Medicine, Chicago, Illinois

KIMBERLY KALLIANOS, MD
Assistant Professor of Clinical Radiology, Department of Radiology and Biomedical Imaging, University of California, San Francisco, San Francisco, California

FLORENCE K. KEANE, MD
Department of Radiation Oncology, Massachusetts General Hospital, Boston, Massachusetts

SETH KLIGERMAN, MD
Professor, Division Chief of Cardiothoracic Radiology, University of California, San Diego, San Diego, California

MICHAEL LANUTI, MD
Department of Surgery, Division of Thoracic Surgery, Massachusetts General Hospital, Boston, Massachusetts

EDWARD Y. LEE, MD, MPH
Department of Radiology, Boston Children's Hospital, Boston, Massachusetts

GREGORY M. LEE, MD
Department of Diagnostic Radiology and Nuclear Medicine, University of Maryland, Baltimore, Maryland

DAVID A. LYNCH, MB, BCh
Professor, Department of Radiology, National Jewish Health, Denver, Colorado

JOSEPH MAMMARAPPALLIL, MD, PhD
Assistant Professor, Department of Radiology, Duke University Medical Center, Durham, North Carolina

H. PAGE MCADAMS, MD
Department of Radiology, Duke University, Duke University Medical Center, Durham, North Carolina

SYDNEY B. MONTESI, MD
Division of Pulmonology and Critical Care Medicine, Massachusetts General Hospital, Boston, Massachusetts

MEGHAN J. MOORADIAN, MD
Massachusetts General Hospital Cancer Center, Boston, Massachusetts

MARK C. MURPHY, MB, BCh, BAO
Department of Radiology, Division of Thoracic
Imaging and Intervention, Massachusetts
General Hospital, Boston, Massachusetts

DAVID P. NAIDICH, MD
Department of Radiology, NYU Langone
Medical Center, New York, New York

HOLLY NICHOLS, MD
Department of Radiology, Duke University,
Duke University Medical Center, Durham,
North Carolina

BRYAN O'SULLIVAN-MURPHY, MD, PhD
Assistant Professor, Department of Radiology,
Duke University Medical Center, Durham,
North Carolina

ANDREA S. OH, MD, Assistant Professor,
Department of Radiology, University of
California, Los Angeles, Los Angeles, California

VANESSA RAMEH, MD
Department of Radiology, Boston Children's
Hospital, Boston, Massachusetts

YASMEEN K. TANDON, MD
Assistant Professor of Radiology, Mayo Clinic
Department of Radiology, Rochester,
Minnesota

SARA O. VARGAS, MD
Department of Pathology, Boston Children's
Hospital, Boston, Massachusetts

CHRISTOPHER M. WALKER, MD
Department of Radiology, University of Kansas
Medical Center, Kansas City, Kansas

LARA WALKOFF, MD
Assistant Professor of Radiology, Mayo Clinic
Department of Radiology, Rochester,
Minnesota

LACEY WASHINGTON, MD
Department of Radiology, Duke University,
Duke University Medical Center, Durham,
North Carolina

ABBEY J. WINANT, MD
Department of Radiology, Boston Children's
Hospital, Boston, Massachusetts

Contents

 Video content accompanies this article at http://www.radiologic.theclinics.com.

The major role of imaging (CT) in usual interstitial pneumonia (UIP)/idiopathic pulmonary fibrosis (IPF) is in the initial diagnosis. We propose several modifications to existing guidelines to help improve the accuracy of this diagnosis and to enhance interobserver agreement. CT detects the common complications and associations that occur with UIP/IPF including acute exacerbation, lung cancer, and dendriform pulmonary ossification and is useful in informing prognosis based on baseline fibrosis severity. Serial CT imaging is a topic of great interest; it may identify disease progression before FVC decline or clinical change.

Interstitial lung abnormalities (ILAs) are specific computed tomography (CT) findings that are potentially compatible with interstitial lung disease (ILD) in patients without clinical suspicion for disease. ILAs are associated with adverse clinical outcomes including increased mortality, imaging progression and lung function decline, and increased lung injury risk with lung cancer therapies. It is expected that identification of ILAs will increase with implementation of lung cancer screening and diagnostic CT imaging for workup of other pathologies. As such, radiologists will play a critical role in the diagnosis and management of ILAs.

Hypersensitivity pneumonia (HP) refers to a heterogeneous group of interstitial lung diseases resulting from a non-IgE immune-mediated reaction to inhaled pathogens in susceptible and sensitized hosts. Environmental and genetic factors are important substrates of disease pathogenesis. A recurrent or ongoing airborne exposure results in activation of humoral and cellular immune responses. This article discusses key clinical, radiologic, and histopathologic features of HP and reviews current recommendations.

The majority of connective tissue diseases (CTDs) are multisystem disorders that are often heterogeneous in their presentation and do not have a single laboratory, histologic, or radiologic feature that is defined as the gold standard to support a specific diagnosis. Given this challenging situation, the diagnosis of CTD is a process that requires the synthesis of multidisciplinary data which may include patient clinical symptoms, serologic evaluation, laboratory testing, and imaging. Pulmonary manifestations of connective tissue disease include interstitial lung disease as well as multicompartmental manifestations. These CT imaging patterns and features of specific diseases will be discussed in this article.

Acute lung injury (ALI) exists on a continuum that includes diffuse alveolar damage, acute fibrinous and organizing pneumonia, and organizing pneumonia. The primary site of injury in ALI is the same, which likely explains similar imaging patterns across the pathologic spectrum. Radiologic outcomes in ALI depend on the degree of injury and the subsequent healing response. Although ALI can heal without permanent injury, development of fibrosis is not uncommon and may be debilitating. ALI is associated with the usual interstitial pneumonia and nonspecific interstitial pneumonia patterns of fibrosis and repeated episodes of ALI are likely a cause of fibrosis progression.

Lung injury associated with smoking tobacco or other substances results in a variety of clinical presentations and imaging patterns, depending on mechanism of injury and substance inhaled. Patients may present in the acute setting, as in the case of acute eosinophilic pneumonia, e-cigarette or vaping product use–associated lung injury, crack lung, or heroin inhalation. They may present with subacute shortness of breath and demonstrate findings of pulmonary Langerhans cell histiocytosis, respiratory bronchiolitis, or desquamative interstitial pneumonia. Alternatively, they may present with chronic dyspnea and demonstrate findings of emphysema or smoking-related interstitial lung fibrosis.

Diffuse cystic lung disease refers to multiple rounded lucencies or low-attenuating areas with well-defined interfaces with normal lung. Parenchymal lucencies, such as cavitary disease, may mimic cystic lung disease. Cystic lung disease generally has a nonspecific presentation. Pulmonary cysts may present in isolation or with ancillary imaging features, such as ground-glass opacities or nodules. Clinical features, such as connective tissue disease, can narrow the differential diagnosis. In cases with indeterminate imaging and clinical features, open lung biopsy should be considered. Ultrarare cystic lung diseases, such as light chain deposition disease, can mimic more common diseases.

Mosaic attenuation pattern is commonly encountered on high-resolution computed tomography and has myriad causes. These diseases may involve small airways, vessels, alveoli, or interstitium, with some involving compartmental combinations. Small airways disease is caused by cellular bronchiolitis, infiltrated by inflammatory cells or constrictive bronchiolitis, resulting in fibrosis of the small airways. Any acute or chronic cause of ground-glass opacity can result in a mosaic pattern. Vascular causes of mosaic attenuation include chronic thromboembolic pulmonary hypertension and rarely other causes of pulmonary arterial hypertension. Ancillary CT findings along with the clinical history help narrow the differential diangosis. Biopsy is uncommonly required for definitiive diagnosis.

Occupational lung diseases (OLDs) encompass a broad group of entities related to the inhalation of a variety of agents in the workplace. OLDs may affect the lung parenchyma, pleura, and/or airways. OLDs can pose a diagnostic challenge for radiologists due to a lack of exposure history and overlap in imaging findings with nonoccupational-related entities. For this reason, it is important for the radiologist to be familiar with the high-resolution computed tomography patterns associated with OLDs and consider OLDs when formulating a differential.

Interstitial lung disease (ILD) including idiopathic pulmonary fibrosis increases the risk of developing lung cancer. Diagnosing and staging lung cancer in patients with ILD is challenging and requires careful interpretation of computed tomography (CT) and fluorodeoxyglucose PET/CT to distinguish nodules from areas of fibrosis. Minimally invasive tissue sampling is preferred but may be technically challenging given tumor location, coexistent fibrosis, and pneumothorax risk. Current treatment options include surgery, radiation therapy, percutaneous thermal ablation, and systemic therapy; however, ILD increases the risks associated with each treatment option, especially acute ILD exacerbation.

Childhood interstitial lung disease (chILD) refers to a diverse group of rare diffuse parenchymal lung diseases affecting infants and children, previously associated with considerable diagnostic confusion due to a lack of information regarding their clinical, imaging, and histopathologic features. Due to improved lung biopsy techniques, established pathologic diagnostic criteria, and a new structured classification system, there has been substantial improvement in the understanding of chILD over the past several years. The main purpose of this article is to review the latest advances in the imaging evaluation of pediatric interstitial lung disease within the framework of the new classification system.

Patients with diffuse lung diseases require thorough medical and social history and physical examinations, coupled with a multitude of laboratory tests, pulmonary function tests, and radiologic imaging to discern and manage the specific disease. This review summarizes the current state of imaging of various diffuse lung diseases by hyperpolarized MR imaging. The potential of hyperpolarized MR imaging as a clinical tool is outlined as a novel imaging approach that enables further understanding of

Diffuse lung diseases are a heterogeneous group of disorders that can be difficult to differentiate by imaging using traditional methods of evaluation. The overlap between various disorders results in difficulty when medical professionals attempt to interpret images. Artificial intelligence offers new tools for the evaluation and quantification of imaging of patients with diffuse lung disease.

PROGRAM OBJECTIVE

The objective of the *Radiologic Clinics of North America* is to keep practicing radiologists and radiology residents up to date with current clinical practice in radiology by providing timely articles reviewing the state of the art in patient care.

TARGET AUDIENCE

Practicing radiologists, radiology residents, and other healthcare professionals who provide patient care utilizing radiologic findings.

LEARNING OBJECTIVES

Upon completion of this activity, participants will be able to:

1. Describe the complexity of interstitial lung disease and how imaging is utilized to help identify abnormalities, make a diagnosis, and creating an appropriate a course of treatment.
2. Discuss the value of a multidisciplinary approach to using imaging techniques, both conventional and novel, to support clinical manifestations of interstitial lung disease and identify mortality risk in patients across the life span.
3. Recognize imaging as a crucial diagnostic, prognostic, tracking disease progression, and management tool for interstitial lung disease.

ACCREDITATION

The Elsevier Office of Continuing Medical Education (EOCME) is accredited by the Accreditation Council for Continuing Medical Education (ACCME) to provide continuing medical education for physicians.

The EOCME designates this journal-based CME activity for a maximum of 13 *AMA PRA Category 1 Credit*(s)™. Physicians should claim only the credit commensurate with the extent of their participation in the activity.

All other healthcare professionals requesting continuing education credit for this enduring material will be issued a certificate of participation.

DISCLOSURE OF CONFLICTS OF INTEREST

The EOCME assesses conflict of interest with its instructors, faculty, planners, and other individuals who are in a position to control the content of CME activities. All relevant conflicts of interest that are identified are thoroughly vetted by EOCME for fair balance, scientific objectivity, and patient care recommendations. EOCME is committed to providing its learners with CME activities that promote improvements or quality in healthcare and not a specific proprietary business or a commercial interest.

The planning committee, staff, authors, and editors listed below have identified no financial relationships or relationships to products or devices they or their spouse/life partner have with commercial interest related to the content of this CME activity:

William F. Auffermann, MD, PhD; Melissa B. Carroll, MD; Cato Chan, MD; Jessica Chan, MD; Apeksha Chaturvedi, MD; Lydia Chelala; Katherine A. Cheng, MD; Jonathan Chung; Olivia DiPrete, MD; Bastiaan Driehuys, PhD; Florian J. Fintelmann, MD; Dane A. Fisher, MD; Jeffrey R. Galvin, MD; Francis G. Girvin, MD; Daniel B. Green, MD; James F. Gruden, MD, FCCP; Travis S. Henry, MD; Stephen B. Hobbs, MD; Kimberly Kallianos, MD; Florence K. Keane, MD; Seth Kligerman, MD; Pradeep Kuttysankaran; Michael Lanuti, MD; Christopher Lee, MD; Edward Y. Lee, MD, MPH; Gregory M. Lee, MD; David A. Lynch, MBBch; Joseph Mammarappallil, MD, PhD; H. Page McAdams, MD; Mark C. Murphy, MBBch, BAO; David P. Naidich, MD; Holly Nichols, MD; Andrea S. Oh, MD; Bryan O'Sullivan-Murphy, MD, PhD; Vanessa Rameh, MD; Yasmeen K. Tandon, MD; Doreen Thomas-Payne, MSN, BSN, RN, PMHNP-BC; Sara O. Vargas, MD; Lara Walkoff, MD; Lacey Washington, MD; Abbey J. Winant, MD.

The planning committee, staff, authors, and editors listed below have identified financial relationships or relationships to products or devices they or their spouse/life partner have with commercial interest related to the content of this CME activity:

Robert W. Hallowell, MD: Consultant: Boehringer Ingelheim, Genentech, Dynamed; Researcher: Boehringer Ingelheim, Regeneron, and Galapagos; Advisor: Boehringer Ingelheim

Lida P. Hariri, MD, PhD: Researcher: Boehringer Ingelheim; Consultant: Boehringer Ingelheim, Pliant Therapeutics, Bioclinica, Biogen Idec

Sydney B. Montesi, MD: Researcher: Merck, United Therapeutics, Pliant Therapeutics; Consultant: DevPro Biopharma, Gilead Sciences, Roche

Meghan J. Mooradian, MD: Consultant/Speaker: AstraZeneca, Bristol Myers Squibb, Istari Oncology, Nektar Therapeutics, Immunai

Christopher M. Walker, MD: Speaker: Boehringer Ingelheim

UNAPPROVED/OFF-LABEL USE DISCLOSURE

The EOCME requires CME faculty to disclose to the participants:

1. When products or procedures being discussed are off-label, unlabelled, experimental, and/or investigational (not US Food and Drug Administration [FDA] approved); and
2. Any limitations on the information presented, such as data that are preliminary or that represent ongoing research, interim analyses, and/or unsupported opinions. Faculty may discuss information about pharmaceutical agents that is outside of FDA-approved labelling. This information is intended solely for CME and is not intended to promote off-label use of these medications. If you have any questions, contact the medical affairs department of the manufacturer for the most recent prescribing information.

TO ENROLL

To enroll in the *Radiologic Clinics of North America* Continuing Medical Education program, call customer service at 1-800-654-2452 or sign up online at http://www.theclinics.com/home/cme. The CME program is available to subscribers for an additional annual fee of USD 356.00.

METHOD OF PARTICIPATION

In order to claim credit, participants must complete the following:
1. Complete enrolment as indicated above.
2. Read the activity.
3. Complete the CME Test and Evaluation. Participants must achieve a score of 70% on the test. All CME Tests and Evaluations must be completed online.

CME INQUIRIES/SPECIAL NEEDS

For all CME inquiries or special needs, please contact elsevierCME@elsevier.com.

RADIOLOGIC CLINICS OF NORTH AMERICA

SERIES OF RELATED INTEREST

Advances in Clinical Radiology
Available at: https://www.advancesinclinicalradiology.com/
Magnetic Resonance Imaging Clinics
Available at: https://www.mri.theclinics.com/
Neuroimaging Clinics
Available at: www.neuroimaging.theclinics.com
PET Clinics
Available at: www.pet.theclinics.com

THE CLINICS ARE AVAILABLE ONLINE!
Access your subscription at:
www.theclinics.com

Preface
Making Sense of Diffuse Lung Disease

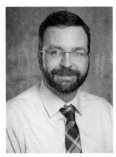

Stephen Hobbs, MD

Editor

Imaging evaluation of diffuse lung disease remains one of the most challenging areas in radiology. In fact, the mere mention of interstitial lung disease (ILD) is enough to turn an untold number of aspiring radiologists away from the entire subspecialty of chest imaging. Challenging cases frequently require multidisciplinary discussion to even arrive at a tentative diagnosis, but one key concept is found even in these difficult cases: imaging is critical. It's so critical that if you could only do one test to further evaluate a particular ILD case, high-resolution computed tomography (HRCT) is almost certainly the test to undergo. This makes a radiologist familiar with these diseases invaluable to their fellow pulmonologists, rheumatologists, and even thoracic surgeons.

This issue of *Radiologic Clinics of North America* updates the reader (both radiologists and nonradiologists alike) about the current concepts and best practices in imaging of ILD in both adults and children. Some diseases, like idiopathic pulmonary fibrosis and hypersensitivity pneumonitis, have recent guideline statements from multiple medical societies that help standardize our interpretation; others rely on decades of expert evaluation and

prior literature to guide our reporting. Some concepts, like that of interstitial lung abnormality, have only been introduced in the past few years, and others, like mosaic attenuation, are challenging for both novice and expert readers to consistently assess. Although HRCT remains the mainstay of evaluating these pathologic conditions for both adults and children, new advancements in MR imaging and machine learning are also addressed. Understanding the key points raised by these internationally recognized authors will give increased confidence to anyone tasked with reviewing these cases, myself included. I am greatly appreciative of the effort that these experts have given to this issue.

Stephen Hobbs, MD, FSCCT
Division of Cardiovascular and Thoracic
Radiology
Department of Radiology
University of Kentucky
800 Rose Street, HX 313B
Lexington, KY 40536, USA

E-mail address:
stephen.hobbs@uky.edu

Radiol Clin N Am 60 (2022) xv
https://doi.org/10.1016/j.rcl.2022.07.001
0033-8389/22/© 2022 Published by Elsevier Inc.

Current Imaging of Idiopathic Pulmonary Fibrosis

James F. Gruden, MD, FCCP[a],*, Daniel B. Green, MD[b], Francis G. Girvin, MD[b],
David P. Naidich, MD[c]

KEYWORDS

- Idiopathic pulmonary fibrosis • Usual interstitial pneumonia • Interstitial lung disease

KEY POINTS

- Current imaging (CT) is important in the initial diagnosis of usual interstitial pneumonia (UIP) (and therefore idiopathic pulmonary fibrosis [IPF]), and accurate, reproducible diagnostic criteria are crucial.
- Honeycombing (HC) and traction bronchiolectasis (Tb) represent a continuous spectrum of advanced fibrosis. Traction bronchiectasis occurs in advanced cases but is not a defining feature in UIP/IPF.
- The fibrosis in UIP/IPF is heterogeneous with normal lung, mild reticulation, and advanced fibrosis (Tb/HC) characteristically seen on the same image.
- CT identifies complications and associations of IPF including acute exacerbation, lung cancer, and dendriform pulmonary ossification.
- Serial CT may show disease progression before clinical or PFT change and could identify "rapid progressors" affecting clinical decision-making in patients with IPF and those with "indeterminate" UIP patterns.

 Video content accompanies this article at http://www.radiologic.theclinics.com.

INTRODUCTION

Idiopathic pulmonary fibrosis (IPF) is a "chronic, progressive, fibrosing interstitial pneumonia of unknown cause, occurring primarily in older adults, limited to the lungs and associated with the histopathological and/or radiological pattern of usual interstitial pneumonia (UIP)".[1] It represents a distinct clinical syndrome (idiopathic UIP) and is the most common of the idiopathic interstitial lung diseases.

UIP is a radiographic and pathologic pattern, not a diagnosis. Other entities associated with the UIP pattern must be excluded before an IPF diagnosis; these include occupational lung disease, connective tissue disorders, chronic hypersensitivity pneumonitis (CHP), or exposure to drugs known to cause pulmonary toxicity.[1] The relationship of CHP to UIP is controversial.

Radiologists have a critical role in the diagnosis and follow-up of patients with known or suspected IPF. This article focuses on the use of current imaging (CT) in the initial diagnosis with modifications to current diagnostic guidelines.[1,2] We will also discuss coincident findings and complications and briefly address the emerging role of serial

a Department of Radiology, University of North Carolina, Chapel Hill, NC 27599, USA; b Department of Radiology, New York Presbyterian-Weill Cornel Medical Center, New York, NY 10065, USA; c Department of Radiology, New York University-Langone Medical Center, 560 First Avenue, New York, NY 10016, USA
* Corresponding author. 101 Manning Drive, CB#7510, Chapel Hill, NC 27599.
E-mail address: james_gruden@med.unc.edu

Radiol Clin N Am 60 (2022) 873–888
https://doi.org/10.1016/j.rcl.2022.06.012

scanning in clinical practice. Focus will be on information new since recent reviews.[3,4]

CLINICAL FEATURES

IPF is more common in men and usually affects adults in their 60s and 70s. The majority are current or former smokers, although familial forms exist with an earlier age at onset and more aggressive clinical course.[5,6] Typical signs and symptoms include progressive dyspnea, dry cough, and bibasilar crackles on chest auscultation. Pulmonary function tests (PFTs) show restriction with reduced lung volumes and diffusing capacity. Disease behavior is variable; most patients have a stable or slowly progressive course, whereas others deteriorate rapidly.[7]

PATHOGENESIS

IPF is characterized by the deposition of fibrous tissue in the interstitium and alveolar walls resulting in reduced lung volume, architectural distortion, and impaired gas exchange. This is a response to repetitive injury from external insults (smoking, gastroesophageal reflux, infection, or others) followed by aberrant tissue repair possibly influenced by age or genetic predisposition.[8,9]

CURRENT IMAGING IN IDIOPATHIC PULMONARY FIBROSIS: TECHNIQUE

Multidetector CT enables volumetric imaging of the lungs during a single breath hold. Contiguous thin sections (1–2 mm) are routine in practice. Both sets of the most recent diagnostic guidelines discuss appropriate CT technique in detail.[1,2]

Prone images are especially important in lower-lung predominant processes such as UIP as dependent atelectasis can mimic or obscure true pathology. . We also routinely obtain sagittal reformatted images to evaluate disease distribution. Expiratory imaging may be helpful in patients with inhalational exposures or who have suspected hypersensitivity pneumonitis but may be confusing in UIP and its utility is not clear (see below).

CURRENT IMAGING IN IDIOPATHIC PULMONARY FIBROSIS: DIAGNOSIS
Current Guidelines for Diagnosis

The current ATS/ERS/JRS/ALAT and Fleischner Society guidelines each propose 4 categories in suspected UIP; the main alteration in both is that the "possible UIP" pattern is replaced with the new categories of "probable" and "indeterminate"

for UIP.[1,2] Both sets of guidelines emphasize the same CT findings with minor differences.

Definite usual interstitial pneumonia
The criteria for "definite" UIP remain essentially unchanged since 2011: CT findings include sub-pleural and basal predominant reticulation with honeycombing (HC) with or without peripheral traction bronchiectasis (TB) or bronchiolectasis (Tb). There should not be findings that suggest an alternative diagnosis (Fig. 1, Video 1).[1,2]

HC is defined by the Fleischner Society as "clustered cystic air spaces in a subpleural location, typically of comparable diameters of the order of 3 to 10 mm, but occasionally as large as 2.5 cm."[10] We suggest updates to this definition to require shared walls and include the vertical stacking of subpleural cysts.[11] Some investigators consider a single subpleural row of 2 to 3 contiguous cysts adequate for diagnosis; both sets of guidelines endorse this definition despite the lack of any proof of accuracy and this can cause difficulties distinguishing HC from paraseptal emphysema (see below).[1,2,12]

Both sets of guidelines now add that the "distribution is often heterogeneous" referring to the zonal distribution (upper, mid, lower). However, it is the actual appearance of the fibrosis on a single image that defines heterogeneity.[3,13] This key diagnostic feature of UIP is addressed in detail below.

Probable usual interstitial pneumonia
The new designation of "probable" UIP recognizes that UIP/IPF is likely when Tb is present with the other features of "definite" UIP in the absence of HC.[14,15] Airway dilatation is predominantly peripheral (outer 1–2 cm) in UIP/IPF and represents predominantly Tb rather than TB. Although TB occurs in advanced cases, Tb is the hallmark of UIP.

The distinction between "definite" and "probable" UIP is subjective. Dilated bronchioles should be separated from one another and from the pleura by lung parenchyma and have no shared walls. However, areas of Tb are pulled together by the advancing fibrosis and may not have a demonstrable connection to the more central airways due to this distortion such that differentiation between severe Tb and mild HC is difficult (Fig. 2). The current guidelines minimize this challenge; surgical biopsy is no longer required for diagnosis of either "definite" or "probable" UIP in the proper clinical setting (although the ATS/ERS/JRS/ALAT guidelines are less definitive in this regard).[1,2,16]

Indeterminate for usual interstitial pneumonia
The pattern of "indeterminate for UIP" is appropriate when CT demonstrates features of fibrosis

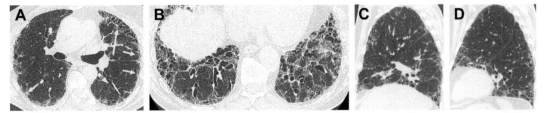

Fig. 1. (A–D) A 78-year-old man with "definite" UIP. Video shows peripheral reticulation (arrows in A) with HC and a basilar predominance. Round subpleural cystic spaces of uniform size with shared walls in vertical stacks of 2 to 3 represent HC (long arrows A, B). Sagittal reformatted images through the right (C) and left (D) lung better demonstrate the peripheral and basilar distribution of HC compared with (B).

but does not meet ""definite" or "probable" UIP criteria and does not suggest a specific alternative diagnosis. It is characterized by peripheral and basal predominant reticulation without "significant" TB/Tb or HC; there may be ground glass opacity (GGO) if it is superimposed on the reticulation (which also represents fibrosis).[2] Some of these cases overlap with the recently defined "early interstitial lung abnormality" (ILA)[17] (Fig. 3). Some may show UIP on surgical biopsy or may

evolve into a ""definite" or "probable" UIP pattern but there is no way to predict clinical course in the individual (Fig. 4).

Alternative diagnosis
Previously labeled as "inconsistent with UIP," the "alternative diagnosis" category includes CT findings that suggest a different specific non-UIP ILD.[18] Other patients have imaging findings that preclude a "typical" or "probable" UIP designation but who also lack other disease-specific ILD

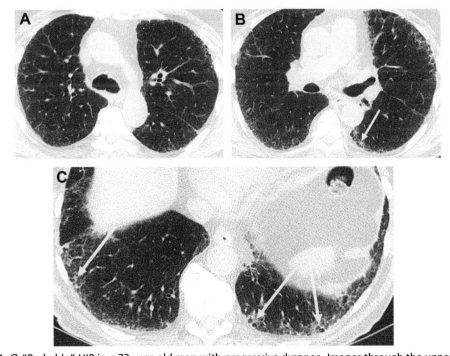

Fig. 2. (A–C) "Probable" UIP in a 72-year-old man with progressive dyspnea. Images through the upper (A), middle (B) and lower (C) lung zones demonstrate peripheral reticulation with a lower zone predominance and areas of Tb; some observers would interpret some areas as HC with 2 or more cystic spaces sharing walls in a horizontal subpleural location (arrows in B, C). This is definition of HC is not universally applied. Tb and HC represent a continuous spectrum of advanced fibrosis.

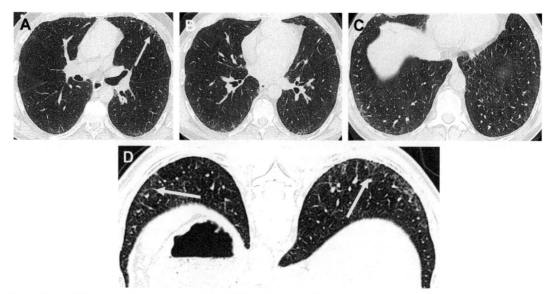

Fig. 3. (*A–D*) CT findings "indeterminate" for UIP in a 59-year-old asymptomatic man with a strong family history of IPF. Images through the upper (*A*), middle (*B, C*), and prone image through the lower (*D*) lung demonstrate very mild peripheral reticulation (*arrow in A*) and both lower lobes confirmed on prone images (*arrows in D*). There is no Tb or HC. Pulmonary function tests were normal. This lies within the spectrum of early interstitial lung abnormality; ultimate clinical course in difficult to predict.

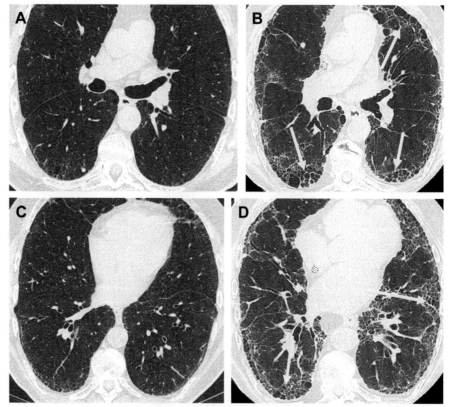

Fig. 4. (*A–D*) Disease progression from 'indeterminate" to "typical" UIP. Images through the middle and lower lung zones at baseline (*A, C*) and 4 years later (*B, D*). At baseline, there is peripheral, bilateral reticulation without HC or Tb and mild centrilobular emphysema. Worsening peripheral reticulation with extensive HC is present (*arrows in B, D*). The patient died of respiratory failure 2 years later.

features.[1,2] These "atypical" findings are subjective, and neither guideline set specifies when a change from "typical" or "probable" UIP to "alternative diagnosis" is appropriate (Video 2).

Guideline Clarifications and Proposed Modifications

A major limitation to guideline application in practice is the variation among readers.[19] We propose modifications that may improve the consistency and reproducibility of CT interpretation and reduce false-negative and false-positive " "definite" or "probable" UIP diagnoses; these criteria are expanded from a prior report[3] (Box 1).

Issue #1: overemphasis on honeycombing and resultant incorrect interpretations

Both guidelines emphasize HC despite confusion in definition. There is poor interobserver agreement as to the presence of HC, including in IPF.[20,21] HC also occurs on other ILDs.

Without emphasis on other imaging features, paraseptal emphysema and bronchiectasis or bronchiolectasis (not ILD-related) can be misinterpreted as HC and result in erroneous characterizations of ""definite" or "probable" UIP (Fig. 5). The distinction between Tb and TB is also important: TB without Tb or HC suggests a diagnosis other than UIP.[22]

Box 1
Current imaging Features of Confident Usual Interstitial Pneumonia

- Peripheral reticulation with lobular distortion and a nonsegmental distribution (crosses fissures).

- There must be some upper lobe involvement[a] but distribution variable and can be lower, diffuse or midzone predominant.

- HC and/or Tb (not TB) in more than one location.

- Heterogeneous appearance.[b]

- Mosaic attenuation or air trapping alone do not exclude confident diagnosis unless this is the dominant finding and other atypical feartures are also present.

[a] The upper lobes are never normal in UIP. A diffuse or midlung predominance of the peripheral fibrosis does not preclude a confident diagnosis. Asymmetry is permitted if "confident" findings are present in each lung. Peribronchovascular fibrosis or more TB than Tb suggests an alternative diagnosis.[b] Within the outer 1 to 2 cm of the parenchyma, where the abnormalities in UIP are located, there is normal lung, mild reticulation, and advanced fibrosis (HC and/or Tb) all on the same image.

Proposed solution HC and Tb represent a continuous spectrum of advanced fibrosis and aberrant repair.[23] Both correlate with the extent of active fibroblastic foci on histology.[24] As IPF progresses, distal bronchioles dilate and become tortuous due to retractile fibrosis resulting in radiographic HC.[25] Staats and colleagues reported that the degree of HC on CT correlates with histopathological Tb in explanted lungs.[26] It is Tb, not TB, that is in the spectrum of advanced fibrosis as HC. This is an important distinction.

We propose strict adherence to the criteria in **Box 1**. All findings must be present to enable confident diagnosis—not just HC or Tb. Hobbs and colleagues also emphasize the importance of other findings of fibrosis to differentiate HC from other entities, especially paraseptal emphysema.[16]

The modified guidelines consolidate "definite" and "probable" UIP into a "confident" UIP category to eliminate the focus on the subjective finding of HC. HC or Tb must be present without distinction between the two. TB is not a defining feature of UIP and is eliminated altogether as a criterion.

The abnormalities are peripheral and basilar predominant but some upper lobe involvement is essential.[13] Hunninghake and colleagues found that the findings most predictive of UIP were basal-predominant HC and reticulation in the upper lobes.[26] The Fleischner guidelines reference "common" upper lobe involvement but not as an essential feature.[2] Nonsegmental involvement (crossing fissures) without regard for bronchopulmonary anatomy is characteristic of UIP. Segmental or multisegmental peripheral scarring, even with a lower lobe predominance, may be related to prior infection or aspiration (Fig. 6). Reticulation must also be associated with lobular distortion (shrunken, triangular instead of polyhedral, not of uniform size or shape).

We emphasize the heterogeneous appearance of the peripheral findings. In the outer 1 to 2 cm of the lung, normal parenchyma alternates with reticulation and areas of Tb/HC (advanced fibrosis). This heterogeneity is characteristic of UIP especially in the setting of IPF[3] (Figs. 7 and 8). The current guidelines emphasize heterogeneity of distribution rather than of appearance.[1,2]

Our proposed modifications apply to UIP specifically due to IPF; some variation in disease patterns are recognized within the broader category of UIP including "exuberant HC" in patients with connective tissue disease compared with IPF[27] (Fig. 9).

Issue #2: guideline subjectivity
Both guidelines use subjective language. The "indeterminate" for UIP pattern, for example, lacks "significant" TB/Tb/HC. There is no clarification

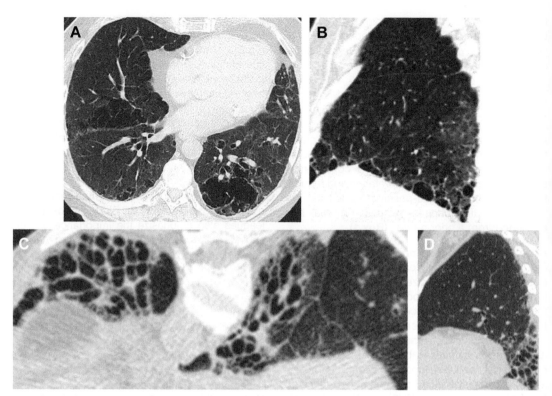

Fig. 5. (*A–D*) Three patients referred with false-positive diagnoses of "definite" UIP suspected basilar HC. Areas of paraseptal emphysema are present in the right middle lobe anterior to the oblique fissure and in both bases (*A*). A sagittal reformatted image in a different patient (*B*) shows paraseptal emphysema (similar to HC, it is peripheral, subpleural thin-walled cystic spaces that share walls) with superimposed homogeneous GGO. This represents smoking-related interstitial fibrosis (also called airspace enlargement with fibrosis). Prone (*C*) and right sagittal reformatted image (*D*) in a 58-year-old man shows cystic bronchiectasis in the posterior basilar segment of both lungs. The patient had a history of severe GERD and chronic acid aspiration. Application of the criteria in **Box 1** would avoid these false-positive diagnoses. GERD, gastroesophageal reflux disease.

regarding the meaning of "significant." Is one image with Tb of HC enough? Other subjective modifiers lead to inconsistency in application. For example, the Fleischner guidelines state that "some degree of upper lung involvement is usual" and "sometimes the craniocaudal distribution may be relatively uniform" and the "distribution may be asymmetric in up to 25% of cases."[2] The lack of clarity in the meaning of these terms and their impact on classification of the individual patient is problematic in clinical practice. We find that more than asymmetry or nonbasilar distribution, it is peribronchovascular involvement often with GGO superimposed on reticulation with TB that suggests an alternative

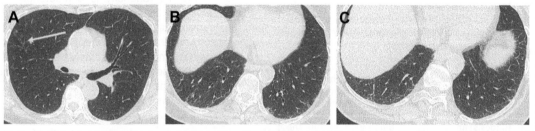

Fig. 6. (*A–C*) False-positive "probable" UIP. Images through the mid (*A*) and lower (*B, C*) zones in a 71-year-old man with a history of GERD and chronic cough. There is mild bronchial and bronchiolar wall thickening (*arrow* in *A*) and bronchial wall thickening and mild bronchiectasis in both lower lobes (*B, C*) with reticulation confined to the posterior basilar segments. This multisegmental distribution is common is patients with chronic gastric acid aspiration. There is no upper lobe reticulation and no Tb or HC.

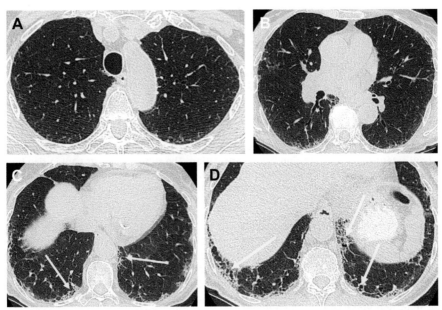

Fig. 7. (*A–D*) "Confident" UIP according to guidelines in **Box 1**. There is peripheral reticulation with lobular distortion with some upper lobe involvement (*A*), a nonsegmental distribution crossing the fissures (*B*), Tb and/or HC with a middle and lower zone predominance (*C, D*), and areas of normal lung, minimal reticulation, and advanced fibrosis (Tb/HC) all on the same image (*C, D*). The distinction between Tb and HC can be difficult (*arrows* in *C, D*) but is not diagnostically relevant.

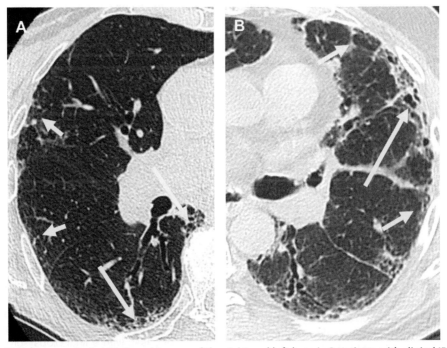

Fig. 8. (*A, B*) Heterogeneity in UIP. Coned images of the right and left lung in 2 patients with clinical IPF (A is the patient in **Fig. 8**). In the outer 1 to 2 cm, where the abnormalities of UIP are located, there is mild of reticulation (*small arrows*), Tb/HC (does not matter which, *long arrows*), and normal lung all on the same image. This heterogeneity—not in distribution but in appearance—is a hallmark of UIP/IPF.

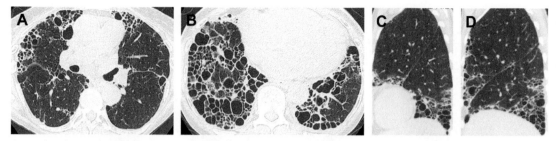

Fig. 9. (*A–D*) A 60-year-old woman with presumed UIP related to rheumatoid arthritis. Images through the lower lungs (*A, B*) show extensive HC without significant reticulation. The subpleural cysts vary in size but are mostly round and have thick walls (unlike paraseptal emphysema). Sagittal reformatted images through the left (*C*) and right (*D*) lungs show the basal and posterior distribution of the HC.

diagnosis especially when in the upper lung zones; this is mentioned in the guidelines but not emphasized or discussed in detail[1,2] (Video 3).

Proposed solution Although not founded in the literature, we propose that Tb/HC should be present at more than one location for a "confident" UIP diagnosis, provided all the other requirements for diagnosis are present (see **Box 1**). The impact of a non-lower zone predilection of the otherwise typical findings remains unclear. Our guidelines allow for asymmetry or a diffuse or midzone predominance on CT if the findings are otherwise characteristic although formal outcome studies in such patients are lacking. Peribronchovascular abnormalities, especially in the upper lobes, preclude a "confident" diagnosis and suggest alternative diagnoses (particularly CHP).

The threshold to move a case from one category to another is difficult to apply in clinical practice. In questionable cases, a repeat CT 6 to 12 months later may be helpful to reassess imaging findings and to identify patients with progression (see later discussion). This is particularly true in patients who have findings of suggestive of UIP but who ack Tb/HC. Patients with peripheral reticulation with some upper lobe involvement, a nonsegmental distribution, and a diffuse, midzone, or lower zone predominance are at high risk for UIP/IPF and likely differ from other patients with "early ILA." Again, further study of such patients is needed.

Issue #3: expiratory scanning, mosaic attenuation, and air trapping
There are many issues with expiratory scanning, and we will focus on a few that are especially problematic. First, there is no consistency in scan performance. Some centers do expiratory images at a few levels; others perform a contiguous low-dose helical acquisition with reduced z-axis coverage. Patient instructions vary. We tell the patient to "blow out a candle" (we find it results in stronger expiratory effort); other centers instruct patients

to "breathe out and hold it." Either way, there is no consistent quality control. The level of expiration varies widely from patient to patient and in the same patient over time.

Second, image interpretation is entirely subjective. Mild, moderate, or severe air trapping are not defined. We are left to analyze expiratory images of variable quality lacking clear interpretative criteria (**Fig. 10**).

Mosaic attenuation, or heterogeneous lung attenuation (HLA), is a finding on inspiratory CT in which the lung parenchyma has different attenuation, often at a lobular level, often associated with differences in the pulmonary arterial caliber between the more lucent and more dense zones. Mosaic attenuation can occur in the setting of pulmonary fibrosis, including UIP/IPF, due to compensatory lobular hyperinflation adjacent to areas of fibrosis (**Fig. 11**). Mosaic attenuation on inspiratory images does not mean that air trapping is present. Air trapping can only be diagnosed on expiratory imaging. The heterogeneous attenuation is accentuated: lobules or zones that trap air should become darker or stay the same density rather become more opaque on expiration.

Mosaic attenuation with air trapping can be present in some patients with features otherwise of "confident" UIP. However, it is not clear what amount of air trapping (if any) justifies a category change to "alternative diagnosis." It should be emphasized that the confident identification of air trapping diminishes as fibrosis becomes more extensive (and more in keeping with the ""definite" UIP pattern).[28] The actual incidence and extent of air trapping in patients with UIP/IPF, especially those who smoke, is unknown.

In a recent study, mosaic attenuation or air trapping was the source of CT-pathologic discordance in 72% of cases with a final biopsy-proven diagnosis of IPF.[28] Many surgical biopsies are being performed simply because mosaic attenuation alone suggests an "alternative" diagnosis.

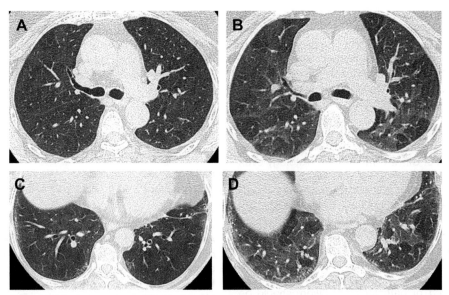

Fig. 10. (*A–D*) Asymptomatic 59-year-old woman with unspecified connective tissue disease. Inspiratory supine image through the midlung (*A*) and prone image through the bases (*C*) demonstrate very mild peripheral reticulation and GGO in the bases (*C*). There is a suggestion of mild mosaic attenuation. Expiratory images (*B, D*) show moderate-to-severe air trapping bilaterally. There was a minimal remote smoking history and PFTs showed mild restriction but no obstruction. The utility of expiratory scanning is controversial (see text).

Proposed solution As with the focus on HC, there is an overemphasis on mosaic attenuation. Quantification of a significant threshold is not well defined, interobserver agreement is poor, expiratory scanning technique is inconsistent, and patient compliance with breathing instructions is variable. Any real clinical value in excluding UIP/IPF is not proven. There should be a clear emphasis that mosaic attenuation (or HLA) on inspiratory images in patients with fibrotic lung disease does not imply air trapping. Most importantly, the presence of mosaic attenuation—with or without air trapping—should not preclude a diagnosis of "confident" UIP in a patient with otherwise

typical imaging findings unless the extent of air trapping is substantial and the dominant finding in comparison to the fibrosis or additional atypical features are present (such as peribronchovascular involvement) (see **Box 1**). Multidisciplinary discussion may be helpful in such instances.

Issue #4: the role of and reliance on surgical lung biopsy
Not all patients with UIP/IPF present with the "confident" CT findings. The Fleischer guidelines state that "up to 60% of cases that have UIP at surgical biopsy did not show a "typical" CT chest imaging pattern."[2] This is largely because of the

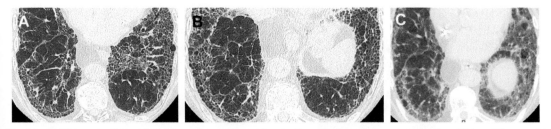

Fig. 11. (*A–C*) Images through the lung bases at end inspiration (*A, B*) and at end expiration (*C*) in a 77-year-old man with known IPF demonstrate peripheral, severe reticulation with Tb/HC with mosaic attenuation (heterogeneous lung attenuation); the secondary lobules adjacent to fibrotic zones seem hyperlucent and enlarged. This can occur in fibrotic lung disease, including IPF; no air trapping is visible on expiration (*C*). Mosaic attenuation does not mean that air trapping is present, and neither should discourage a "confident" UIP diagnosis (see Box 1).

confusion created by the Tb/HC distinction, atypical disease distribution, and the confusion surrounding mosaic attenuation and/or air trapping. These guidelines also state that "in the correct clinical setting, a diagnosis of IPF is not excluded by CT appearances more suggestive of other interstitial lung diseases such as nonspecific interstitial pneumonia (NSIP), CHP, or sarcoidosis."[2] This is confusing and implies that UIP can look like anything at all; the ATS guidelines also allow a diagnosis of UIP/IPF with proper histology even if the CT is not consistent with the diagnosis.[1] It is not at all clear that a CT diagnosis of sarcoidosis, for example, should be reclassified as IPF because a lung biopsy is interpreted as UIP. There is an over-reliance on the accuracy of the surgical lung biospy.

The ATS/ERS/JRS/ALAT guidelines do make an important point: the diagnosis of IPF, whether based on CT or pathologic condition, should be frequently reevaluated especially if clinical or radiographic findings are inconsistent with the diagnosis[1] (Fig. 12).

Proposed solution Multidisciplinary discussion may help in these problematic cases, although expertise in radiology, pathology, and clinical ILD is not uniformly available. These difficult cases are best described as "radiologically and pathologically discordant." Serial CT may be of benefit as patterns evolve with time and may become more diagnostically apparent. We hope that by using the guidelines in Box 1 and clarifying the issues above, a "confident" and accurate CT diagnosis of UIP will be more often possible.

CURRENT IMAGING IN IDIOPATHIC PULMONARY FIBROSIS: COMPLICATIONS AND ASSOCIATIONS

A thorough overview of the parenchymal complications of IPF is available.[29] We highlight a few of these that are common of particular importance.

Acute Exacerbations

Acute exacerbation (AE) is an acute respiratory deterioration due to an acceleration of IPF or as a response to external insult (infection, aspiration).[30] It can occur in patients with mild, moderate, or severe fibrosis at baseline. The histology of AE is diffuse alveolar damage.[30] Analysis of the placebo arms from 3 clinical trials showed that AE occurred only in patients not on antiacid therapy.[31] Mortality following AE is estimated to be more than 50%.[30]

CT shows areas of GGO and/or consolidation away from the fibrotic zones. The typical findings of UIP/IPF may be obscured by the acute process; occasionally, patients with IPF may initially present with AE.[32]

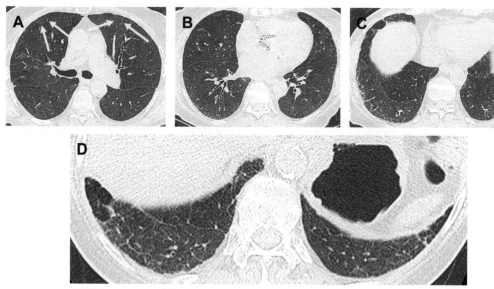

Fig. 12. (A–D) Supine images in an 86-year-old woman with clinical IPF after open lung biopsy showed UIP 15 years earlier. The upper lobe (A) shows bronchial wall thickening and mild interlobular septal thickening (arrows); the secondary lobules are normal in size and shape and not distorted. This could represent mild interstitial edema; she has coronary disease and recent transcatheter aortic valve replacement. Mild peripheral reticulation in the lower lobes (B–D) is confined to the posterior and lateral basilar segments. There is no Tb or HC. The findings are nonspecific and confined to the lung bases. Diagnoses of UIP/IPF should be periodically reevaluated.

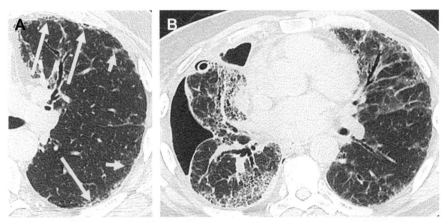

Fig. 13. (A, B) AE after lung biopsy in a 62-year-old man. Supine video through both lungs demonstrates marked asymmetry with minimal peripheral reticulation in the left lung with a few areas of Tb. Areas of GGO on the right are superimposed on intralobular lines and mild Tb indicating fibrosis. Despite the asymmetry, findings of "confident" UIP are present on the left (A). There is a heterogenous appearance with normal lung, mild reticulation (*small arrows*), and advanced fibrosis (in this case Tb, *large arrows*) all on the same image (A). Surgical biopsy showed UIP, and the clinical diagnosis was IPF. He developed AE and a chronic air leak on the right with subsequent empyema and had a prolonged hospital stay (B).

Acute respiratory deterioration after lung cancer resection in patients with IPF occurs in 7% to 32% of patients.[30] AE can also occur after surgical lung biopsy possibly related to the duration of the surgery, the use of high levels of oxygen, or barotrauma. The risk of postoperative AE should always be considered when referring patients with IPF to surgery (**Fig. 13**, Video 4).

Lung Cancer

Several factors may increase the risk of lung cancer in patients with IPF: age, gender, smoking status, and coexistent emphysema are associated with elevated risk.[33,34] Most cancers arise in a peripheral location either in the zones of fibrosis or in the immediately subjacent parenchyma, which may lead to a delay in recognition of these malignancies.[35]

The CT appearance, typically lobulated or spiculated nodules or areas of irregular consolidation or GGO, is difficult to distinguish from the progression of the underlying disease or superimposed infection or aspiration. Adenocarcinoma and squamous cell carcinoma are equally represented.[33] It is important to thoroughly analyze the peripheral zones of fibrosis for any new or progressive abnormalities; multiplanar reformatted images may be helpful in this regard (**Fig. 14**, Video 5).

Dendriform Pulmonary Ossification

Small dense (ossified) nodules within the areas of fibrosis may be present, located in the interlobular

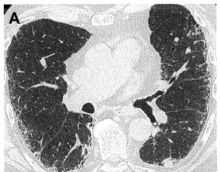
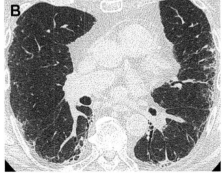

Fig. 14. (A, B) Video through both lungs in a 74-year-old man with IPF showing the difficulty detecting lung cancer that occurs in the zones of fibrosis. There is an adenocarcinoma in the posterior left lower lobe (A) that was overlooked on a prior 1 year earlier (B).

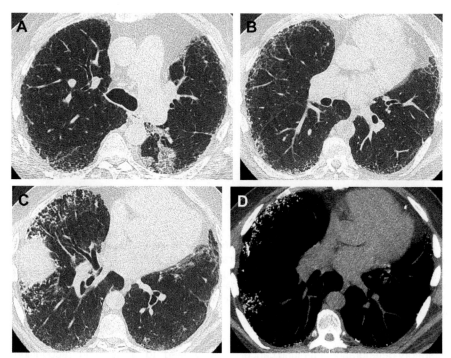

Fig. 15. (*A–D*) Lung cancer and DPO in an 80-year-old man with IPF. Axial (*A–C*) images show peripheral reticulation with a nonsegmental distribution; Tb/HC was present in the lower lugs (not shown). There is a nonsolid adenocarcinoma in the left lower lobe (*A*). Maximum intensity projection image with 8 mm collimation (*D*) demonstrates high attenuation micronodules in the subpleural region and interlobular septa. DPO occurs more frequently in UIP/IPF than in other ILDs.

septa and subpleural and perifissural regions.[36] These are more common in patients with UIP/IPF than other fibrotic lung diseases and are thought to represent a response to local acidosis or tissue injury; pulmonary macrophages or fibroblasts differentiate into osteoclasts and lay down mature bone (with marrow elements) in the peripheral pulmonary interstitium.[37] DPO in UIP/IPF is not clearly associated with severity or prognosis but its presence may be helpful in differential diagnosis (**Fig. 15**, Video 6). DPO also occurs without fibrosis in the setting of chronic gastric acid aspiration, and in some IPF patients, acid aspiration may also contribute to the presence of DPO, especially if the distribution of the dense nodules is asymmetric or in the lung bases rather than more diffusely in the lung periphery.[36]

CURRENT IMAGING IN IDIOPATHIC PULMONARY FIBROSIS: BASELINE DISEASE STAGING

Accurate assessment of disease severity in IPF is clinically and prognostically important but there is no staging system in clinical use. In general, the more severe the fibrosis (HC/Tb), the worse

the prognosis.[25,38–41] The overall "global assessment of interstitial abnormalities" also correlates with increased mortality.[42]

Unlike in oncology, where image-based staging dictates management strategy, CT-based staging is not yet routinely used in IPF; a staging system could improve the quality of information given to patients and may identify thresholds for initiating therapy with antifibrotic agents or listing for lung transplantation.[43] The problem is that in IPF, disease course in the individual patient is unpredictable based on a single CT examination.

CURRENT IMAGING IN IDIOPATHIC PULMONARY FIBROSIS: SERIAL CURRENT IMAGING AS A BIOMARKER

IPF is a disease that progresses in an unpredictable manner. pulmonary function tests (PFTs) are used to monitor and predict prognosis; an absolute decline in forced vital capacity (FVC) of 10% or greater or in diffusiing capacity (DLCO) of 15% or greater during 6 months defines "significant" disease progression.[44] A decline in FVC of 5% to 10% indicates possible progression but is within the range of measurement error. Limitations of pulmonary function testing include effort dependence and coexistent cardiopulmonary pathologic condition, particularly emphysema, present in a significant number of patients with IPF.

Serial change in CT features such as reticulation with architectural distortion and TB/Tb are predictors of mortality in patients with IPF[45,46] (Video 7). Oda and colleagues studied 98 patients with IPF using baseline CT and then at CT and PFTs 6 and 12 months later.[47] Two observers quantified the CT findings: reticulation, TB/Tb, HC, and normal lung. Scores were assigned with 1 for normal lung, 2 for reticulation, 3 for TB/Tb, and 4 for HC. The readers assessed upper, middle, and lower lung zones at predefined levels. In patients with no significant FVC decline, a CT fibrosis score higher than that at baseline heralded a worse prognosis. This is the first study showing that CT can identify a subset of patients with a stable FVC at 6 months with significant disease progression.[47] Serial change in Tb was found to predict mortality independent of FVC decline in another more recent investigation.[48] The overall extent of visible fibrosis and/or progression in severity (increasing Tb/HC) may be important biomarkers in patients with IPF indicating the need for antifibrotic therapy (in relatively mild disease) or placement on lung transplantation lists (**Fig. 16**). Further study is needed to determine if the rate of such change on CT is also important.

The precision, sensitivity, and absence of interobserver variability make quantitative CT (QCT) a logical substitute for subjective visual analysis. Quantifying subtle changes in CT features using computer analysis is also an attractive concept in an era of newly emerging drug therapies and is a topic for its own review.[49]

Current QCT has several limitations. It cannot effectively separate HC from TB, Tb, or emphysema (especially paraseptal) or bronchiectasis.. Therefore, the quantification of Tb/HC, the most important predictor of mortality and progression in IPF, remains a challenge. The distinction between true GGO and dependent atelectasis is problematic; prone images are not routinely used in QCT studies. The key contribution of QCT may be to identify subtle serial changes difficult for the radiologist to identify but the clinical significance of detecting such minimal change in a disease that has a natural history of progression remains unclear. Despite an overwhelming increase in published articles on this topic, QCT is not currently used in clinical practice. The appropriate focus of QCT—whether GGO, reticulation,

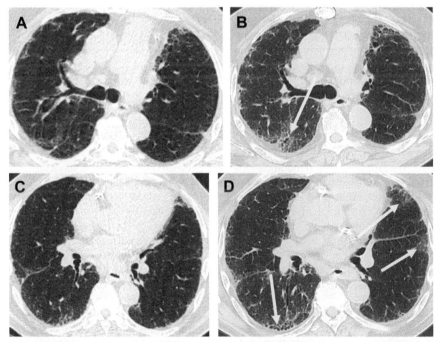

Fig. 16. (*A–D*) Rapid progression in a 64-year-old man with stable clinical symptoms and a marginal (5%) FVC decline. Baseline images (*A, C*) (3 mm collimation, standard reconstruction algorithm) and images 8 months later (*B, D*) show worsening reticulation and Tb in the posterior right lung (*arrows A and B*), and peripheral left lung and right base (*arrows in B and D*). Such rapid progression may indicate a poor prognosis and inform clinical management (see text).

Tb/HC, overall airway or lung volume, or another parameter—has also yet to be defined.

NEW DEVELOPMENT: THE PROGRESSIVE FIBROSING PHENOTYPE

ILDs other than IPF can cause progressive respiratory decline, recently termed the "progressive fibrosing phenotype."[50] IPF and other progressive fibrotic ILDs (PFILDs) may share similar self-sustaining patterns of fibrosis despite different initial insults. Patients with PFILD may have atypical imaging findings for UIP/IPF but also lack specific features diagnostic of other ILD. In clinical practice, a working diagnosis of either IPF or PFILD is currently sufficient for the prescription of antifibrotic therapy. Nintedanib and pirfenidone are the antifibrotic agents currently approved for the treatment of IPF; both slow the decline in FVC compared with placebo although neither reverses the disease. Nintedanib also showed a significant benefit in a clinical trial of patients with non-UIP/IPF PFILD and is now approved for the treatment of scleroderma-associated ILD and non-IPF PFILD[51]; the pirfenidone trial also showed benefit that was not quite statistically significant but this agent may alsoslow disease progression in non-IPF PFILD.[52] Lumping patients with similar disease behavior simplifies clinical management but further study is needed in this area, especially regarding long-term outcomes based on imaging patterns. The definition of IPF (requiring the UIP pattern) may undergo modification in the future possibly "lumping" IPF with other forms of PFILD with variable no documented histologic documentation.[52,53]

SUMMARY

The major current role of CT in UIP/IPF is in the initial diagnosis. We propose several modifications to existing guidelines to help improve accuracy of diagnosis and interobserver agreement and potentially reduce the need for surgical lung biopsies (see **Box 1**). CT detects the common complications and associations that occur with UIP/IPF including AE, lung cancer, and DPO and is useful in informing prognosis based on baseline fibrosis severity. Serial CT imaging is a topic of great interest; it may identify disease progression before FVC decline or clinical change. Evolving CT patterns in the short term may help serve as a biomarker identifying adverse long-term outcomes and informing clinical management, especially in patients with "indeterminate" patterns. The role and appropriate focus of QCT remains to be determined.

CRITICAL CARE POINTS

- The radiologist plays a key role in the initial diagnosis of UIP/IPF, and current guidelines are not always straightforward to apply in practice.
- False positive confident diagnoses must be avoided.
- CT is useful in monitoring patients with UIP/IPF, although the frequency and timing of such examinations is not established.

DISCLOSURE

The authors have nothing to disclose relevant to this project.

SUPPLEMENTARY DATA

Supplementary data related to this article can be found online at https://doi.org/10.1016/j.rcl.2022.06.012.

Note: all axial images are at 1.25 mm collimation using a high-frequency reconstruction algorithm unless otherwise specified; sagittal reformatted images are at 2.5 mm collimation with a standard (soft tissue) kernel.

REFERENCES

1. Raghu G, Remy-Jardin M, Myers JL, et al. American Thoracic Society, European Respiratory Society, Japanese Respiratory Society, and Latin American Thoracic Society. Diagnosis of idiopathic pulmonary fibrosis. An official ATS/ERS/JRS/ALAT clinical practice guideline. Am J Respir Crit Care Med 2018; 198(5):e44–68.
2. Lynch DA, Sverzellati N, Travis WD, et al. Diagnostic criteria for idiopathic pulmonary fibrosis: a Fleischner Society White Paper. Lancet Respir Med 2018; 6(2):138–53.
3. Gruden JF. CT in idiopathic pulmonary fibrosis: diagnosis and beyond. AJR Am J Roentgenol 2016;206(3):495–507.
4. Mohning MP, Richards JC, Huie TJ. Idiopathic pulmonary fibrosis: the radiologist's role in making the diagnosis. Br J Radiol 2019;92(1099):20181003.
5. Lee H-L, Ryu JH, Wittmer MH, et al. Familial idiopathic pulmonary fibrosis: clinical features and outcome. Chest 2005;127(6):2034–41.
6. Krauss E, Gehrken G, Drakopanagiotakis F, et al. Clinical characteristics of patients with familial idiopathic pulmonary fibrosis (f-IPF). BMC Pulm Med 2019;19:130.

7. Kim HJ, Perlman D, Tomic R. Natural history of idiopathic pulmonary fibrosis. Respir Med 2015;109(6): 661–70.

8. Wuyts WA, Agostini C, Antoniou KM, et al. The pathogenesis of pulmonary fibrosis: a moving target. Eur Respir J 2013;41(5):1207–18.

9. Lederer DJ, Martinez FJ. Idiopathic Pulmonary Fibrosis. N Engl J Med 2018;378:1811–23.

10. Hansell DM, Bankier AA, MacMahon H, et al. Fleischner Society: glossary of terms for thoracic imaging. Radiology 2008;246(3):697–722.

11. Johkoh T, Sakai F, Noma S, et al. Honeycombing on CT: its definitions, pathologic correlation, and future direction of its diagnosis. Eur J Radiol 2014;83: 27–31.

12. Jacob J, Hansell DM. HRCT of fibrosing lung disease. Respirology 2015;20(6):859–72.

13. Gruden JF, Panse PM, Leslie KO, et al. UIP diagnosed at surgical lung biopsy, 2000-2009: HRCT patterns and proposed classification system. AJR Am J Roentgenol 2013;200(5):W458–67.

14. Chung JH, Chawla A, Peljto AL, et al. CT scan findings of probable usual interstitial pneumonitis have a high predictive value for histologic usual interstitial pneumonitis. Chest 2015;147(2):450–9.

15. Gruden JF, Panse PM, Gotway MB, et al. Diagnosis of usual interstitial pneumonitis in the absence of honeycombing: evaluation of specific CT criteria with clinical follow-up in 38 patients. AJR Am J Roentgenol 2016;206(3):472–80.

16. Hobbs S, Chung JH, Leb J, et al. Practical imaging interpretation in patients suspected of having idiopathic pulmonary fibrosis: official recommendations from the Radiology Working Group of the Pulmonary Fibrosis Foundation. Radiol Cardiothorac Imaging 2021;3(1):e200279.

17. Hatabu H, Hunninghake GM, Richeldi L, et al. Interstitial Lung Abnormality (ILA) incidentally detected on CT: position paper from the Fleischner Society. Lancet Respir Med 2020;8(7):726–37.

18. Gruden JF, Naidich DP, Machnicki SC, et al. An algorithmic approach to the interpretation of diffuse lung disease on chest CT imaging: a theory of almost everything. Chest 2020;157(3):612–35.

19. Shih AR, Nitiwarangkul C, Little BP, et al. Practical application and validation of the 2018 ATS/ERS/JRS/ALAT and Fleischner Society guidelines for the diagnosis of idiopathic pulmonary fibrosis. Respir Res 2021;22(1):124.

20. Watadani T, Sakai F, Johkoh T, et al. Interobserver variability in the CT assessment of honeycombing in the lungs. Radiology 2013;266(3):936–44.

21. Lynch DA, Godwin JD, Safrin S, et al. Idiopathic pulmonary fibrosis study group. High-resolution computed tomography in idiopathic pulmonary fibrosis: diagnosis and prognosis. Am J Respir Crit Care Med 2005;172(4):488–93.

22. Hunninghake GW, Lynch DA, Galvin JR, et al. Radiologic findings are strongly associated with a pathologic diagnosis of usual interstitial pneumonia. Chest 2003;124(4):1215–23.

23. Piciucchi S, Tomassetti S, Ravaglia C, et al. From "traction bronchiectasis" to honeycombing in idiopathic pulmonary fibrosis: a spectrum of bronchiolar remodeling also in radiology? BMC Pulm Med 2016;16(1):87.

24. Walsh SL, Wells AU, Sverzellati N, et al. Relationship between fibroblastic foci profusion and high resolution CT morphology in fibrotic lung disease. BMC Med 2015;13:241.

25. McDonough JE, Verleden SE, Verschakelen J, et al. The structural origin of honeycomb cysts in IPF. Am J Respir Crit Care Med 2018;197:A6388.

26. Staats P, Kligerman S, Todd N, et al. A comparative study of honeycombing on high resolution computed tomography with histologic lung remodeling in explants with usual interstitial pneumonia. Pathol Res Pract 2015;211(1):55–61.

27. Chung JH, Cox CW, Montner SM, et al. CT features of the Usual interstitial Pneumonia pattern: differentiating connective tissue disease-associated interstitial lung disease from idiopathic pulmonary fibrosis. AJR Am J Roentgenol 2018;210(2):307–13.

28. Yagihashi K, Huckleberry J, Colby TV, et al. Idiopathic Pulmonary Fibrosis Clinical Research Network (IPFnet). Radiologic-pathologic discordance in biopsy-proven usual interstitial pneumonia. Eur Respir J 2016;47(4):1189–97.

29. Baratella E, Fiorese I, Marrocchio C, et al. Imaging review of the lung parenchymal complications in patients with IPF. Medicina 2019;55(10):613.

30. Collard HR, Ryerson CJ, Corte TJ, et al. Acute exacerbation of idiopathic pulmonary fibrosis. An international working group report. Am J Respir Crit Care Med 2016;194(3):265–75.

31. Lee JS, Collard HR, Anstrom KJ, et al. Anti-acid treatment and disease progression in idiopathic pulmonary fibrosis: an analysis of data from three randomised controlled trials. Lancet Respir Med 2013;1: 369–76.

32. Akira M, Kozuka T, Yamamoto S, et al. Computed tomography findings in acute exacerbation of idiopathic pulmonary fibrosis. Am J Respir Crit Care Med 2008;178:372–8.

33. Aubry MC, Myers JL, Douglas WW, et al. Primary pulmonary carcinoma in patients with idiopathic pulmonary fibrosis. Mayo Clin Proc 2002;77(8):763–70.

34. Kato E, Takayanagi N, Takaku Y, et al. Incidence and predictive factors of lung cancer in patients with idiopathic pulmonary fibrosis. ERJ Open Res 2018; 4(1):00111-2016.

35. Kishi K, Homma S, Kurosaki A, et al. High-resolution computed tomography findings of lung cancer associated with idiopathic pulmonary fibrosis. J Comput Assist Tomogr 2006;30:95–9.

36. Gruden JF, Green DB, Legasto AC, et al. Dendriform pulmonary ossification in the absence of usual interstitial pneumonia: CT features and possible association with recurrent acid aspiration. AJR Am J Roentgenol 2017;209(6):1209–15.

37. Egashira R, Jacob J, Kokosi MA, et al. Diffuse pulmonary ossification in fibrosing interstitial lung diseases: prevalence and associations. Radiology 2017;284:255–63.

38. Sumikawa H, Johkoh T, Colby TV, et al. Computed tomography findings in pathological usual interstitial pneumonia: relationship to survival. Am J Respir Crit Care Med 2008;177(4):433–9.

39. Nakagawa H, Ogawa E, Fukunaga K, et al. Quantitative CT analysis of honeycombing area predicts mortality in idiopathic pulmonary fibrosis with definite usual interstitial pneumonia pattern: A retrospective cohort study [published correction appears in. PLoS One 2019;14(12):e0226214.

40. Sverzellati N, Silva M, Seletti V, et al. Stratification of long-term outcome in stable idiopathic pulmonary fibrosis by combining longitudinal computed tomography and forced vital capacity. Eur Radiol 2020; 30(5):2669–79.

41. Arcadu A, Byrne SC, Pirina P, et al. Correlation of pulmonary function and usual interstitial pneumonia computed tomography patterns in idiopathic pulmonary fibrosis. Respir Med 2017;129:152–7.

42. Fraser E, St Noble V, Hoyles RK, et al. Readily accessible CT scoring method to quantify fibrosis in IPF. BMJ Open Respir Res 2020;7(1):e000584.

43. Robbie H, Daccord C, Chua F, et al. Evaluating disease severity in idiopathic pulmonary fibrosis. Eur Respir Rev 2017;26(145):170051.

44. du Bois RM, Weycker D, Albera C, et al. Forced vital capacity in patients with idiopathic pulmonary fibrosis: test properties and minimal clinically important difference. Am J Respir Crit Care Med 2011; 184(12):1382–9.

45. Kim GHJ, Weigt SS, Belperio JA, et al. Prediction of idiopathic pulmonary fibrosis progression using early quantitative changes on CT imaging for a short term of clinical 18-24-month follow-ups. Eur Radiol 2020;30(2):726–34.

46. Hansell DM, Goldin JG, King TE Jr, et al. CT staging and monitoring of fibrotic interstitial lung diseases in clinical practice and treatment trials: a position paper from the Fleischner Society. Lancet Respir Med 2015;3(6):483–96.

47. Oda K, Ishimoto H, Yatera K, et al. High-resolution CT scoring system-based grading scale predicts the clinical outcomes in patients with idiopathic pulmonary fibrosis. Respir Res 2014;15:10.

48. Jacob J, Aksman L, Mogulkoc N, et al. Serial CT analysis in idiopathic pulmonary fibrosis: comparison of visual features that determine patient outcome. Thorax 2020;75(8):648–54.

49. Wu X, Kim GH, Salisbury ML, et al. Computed tomographic biomarkers in idiopathic pulmonary fibrosis. the future of quantitative analysis. Am J Respir Crit Care Med 2019;199(1):12–21.

50. Cottin V, Hirani NA, Hotchkin DL, et al. Presentation, diagnosis and clinical course of the spectrum of progressive-fibrosing interstitial lung diseases. Eur Respir Rev 2018;27(150):180076.

51. Flaherty KR, Wells AU, Cottin V, et al. Nintedanib in progressive fibrosing interstitial lung diseases. N Engl J Med 2019;381(18):1718–27.

52. Behr J, Prasse A, Kreuter M, et al. RELIEF investigators. Pirfenidone in patients with progressive fibrotic interstitial lung diseases other than idiopathic pulmonary fibrosis (RELIEF): a double-blind, randomised, placebo-controlled, phase 2b trial. Lancet Respir Med 2021;9(5):476–86.

53. Wells AU, Brown KK, Flaherty KR, et al, IPF Consensus Working Group. What's in a name? That which we call IPF, by any other name would act the same. Eur Respir J 2018;51:1800692.

Interstitial Lung Abnormality—Why Should I Care and What Should I Do About It?

Andrea S. Oh, MD[a], David A. Lynch, MB BCh[b],*

KEYWORDS

- Interstitial lung abnormalities (ILA) • Interstitial lung disease (ILD) • Preclinical ILD
- Computed tomography • Pulmonary fibrosis

KEY POINTS

- Interstitial lung abnormalities (ILAs) are a purely radiological finding based on incidental computed tomography abnormalities.
- ILAs are associated with adverse clinical outcomes including respiratory impairment, incident lung cancer, and increased mortality.
- ILAs are more common than clinical interstitial lung disease (ILD), although a subset of patients with ILA will progress to ILD.
- Risk of progression can be stratified by clinical and imaging characteristics; those with fibrotic subtypes should be actively monitored for disease progression.

INTRODUCTION

Interstitial lung abnormalities (ILAs) are incidental computed tomography (CT) findings that are potentially compatible with interstitial lung disease (ILD) in patients without clinical suspicion for ILD.[1–8] ILAs are differentiated from ILDs based on clinical assessment. ILAs are not uncommon, with systematic evaluation of large research cohorts showing a prevalence of up to 17% in smokers older than 60 years and up to 10% in general population–based cohorts where the mean age of participants was ~70 years.[3,9–11] With the implementation of lung cancer screening and growing use of CT imaging for diagnostic purposes, ILAs will be increasingly identified. Moreover, as ILAs are associated with increased risk of mortality, functional impairment, and disease progression, appropriate identification and characterization by radiologists is important for management of patients with ILAs.

RISK FACTORS

Risk factors associated with ILAs overlap with many of the risk factors for ILD, specifically idiopathic pulmonary fibrosis (IPF) (Table 1). Increasing age is a cardinal risk factor for the presence of ILAs. In both smoking and general population–based cohort studies, participants with ILAs are older than those without ILAs.[2,12] In the Framingham Heart Study, there was an increasing prevalence of ILAs by age group; 4% in those younger than 60 years versus 47% in those older than 70 years.[13] Cigarette smoking, including current smoking status and quantity, is also strongly correlated with ILAs.[2,9,11] Among populations of smokers including lung cancer screening cohorts, the prevalence of ILAs is similar to prevalence rates in the general population–based cohorts; however, the mean age of participants with ILA in the cohorts of smokers is on average approximately 10 years younger than in

[a] Department of Radiology, University of California Los Angeles, 757 Westwood Plaza, Box 957437, Los Angeles, CA 90095-7437, USA; [b] Department of Radiology, National Jewish Health, 1400 Jackson Street, Room K012f, Denver, CO 80206, USA
* Corresponding author.
E-mail address: lynchd@njhealth.org

Radiol Clin N Am 60 (2022) 889–899
https://doi.org/10.1016/j.rcl.2022.06.002
0033-8389/22/© 2022 Elsevier Inc. All rights reserved.

Table 1
Risk factors associated with interstitial lung abnormalities and interstitial lung abnormality progression

Radiologic	Clinical
Subpleural reticulations	Older age
Lower lobe predominance	Male sex
Traction bronchiectasis	Cigarette smoking
Honeycombing	Inhalational exposures (air pollution, occupational exposures)
Nonemphysematous cysts	rs35705950 promoter polymorphism of the MUC5B gene
Subpleural fibrotic subtype (UIP and probable UIP patterns)	Medications (ie, chemotherapy, immunotherapy)
—	Radiation therapy
—	Thoracic surgery

the general population–based cohorts.[2,3,10,12,14,15] Additional risk factors for the presence of ILAs include male sex, air pollution due to elemental carbon and nitrogen oxides, and occupational exposure to vapors, gas, dust, and fumes.[2,11,16,17]

In terms of genetics, the rs35705950 promoter polymorphism of the MUC5B gene, an established genetic risk factor for IPF and familial interstitial pneumonia, has been shown to be strongly associated with the presence and progression of ILAs and preclinical ILD in high-risk populations.[9,18–20] More recently, genome-wide association studies of ILAs in 6 different cohorts also confirmed the relationship with the MUC5B promoter variant and described novel associations near IPO11 (rs6886640) and FCF1P3 (rs73199442) with ILA but not IPF and near HTRE1 (rs7744971) with subpleural-predominant ILA.[21]

CLINICAL ASSOCIATIONS AND OUTCOMES
Mortality

ILAs are associated with increased respiratory, lung cancer, and all-cause mortality. Research cohorts constituting general population samples, longitudinal birth cohorts, lung cancer screening populations, and smokers enriched for chronic obstructive pulmonary disease (COPD) have shown greater risk of mortality in the presence of ILAs.

In the Age, Gene/Environment Susceptibility (AGES)-Reykjavik Study on a longitudinal birth cohort of men and women born in Reykjavik, Iceland, participants with ILAs had increased all-cause and respiratory mortality compared with those without ILAs.[2,22] Of those who died of a respiratory cause, ILAs were associated with an increased rate of death from pulmonary fibrosis.[2] Because ILAs are potentially compatible with ILDs, it is feasible to conclude that mortality is attributable to pulmonary fibrosis; however, several cohorts have shown increased mortality rates beyond the expected rate of progression to clinically significant pulmonary fibrosis, suggesting that fibrosis is not the sole cause.[1]

In a study looking at ILAs in patients undergoing transcatheter aortic valve replacement, those with ILAs had increased mortality compared with non-ILA controls.[23] Several studies have also demonstrated increased mortality risk in association with specific ILA imaging patterns and imaging progression.[5,22,24] A recent study looking at traction bronchiectasis, a marker of fibrosis, in participants with ILA from the AGES-Reykjavik Study, found that baseline presence and interval progression of traction bronchiectasis was associated with shorter survival.[24] In the Framingham Heart Study, participants with ILA imaging progression over ~5 years were more likely to die in a subsequent 4-year follow-up interval.[5]

Prior and more recent studies in patients with early and late-stage lung cancers have found significant associations between the presence of ILAs and shorter overall survival.[25–27] Lung cancer screening and birth cohort studies, specifically the Danish Lung Cancer Screening Trial, National Lung Screening Trial, and AGES-Reykjavik Study, have also shown an association with increased lung cancer–related mortality.[3,15,28]

Progression

Estimates of ILA progression in longitudinal studies are variable with reports of up to 76% of participants with ILA at baseline progressing over 5 to 6 years of follow-up.[5,22] Studies with a follow-up of 2 years, albeit with younger patients, have found a much lower proportion of participants progressing over that time.[10] Although all cases of ILA do not progress, progression is more likely when patients are followed-up over a longer period of time and in those with specific clinical and imaging risk factors (**Figs. 1** and **2**, see **Table 1**).

Risk of ILA progression is associated with several features such as increasing age, active smoking, ambient air pollution (ie, elemental

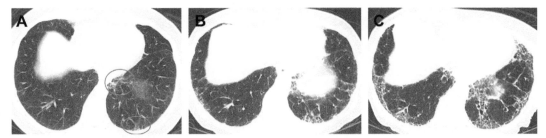

Fig. 1. ILA progression. (*A*) Subpleural nonfibrotic ILA. Baseline CT in an asymptomatic patient shows mild left lower lobe subpleural reticulations (*circled*). (*B*) The patient developed increased symptoms, and follow-up CT 7 years after baseline showed increased extent of reticulations and development of fibrosis with traction bronchiectasis. (*C*) The patient became oxygen dependent, and follow-up CT 14 years after baseline shows a UIP pattern of fibrosis.

carbon), vascular pruning on CT, and the rs35705950 promoter polymorphism of the MUC5B gene.[5,22,29,30] Putman and colleagues identified imaging patterns associated with disease progression including subpleural reticulations, lower lobe predominant changes, traction bronchiectasis, honeycombing, and nonemphysematous cysts, which remained significant predictors even after adjustment for potential confounders (ie, smoking, age, MUC5B genotype).[22] A recent study by Chae and colleagues looking at radiologic-pathologic correlations of ILA found that subpleural fibrotic subtypes of ILA, which correlated with a usual interstitial pneumonia (UIP) pattern on histopathology, were associated with ILA progression and mortality.[31]

Clinical consequences of imaging progression of ILA include accelerated pulmonary function decline over time and increased mortality. In the Framingham Heart Study, participants with ILA progression had an accelerated decline in their measure of forced vital capacity (FVC) compared with those without ILA or nonprogressive ILA.[5] This lung function decline coincided with the period of progressive imaging changes. Moreover, participants in the study who progressed were

more likely to die in a subsequent 4-year follow-up interval. A recent study of patients with COPD with ILA demonstrated a higher rate of annual decline in FVC and forced expiratory volume in 1 second in patients with ILA progression versus those without progression.[4]

Lung Cancer

Lung cancer screening studies and retrospective studies of patients with lung cancer have consistently demonstrated an increased incidence of lung cancer and lung cancer–associated mortality in participants with ILAs.[3,15,25–27,32] Findings from the AGES-Reykjavik Study involving a general population cohort further support these findings.[28] Although ILAs and lung cancer share overlapping risk factors (ie, age and smoking), the association between these conditions persists even after accounting for confounding factors.

Preexisting ILAs are also risk factors for increased morbidity and complications in patients with lung cancer receiving treatment (**Figs. 3** and **4**). Im and colleagues assessed patients undergoing lung resection for early stage non–small cell lung cancer and showed that preexisting ILAs on

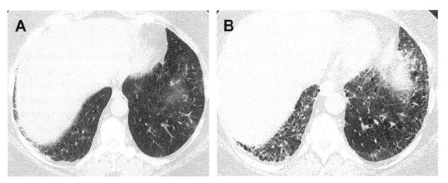

Fig. 2. ILA progression. (*A*) Baseline CT with reticular abnormality. (*B*) Follow-up CT 5 years after baseline, following COVID infection, shows UIP pattern of fibrosis.

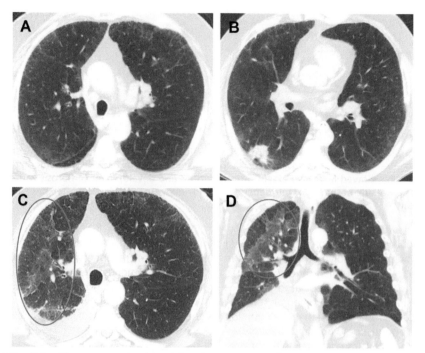

Fig. 3. Preexisting ILA with postoperative lung injury in a patient with adenocarcinoma. (*A*) Nonsubpleural ILA characterized by patchy groundglass abnormality. (*B*) Biopsy-proven lung adenocarcinoma in the right lower lobe. (*C, D*) Axial and coronal images postlobectomy show groundglass abnormality (*circled*) presumed to be acute lung injury.

CT were an independent risk factor for postoperative acute respiratory distress syndrome, pneumonia, and respiratory failure.[33] In patients with small cell lung cancer receiving radiation therapy, preexisting ILAs were associated with increased risk of radiation pneumonitis.[7,34] Finally, in patients with lung cancer and other malignancies receiving immunotherapy, the presence of pretreatment ILAs was a significant risk factor for immune checkpoint inhibitor–related ILD.[6,8]

IMAGING
Computed Tomography Protocol

When ILAs are detected, a dedicated chest CT examination may be needed to confirm and characterize the abnormality, for example, if the initial scan of the lungs was incomplete (ie, abdominal CT), dependent atelectasis is suspected, or if the scan was done without thin axial sections.[1] If a dedicated chest CT is performed, a similar protocol as used for ILD assessment can be considered, specifically, CT with thin sections (<2 mm) and high spatial resolution reconstruction.[35] Supine images should be obtained at full inspiration to total lung capacity. Prone imaging may be useful when there is a need to distinguish dependent atelectasis from true interstitial abnormality.[36]

Expiratory imaging could potentially identify lobular air trapping, a feature that suggests hypersensitivity pneumonitis. Prone and expiratory images can be done with noncontiguous imaging and at lower doses than the inspiratory CT. Follow-up CTs to assess progression should use similar scanning protocols.

Radiologic Definition of Interstitial Lung Abnormalities

ILAs are defined as nondependent imaging findings that affect more than 5% of a lung zone (ie, upper, middle, lower) and include groundglass or reticulations, parenchymal distortion, nonemphysematous cysts, honeycombing, and/or traction bronchiectasis.[1] Diffuse centrilobular nodularity was previously part of the radiologic definition but was ultimately removed from the Fleischner Society Position Paper because studies found it to be a common finding in smokers and not associated with fibrosis or disease progression.[12,22] In addition to the individual imaging features, the distribution of ILAs in the craniocaudal and axial planes should be communicated, as they may have prognostic significance.[22] Dependent lung atelectasis, osteophyte-related paraspinal fibrosis, interlobular septal thickening due to

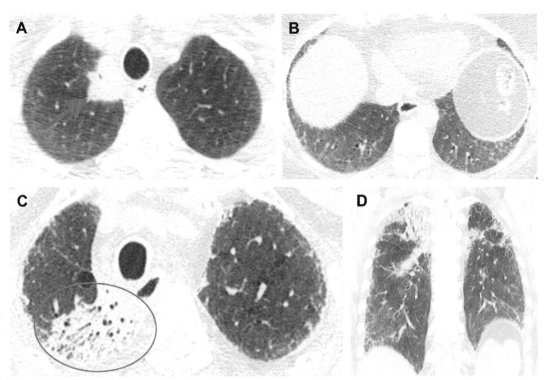

Fig. 4. Preexisting ILA in a patient with a right apical squamous cell carcinoma. (A) Axial image with right apical mass compatible with biopsy-proven squamous cell carcinoma (*arrow*). (B) Subpleural fibrotic ILA in the lung bases with groundglass, reticulations, and traction bronchiectasis. (C) Axial image 9 months postchemoradiation therapy demonstrating extensive radiation fibrosis (*circle*). (D) Coronal image showing radiation fibrosis and progression of background fibrosis.

interstitial edema, and focal or unilateral abnormality such as aspiration are not considered ILAs (**Fig. 5**).

In high-risk population groups undergoing CT screening for potential ILD, identified imaging abnormalities are not considered ILAs because they are not incidental. For example, in patients with a family history of familial ILD, a known diagnosis of connective tissue disease such as rheumatoid arthritis or systemic sclerosis, or a significant occupational exposure with a known association with ILD, CT abnormalities can be considered preclinical ILD.[1,37]

Computed Tomography Subtypes

ILAs are classified based on imaging features and distribution, as certain patterns are associated with imaging progression and mortality. The 3 ILA subcategories are nonsubpleural, subpleural nonfibrotic, and subpleural fibrotic (**Figs. 6 and 7**).

Nonsubpleural ILAs usually do not progress and are not associated with increased mortality.[22] Subpleural ILAs may be more significant and are further subdivided into nonfibrotic and fibrotic types.[1] Fibrotic ILAs, which are characterized by

the presence of architectural distortion and reticulations or groundglass with traction bronchiectasis and/or honeycombing, are associated with disease progression and increased mortality.[22,24] In fibrotic cases, the pattern can be classified according to the 2018 Fleischner and American Thoracic Society, European Respiratory Society, Japanese Respiratory Society, and Latin American Thoracic Society criteria for UIP.[35,38] A definite fibrotic pattern including UIP and probable UIP patterns in the AGES-Reykjavik population–based cohort was associated not only with progression on subsequent imaging but also with a 70% increase in the risk of death compared with those without definite fibrosis.[22] Of note, in the same study by Putman and colleagues, an increased risk of ILA progression and mortality was associated with nonemphysematous cysts, albeit not as strongly as other features such as reticulations and traction bronchiectasis.[22] These cysts are described as irregular, thin-walled airspaces often seen in cigarette smokers and usually correlate with smoking-related interstitial fibrosis on histology (**Fig. 8**).[39,40] Ultimately, accurate characterization of ILAs, especially those with

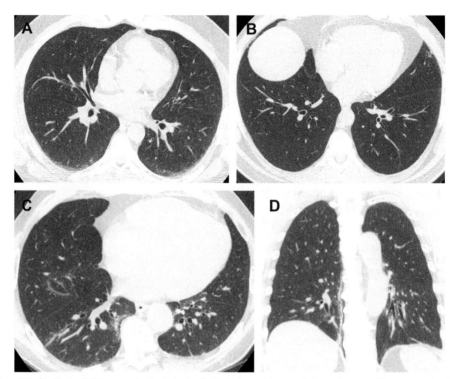

Fig. 5. Non-ILA findings. (*A*) Dependent atelectasis. Subpleural groundglass abnormality on supine inspiratory imaging. (*B*) Prone imaging demonstrates clearance of the groundglass. (*C*) Osteophyte-related paraspinal fibrosis. Localized groundglass and irregular linear opacities in the paraspinal right lower lobe. (*D*) Coronal image showing intimate association with thoracic osteophytes.

fibrotic features, is essential for the radiologist who acts as the gatekeeper in properly triaging these patients.

Deep learning approaches have been shown to be sensitive enough to detect preclinical ILD in high-risk patients (**Fig. 9**). A study in first-degree

Quantitative Imaging

Quantitative imaging offers an objective assessment of regional disease pattern of the lung that can increase the diagnostic reliability and severity assessment of ILD.[1] CT-based approaches for quantitative evaluation of interstitial features include densitometry of high attenuation areas, histogram analysis, texture-based analysis, and deep learning methods.[41–45] Quantitative CT methods used in ILD cohorts seem to be reliable, reproducible, and associated with clinical outcomes.[46] Similarly, when applied to ILA cohorts, these approaches provide increased sensitivity and clinical prognostic information. A study by Ash and colleagues applied a histogram-based method to a cohort of smokers with ILA and showed that an increase in quantitative interstitial changes on CT was associated with impaired lung function, worse quality of life, increased mortality, and more copies of a MUC5B promoter polymorphism.[47]

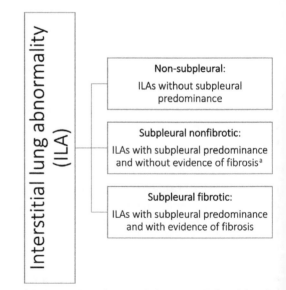

Fig. 6. ILA CT subtypes. [a]Fibrosis is defined by the presence of architectural distortion, traction bronchiectasis, and/or honeycombing.

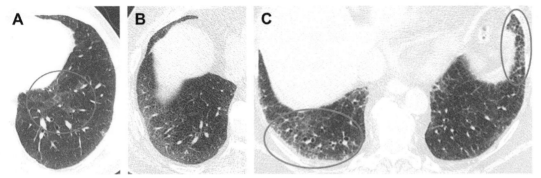

Fig. 7. ILA subtypes. (A) Nonsubpleural ILA. Groundglass abnormality (circled), patchy in the axial plane. (B) Subpleural nonfibrotic ILA. Peripheral groundglass abnormality without fibrosis. (C) Subpleural fibrotic ILA. Peripheral reticulations and mild traction bronchiolectasis (circled).

relatives of patients with familial ILD showed that a texture-based deep learning method was capable of detecting interstitial features in at-risk relatives with a sensitivity of 84% and specificity of 86%.[18] Another recently published study applying the same deep learning method in patients with rheumatoid arthritis without a prior diagnosis of ILD demonstrated an association between higher quantitative fibrosis scores and decreased lung function.[48] Much potential remains for quantitative CT analysis to reliably characterize and quantify parenchymal abnormalities in patients with ILAs, and it is likely that quantitative CT will be helpful to identify progressive ILA. However, further validation is needed.

MANAGEMENT AND FOLLOW-UP

Long-term prospective studies on ILA management and follow-up do not currently exist. The Fleischner Society position paper, however, provides a multidisciplinary perspective on management as outlined in **Fig. 10.**[1]

Patients with clinically significant disease must first be separated from those without clinical disease. Once ILD is excluded, patients with ILAs can be stratified into those at higher risk of progression and those at lower risk. Individuals without risk factors should follow expectant management and return for evaluation if they develop symptoms of respiratory impairment. Patients with risk factors should be actively monitored with symptom assessment and pulmonary function testing at 3 to 12 months. Continued long-term follow-up is also suggested, although the frequency and duration are unknown. Follow-up CT scans should also be performed and might include a scan at 12 to 24 months in high-risk patients. If signs and symptoms of progression develop before the interval, a CT scan can be performed sooner. A recent survey of 44 pulmonologists and radiologists with expertise in ILD found overall agreement with these suggestions.[49] There was also agreement that honeycombing detected during lung cancer screening should be reported as a

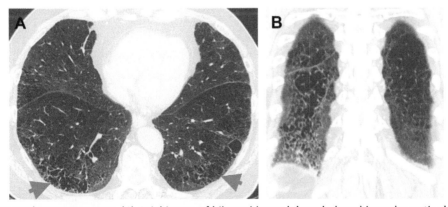

Fig. 8. Nonemphysematous cysts. (A) Axial image of bilateral lower lobe subpleural irregular cystic abnormality (arrows). (B) Coronal image showing confluent nonemphysematous cysts in the lower lobes.

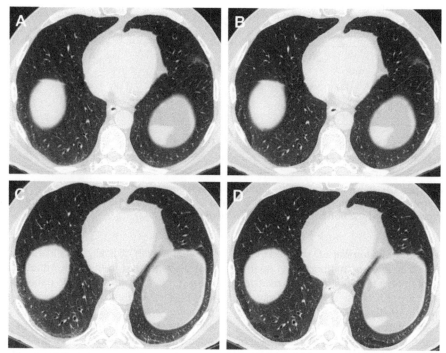

Fig. 9. Quantitative imaging in ILA. (*A*) Baseline CT scan shows subpleural nonfibrotic ILA with minimal ground-glass and reticular abnormality. (*B*) Data-driven textural analysis quantified the reticular abnormality at 1.2%. (*C*) Follow-up CT 18 months after baseline shows progression. (*D*) Data-driven textural analysis quantified the reticular/fibrotic abnormality at 2.6%.

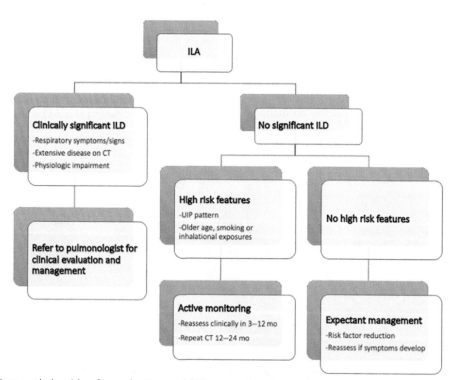

Fig. 10. Proposed algorithm for evaluation and follow-up of patients with ILA.

potentially significant finding as part of the screening.

As there are no recommendations for treatment initiation, management should focus on risk reduction and shared decision-making, such as smoking cessation, respiratory protection for ongoing inhalational exposures, and avoidance of pneumotoxic medications.[50] Lung cancer screening should be encouraged in patients who meet criteria, given the increased risk in this population. In patients with ILAs undergoing surgery or lung cancer therapy, the increased risk of acute lung injury and exacerbations warrant appropriate planning and close monitoring of these patients.

SUMMARY

The presence of ILAs, specifically subpleural fibrotic ILA, is associated with adverse clinical outcomes including increased mortality. ILAs share risk factors with ILD and in some cases may represent a precursor of ILD. Radiologists play a vital role in ILA assessment and risk stratification, as they are the first to identify and characterize these abnormalities. Individuals with ILA and high-risk features should undergo clinical evaluation for ILD and should be actively monitored for disease progression.

CLINICS CARE POINTS

- Incidentally detected interstitial lung abnormalities (ILA) are associated with increased mortality risk.
- ILA should be categorized as non-subpleural, subpleural non-fibrotic, and subpleural fibrotic.
- Progression and mortality are most likely in subjects with fibrotic ILA.
- Patients with ILA who experience lung injury from radiation, chemotherapy, or other factors are at increased risk of interstitial lung disease.

DISCLOSURE

The authors have nothing to disclose.

REFERENCES

1. Hatabu H, Hunninghake GM, Richeldi L, et al. Interstitial lung abnormalities detected incidentally on CT: a Position Paper from the Fleischner Society. Lancet Respir Med 2020;8(7):726–37.

2. Putman RK, Hatabu H, Araki T, et al. Association Between Interstitial Lung Abnormalities and All-Cause Mortality. JAMA 2016;315(7):672–81.

3. Hoyer N, Wille MMW, Thomsen LH, et al. Interstitial lung abnormalities are associated with increased mortality in smokers. Respir Med 2018;136:77–82.

4. Lee TS, Jin KN, Lee HW, et al. Interstitial Lung Abnormalities and the Clinical Course in Patients With COPD. Chest 2021;159(1):128–37.

5. Araki T, Putman RK, Hatabu H, et al. Development and Progression of Interstitial Lung Abnormalities in the Framingham Heart Study. Am J Respir Crit Care Med 2016;194(12):1514–22.

6. Nakanishi Y, Masuda T, Yamaguchi K, et al. Pre-existing interstitial lung abnormalities are risk factors for immune checkpoint inhibitor-induced interstitial lung disease in non-small cell lung cancer. Respir Investig 2019;57(5):451–9.

7. Li F, Zhou Z, Wu A, et al. Preexisting radiological interstitial lung abnormalities are a risk factor for severe radiation pneumonitis in patients with small-cell lung cancer after thoracic radiation therapy. Radiat Oncol 2018;13(1):1–9.

8. Shimoji K, Masuda T, Yamaguchi K, et al. Association of Preexisting Interstitial Lung Abnormalities With Immune Checkpoint Inhibitor–Induced Interstitial Lung Disease Among Patients With Nonlung Cancers. JAMA Netw Open 2020;3(11):e2022906.

9. Hunninghake GM, Hatabu H, Okajima Y, et al. MUC5B Promoter Polymorphism and Interstitial Lung Abnormalities. N Engl J Med 2013;368(23):2192–200.

10. Jin GY, Lynch D, Chawla A, et al. Interstitial Lung Abnormalities in a CT Lung Cancer Screening Population: Prevalence and Progression Rate. Radiology 2013;268(2):563–71.

11. Buendía-Roldán I, Fernandez R, Mejía M, et al. Risk factors associated with the development of interstitial lung abnormalities. Eur Respir J 2021;58(2). https://doi.org/10.1183/13993003.03005-2020.

12. Washko GR, Hunninghake GM, Fernandez IE, et al. Lung volumes and emphysema in smokers with interstitial lung abnormalities. N Engl J Med 2013;364(10):897–906.

13. Sanders JL, Putman RK, Dupuis J, et al. The Association of Aging Biomarkers, Interstitial Lung Abnormalities, and Mortality. Am J Respir Crit Care Med 2021;203(9):1149–57.

14. Sverzellati N, Guerci L, Randi G, et al. Interstitial lung diseases in a lung cancer screening trial. Eur Respir J 2011;38(2):392–400.

15. Whittaker Brown SA, Padilla M, Mhango G, et al. Interstitial Lung Abnormalities and Lung Cancer Risk in the National Lung Screening Trial. Chest 2019;156(6):1195–203.

16. Sack C, Vedal S, Sheppard L, et al. Air pollution and subclinical interstitial lung disease: the Multi-Ethnic

Study of Atherosclerosis (MESA) air–lung study. Eur Respir J 2017;50(6). https://doi.org/10.1183/13993003.00559-2017.

17. Sack CS, Doney BC, Podolanczuk AJ, et al. Occupational Exposures and Subclinical Interstitial Lung Disease. The MESA (Multi-Ethnic Study of Atherosclerosis) Air and Lung Studies. Am J Respir Crit Care Med 2017;196(8):1031–9.

18. Mathai SK, Humphries SM, Kropski JA, et al. MUC5B variant is associated with visually and quantitatively detected preclinical pulmonary fibrosis. Thorax 2019;74(12):1131–9.

19. Seibold MA, Wise AL, Speer MC, et al. A Common MUC5B Promoter Polymorphism and Pulmonary Fibrosis. https://doi.org.proxy.hsl.ucdenver.edu/10.1056/NEJMoa1013660.

20. Putman RK, Gudmundsson G, Araki T, et al. The MUC5B Promoter Polymorphism Is Associated with Specific Interstitial Lung Abnormality Subtypes. Eur Respir J 2017;50(3):1700537.

21. Hobbs BD, Putman RK, Araki T, et al. Overlap of Genetic Risk between Interstitial Lung Abnormalities and Idiopathic Pulmonary Fibrosis. Am J Respir Crit Care Med 2019;200(11):1402–13.

22. Putman RK, Gudmundsson G, Axelsson GT, et al. Imaging Patterns Are Associated with Interstitial Lung Abnormality Progression and Mortality. Am J Respir Crit Care Med 2019;200(2):175–83.

23. Kadoch M, Kitich A, Alqalyoobi S, et al. Interstitial Lung Abnormality is Prevalent and Associated with Worse Outcome in Patients Undergoing Transcatheter Aortic Valve Replacement. Respir Med 2018;137:55–60.

24. Hino T, Hida T, Nishino M, et al. Progression of traction bronchiectasis/bronchiolectasis in interstitial lung abnormalities is associated with increased all-cause mortality: Age Gene/Environment Susceptibility-Reykjavik Study. Eur J Radiol Open 2021;8:100334.

25. Hida T, Hata A, Lu J, et al. Interstitial lung abnormalities in patients with stage I non-small cell lung cancer are associated with shorter overall survival: the Boston lung cancer study. Cancer Imaging 2021;21:14.

26. Araki T, Dahlberg SE, Hida T, et al. Interstitial lung abnormality in stage IV non-small cell lung cancer: A validation study for the association with poor clinical outcome. Eur J Radiol Open 2019;6:128–31.

27. Nishino M, Cardarella S, Dahlberg SE, et al. Interstitial lung abnormalities in treatment-naïve advanced non-small-cell lung cancer patients are associated with shorter survival. Eur J Radiol 2015;84(5):998–1004.

28. Axelsson GT, Putman RK, Aspelund T, et al. The Associations of Interstitial Lung Abnormalities with Cancer Diagnoses and Mortality. Eur Respir J 2020;56(6):1902154.

29. Rice MB, Li W, Schwartz J, et al. Ambient air pollution exposure and risk and progression of interstitial lung abnormalities: the Framingham Heart Study. Thorax 2019;74(11):1063–9.

30. Synn AJ, Li W, Hunninghake GM, et al. Vascular Pruning on Computed Tomography and Interstitial Lung Abnormalities in the Framingham Heart Study. CHEST 2020;0(0). https://doi.org/10.1016/j.chest.2020.07.082.

31. Chae KJ, Chung MJ, Jin GY, et al. Radiologic-pathologic correlation of interstitial lung abnormalities and predictors for progression and survival. Eur Radiol 2022. https://doi.org/10.1007/s00330-021-08378-8.

32. Hoyer N, Thomsen LH, Wille MMW, et al. Increased respiratory morbidity in individuals with interstitial lung abnormalities. BMC Pulm Med 2020;20:67. https://doi.org/10.1186/s12890-020-1107-0.

33. Im Y, Park HY, Shin S, et al. Prevalence of and risk factors for pulmonary complications after curative resection in otherwise healthy elderly patients with early stage lung cancer. Respir Res 2019;20(1):1–9.

34. Kobayashi H, Wakuda K, Naito T, et al. Chemoradiotherapy for limited-stage small-cell lung cancer and interstitial lung abnormalities. Radiat Oncol 2021;16(1):1–9.

35. Lynch DA, Sverzellati N, Travis WD, et al. Diagnostic criteria for idiopathic pulmonary fibrosis: a Fleischner Society White Paper. Lancet Respir Med 2018;6(2):138–53.

36. Hansell DM. Thin-Section CT of the Lungs: The Hinterland of Normal. Radiology 2010;256(3):695–711.

37. Hata A, Schiebler ML, Lynch DA, et al. Interstitial Lung Abnormalities: State of the Art. Radiology 2021;301(1):19–34.

38. Raghu G, Remy-Jardin M, Myers JL, et al. Diagnosis of Idiopathic Pulmonary Fibrosis. An Official ATS/ERS/JRS/ALAT Clinical Practice Guideline. Am J Respir Crit Care Med 2018;198(5):e44–68.

39. Otani H, Tanaka T, Murata K, et al. Smoking-related interstitial fibrosis combined with pulmonary emphysema: computed tomography-pathologic correlative study using lobectomy specimens. Int J Chron Obstruct Pulmon Dis 2016;11:1521–32. https://doi.org/10.2147/COPD.S107938.

40. Watanabe Y, Kawabata Y, Kanauchi T, et al. Multiple, thin-walled cysts are one of the HRCT features of airspace enlargement with fibrosis. Eur J Radiol 2015;84(5):986–92.

41. Uppaluri R, Hoffman EA, Sonka M, et al. Interstitial Lung Disease. Am J Respir Crit Care Med 1999;159(2):519–25.

42. Bartholmai BJ, Raghunath S, Karwoski RA, et al. Quantitative CT Imaging of Interstitial Lung Diseases. J Thorac Imaging 2013;28(5):10, 1097/RTI.0b013e3182a21969.

43. Ash SY, Harmouche R, Ross JC, et al. The Objective Identification and Quantification of Interstitial Lung Abnormalities in Smokers. Acad Radiol 2017;24(8): 941–6.

44. Humphries SM, Yagihashi K, Huckleberry J, et al. Idiopathic Pulmonary Fibrosis: Data-driven Textural Analysis of Extent of Fibrosis at Baseline and 15-Month Follow-up. Radiology 2017;285(1):270–8.

45. Christodoulidis S, Anthimopoulos M, Ebner L, et al. Multisource Transfer Learning With Convolutional Neural Networks for Lung Pattern Analysis. IEEE J Biomed Health Inform 2017;21(1):76–84.

46. Wu X, Kim GH, Salisbury ML, et al. Computed Tomographic Biomarkers in Idiopathic Pulmonary Fibrosis. The Future of Quantitative Analysis. Am J Respir Crit Care Med 2018;199(1):12–21.

47. Ash SY, Harmouche R, Putman RK, et al. Clinical and Genetic Associations of Objectively Identified Interstitial Changes in Smokers. Chest 2017;152(4):780–91.

48. Matson SM, Deane KD, Peljto AL, et al. Prospective Identification of Subclinical Interstitial Lung Disease in Rheumatoid Arthritis Cohort is Associated with the MUC5B Promoter Variant. Am J Respir Crit Care Med 2021. rccm.202109–2087LE.

49. Hunninghake GM, Goldin JG, Kadoch MA, et al. Detection and Early Referral of Patients With Interstitial Lung Abnormalities: An Expert Survey Initiative. Chest 2021. https://doi.org/10.1016/j.chest.2021.06.035.

50. Podolanczuk AJ, Putman RK. Clinical Relevance and Management of "Pre–Interstitial Lung Disease.". Clin Chest Med 2021;42(2):241–9.

Updated Imaging Classification of Hypersensitivity Pneumonitis

Lydia Chelala, MD*, Ayodeji Adegunsoye, MD, Brittany A. Cody, MD, Aliya N. Husain, MD, Jonathan H. Chung, MD

KEYWORDS

- Fibrotic hypersensitivity pneumonitis • non-fibrotic hypersensitivity pneumonitis
- interstitial lung disease • high-resolution CT • histopathology

KEY POINTS

- Hypersensitivity pneumonia (HP) should be suspected in any patient presenting with interstitial lung disease in the appropriate clinical context
- A detailed investigation of potential exposures is necessary. The absence of an identifiable causative antigen does not exclude HP.
- There is a significant overlap in the clinical presentation and radiologic appearance of fibrotic HP and usual interstitial pneumonia/idiopathic pulmonary fibrosis.
- Fibrotic HP carries a worse prognosis when compared with non-fibrotic HP.

Abbreviations	
IgE	Immunoglobulin
ECT	Computed Tomography
UIP	Usual Interstitial Pneumonia
NSIP	Non-Specific Interstitial Pneumonia

INTRODUCTION

History

Bernardino Ramazzini, an Italian researcher regarded by many as the father of occupational medicine, recognized the high prevalence of respiratory failure and reduced life expectancy among grain workers in 1713.[1] He subsequently provided the first description of the inhalational disease now known as hypersensitivity pneumonia (HP). In the early 1900s, further detailed accounts of the disease were made in workers exposed to fungal spores, notably bark peelers in whom removal from the work environment prompted clinical and radiographic improvement.[2] Numerous airborne organic and inorganic antigens have since been incriminated in the development of HP also previously termed "extrinsic allergic alveolitis."

Definition

HP refers to a heterogeneous group of interstitial lung diseases (ILDs) resulting from a non-IgE immune-mediated reaction to inhaled pathogens in susceptible and sensitized hosts.[3] Environmental and genetic factors are important substrates of disease pathogenesis. A recurrent or ongoing airborne exposure results in activation of humoral and cellular immune responses. HP is characterized by the ensuing parenchymal inflammation, leading to fibrosis in a subset of patients.[4] Specific disease designations may occasionally

The authors have nothing to disclose.
The University of Chicago Medicine, 5841 South Maryland Avenue, Chicago, IL 60637, USA
* Corresponding author.
E-mail address: LChelala@radiology.bsd.uchicago.edu

radiologic.theclinics.com

be used on the identification of particular inciting agents (eg, "bird fancier lung" resulting from repeated exposure to avian antigens).[5] Because previously defined disease categories relying on the duration of symptoms (ie, acute, subacute, and chronic) overlapped and did not translate into distinct prognostic groups, this nomenclature has been abandoned in the most recently updated categorization schemes. HP is currently divided into non-fibrotic and fibrotic subtypes giving greater weight to radiologic and histologic findings and bearing prognostic significance.[6,7] Inflammation is the hallmark of non-fibrotic HP. Fibrosis with or without inflammation is characteristic of fibrotic HP.

Background

The diagnosis of HP may be challenging in clinical practice. The great variability in the prevalence and forms of the disease stemming from geographic and occupational factors contributed in past years to a lack of consensus regarding disease definition and the optimal diagnostic approach.[8–10] Furthermore, the culprit antigen may frequently remain unknown despite thorough investigation, lowering clinicians' diagnostic confidence. The proportion of the patients without identifiable exposure exceeds 50% in some reports.[11] HP also shares common clinical and radiologic features with other types of ILD which may contribute to the delayed or misdiagnosis and adverse patient outcomes.[12] It is therefore imperative to consider the diagnosis of HP in any patient presenting with ILD. Accurate and timely diagnosis is crucial in altering the disease course, directing treatment and improving prognosis. The American Thoracic Society/Japanese Respiratory Society/Asociación Latino americana del Tórax (ATS/JRS/ALAT) and the American College of Chest Physicians (ACCP) have therefore recently provided updated guidelines to optimize the diagnostic approach and management of HP patients with special emphasis placed on the importance of a multidisciplinary approach.[6,7] Multidisciplinary discussions (MDD) should rely on clinical and radiological findings as well as bronchoalveolar lavage (BAL) and histopathology results when appropriate. This article discusses key clinical, radiologic, and histopathologic features of HP and reviews current recommendations.

DISCUSSION
Considerations

The development of HP is governed by exposure and host-specific factors. The type, duration, and severity of the inciting exposure may impact the clinical presentation and course of the disease. Exposure may be domestic, occupational, or recreational. Inciting allergens include an ever-growing list of microbes, protein allergens, and inorganic chemicals.[4] Antigens, many of which remain unrecognized, may also share common epitopes, resulting in cross-sensitization to several other agents following one specific exposure.[13] The absence of an identifiable inciting antigen does not exclude HP, as it may remain unknown even after thorough investigation.[11] Patients with fibrotic HP are less likely to have a recognized inciting exposure.[14]

Interestingly, only a small proportion of individuals with known inhalational exposures develop HP.[5] For example, the proportion of HP among farmers with known exposures is 12% or less in certain populations.[15] In addition, there is variable disease expression in individuals with similar exposure histories. Such observations have prompted discussions about predisposing factors in susceptible hosts. HP has been known to occur with greater frequency in nonsmokers, presumably due to the inhibitory effect of nicotine on alveolar macrophages.[16] The absence of a smoking history therefore increases the likelihood of an HP diagnosis. Nonetheless, a history of smoking usually portends a worse prognosis.[17] Cigarette smoking may alter the clinical features of the disease and delay the diagnosis.[18] Certain genetic polymorphisms known to promote fibrotic pathways have also been associated with HP, such as the MUC5B promoter polymorphism and telomere-related mutations. Such polymorphisms have previously been implicated in other types of fibrotic lung diseases, most notably idiopathic pulmonary fibrosis (IPF), possibly accounting for overlapping presentations in some of these patients.[15] HP is also more frequent among older adults, the same age group affected by IPF.[9] A high index of suspicion for HP should therefore be maintained in any patient presenting with ILD. A familial form of HP has also been described.[19]

Evaluation

Evaluation relies on a detailed clinical assessment, including a thorough investigation of patients' exposures and a detailed radiologic assessment. Frequently, evaluation will also rely on the analysis of bronchoscopic and histopathologic specimens. The ATS/JRS/ALAT and ACCP guidelines provide diagnostic algorithms based on current evidence aiming at optimization and improved standardization of the diagnostic approach.[6,7]

Clinical evaluation

The clinical presentation may be acute (ie, hours to days), subacute (ie, days to weeks), or chronic (ie, weeks to months).[12] The duration of symptoms is not clearly correlated to disease outcomes or the presence or absence of fibrosis.[20] An insidious onset of symptoms in fibrotic HP can mimic IPF. Presenting symptoms are nonspecific, including exertional dyspnea, cough, and chest tightness. Patient may occasionally present with constitutional symptoms (eg, fevers, chills, malaise, and headache). On physical examination, mid-inspiratory rales, bibasilar crackles, wheezing, and cyanosis may be observed.

A detailed history is of utmost importance in identifying a potential exposure and establishing a temporal relationship to the patient's symptoms thereby improving outcomes.[17] Serum testing for precipitating immunoglobulin G (IgG) against culprit antigens is suggested by the ATS/JRS/ALAT in suspected fibrotic or non-fibrotic HP.[7] Serum IgG test-positivity supports previous antigenic exposure, and increasingly positive serology titers seem to be the predictive of HP diagnosis.[21] Although this test is fairly sensitive, its specificity is suboptimal; therefore, test positivity does not prove causation of ILD and may not confirm or exclude a diagnosis of HP. Use of this test in clinical practice is also limited by the absence of a universal standardized HP panel and the overall suboptimal performance of available test kits.[5,22] Specific inhalational bronchial challenges may occasionally be attempted, in which patients are exposed to a suspected antigen in a controlled environment. These tests may be considered in patients who are unable or reluctant to pursue histopathologic diagnosis. Their use is also limited by a lack of standardization and restricted availability to specific experienced centers.[23]

Pulmonary function tests have limited value in discriminating HP from other ILDs, although they could be helpful in assessing the extent of functional impairment at diagnosis and follow-up. Restrictive or mixed restrictive/obstructive physiology may be present.[24] Restriction is less likely in smokers when compared with nonsmokers and more significant in fibrotic HP when compared with non-fibrotic HP.[14,18] A reduction in the diffusion capacity for carbon monoxide is characteristic and typically more pronounced in fibrotic HP and in smokers.

BAL lymphocytic analysis is key in aiding the diagnosis of suspected HP. The demonstration of an elevated proportion of lymphocytes in BAL fluid ($\geq$30%) increases the likelihood of HP, especially favoring this diagnosis over IPF or sarcoidosis.[7,20] The absence of lymphocytosis may,

however, occasionally confound the diagnosis of fibrotic HP and cannot be used to exclude the diagnosis.[5] The ATS/JRS/ALAT guidelines recommend using BAL analysis in the workup of any suspected fibrotic or non-fibrotic HP when possible. As per these guidelines, without histopathological evaluation, the diagnostic confidence is at most moderate in the absence of BAL analysis or BAL lymphocytosis.[7] BAL fluid analysis may also help exclude other causes of ILD in non-fibrotic forms. Conversely, the need for bronchoscopic evaluation is obviated in the presence of a known exposure and typical high-resolution CT (HRCT) findings as per the ACCP.[6]

High-resolution CT evaluation

HRCT evaluation is central to the diagnostic workup in any patient presenting with ILD. HRCT is typically a noncontrast evaluation using dose optimization techniques and including supine inspiratory and expiratory acquisitions as well as a prone inspiratory acquisition if deemed appropriate. Volumetric acquisition is recommended for the supine inspiratory sequence. Expiratory and prone imaging may be obtained using volumetric or sequential acquisitions. Thin-section reconstructions of $\leq$1.5 mm should use a high spatial frequency algorithm and iterative reconstructions when possible.[7]

An important initial determination to include or exclude the presence of fibrosis is crucial, as it will carry both diagnostic and prognostic implications.[6,7] HRCT categorization schemes are suggested by the ATS/JRS/ALAT and ACCP for both fibrotic and non-fibrotic HP, in which typical and compatible HRCT patterns are described. An indeterminate HRCT pattern is also described for fibrotic HP. **Tables 1** and **2** summarize the diagnostic HRCT criteria for both categorization schemes in non-fibrotic and fibrotic HP, respectively. A typical HRCT pattern is suggestive of the diagnosis, and a compatible HRCT pattern is consistent with HP when supported by the MDD. An indeterminate HRCT pattern suggests an alternative diagnosis. A greater confidence level for HP is achieved overall when a higher HRCT confidence level is possible.

Non-fibrotic HP: In the ATS/JRS/ALAT algorithm, a typical HRCT pattern implies the presence of diffuse parenchymal infiltration in association with features of small airway disease (SAD; **Figs. 1** and **2**).[7] A diffuse distribution of radiographic abnormalities is key, both in the craniocaudal and axial planes. Parenchymal infiltration may manifest as ground-glass opacity (GGO) or mosaicism. SAD features include air trapping and the presence of ill-defined centrilobular nodules (CLNs) measuring

Table 1
Summary of the American Thoracic Society/Japanese Respiratory Society/Asociación Latino americana del Tórax and the American College of Chest Physicians diagnostic CT categories of non-fibrotic hypersensitivity pneumonia on high-resolution CT

HRCT Pattern	Typical HP	Compatible with HP
ATS/JRS/ALAT	≥1 feature of parenchymal infiltration • Ground-glass opacity • Mosaicism *AND* ≥1 feature of small airway disease: • Ill-defined centrilobular nodules • Air trapping *AND* Diffuse distribution	Nonspecific parenchymal abnormalities • Uniform and subtle ground-glass opacity • Consolidation • Cysts *AND* Diffuse distribution *OR* Variant distribution: • Craniocaudal: lower lung predominant • Axial: peribronchovascular
ACCP	• Profuse and diffuse ill-defined centrilobular ground-glass nodules *OR* • Mosaicism with either air trapping and centrilobular nodules or three-density sign *AND* • Lack of features to support an alternative diagnosis	• Non-profuse, non-diffuse ill-defined centrilobular ground-glass nodules *OR* • Mosaicism or air trapping *OR* • Patchy and diffuse ground-glass opacity *AND* • Lack of features to support an alternative diagnosis

up to 5 mm. Mosaicism and air trapping are distinct terms which should not be used interchangeably. Mosaicism refers to the juxtaposition of regions of varying attenuation on inspiratory CT, which may indicate SAD, small vessel disease or parenchymal infiltration. Air trapping is a specific term relevant to expiratory imaging. It refers to relative regional hypoattenuation distal to airway obstruction. Basic HRCT descriptors of common use in HP are summarized in **Table 3**. Nonspecific isolated abnormalities such as subtle and uniform GGO, consolidation or cysts could occasionally be encountered in non-fibrotic HP (**Fig. 3**). Such findings may be deemed compatible with HRCT when diffusely distributed. A lower lobe or peribronchovascular predominance of these abnormalities may also be accepted in the compatible ATS/JRS/ALAT category. The ACCP description differs in that it does not rely as strongly on distribution and does not strictly necessitate a combination of airway and parenchymal abnormality to reach a higher degree of HRCT confidence.[6] As per the ACCP description of a typical HRCT pattern, SAD manifesting as diffuse CLNs may suffice in the absence of features to suggest alternative diagnoses. Typical HRCT patterns also include the presence of mosaicism with either air trapping and CLNs or the three-density sign. The three-

density sign (previously headcheese sign) refers to juxtaposed regions of low, intermediate, and high attenuation, respectively, reflective of air trapping, spared lung, and parenchymal infiltration. The use of this term is conversely limited to the fibrotic form of the disease in the ATS/JRS/ALAT guidelines.

Fibrotic HP: In the ATS/JRS/ALAT algorithm, typical and compatible HRCT patterns imply the combination of fibrosis and SAD in specific distributions. In typical HP, coarse reticulation predominates. Although honeycombing and traction bronchiectasis may be present, they should not be the dominant feature. Distribution may be diffuse in both craniocaudal and axial planes, which predominantly involve the mid-lung zones or spare the lung bases. In the compatible HP category, variant fibrotic and distribution patterns are accepted. A typical UIP pattern (ie, lower lobe and subpleural predominant honeycombing) and subtle fibrosis superimposed on extensive GGO are described as potential variant patterns of fibrosis. Honeycombing the radiologic hallmark feature of a typical UIP pattern is frequently present and may be seen in up to 42% of patients with fibrotic HP [PMID: 30653927]. The distribution of these abnormalities may be upper lobe predominant craniocaudally and/or peribronchovascular or subpleural

Table 2
Summary of the American Thoracic Society/Japanese Respiratory Society/Asociación Latino americana del Tórax and American College of Chest Physicians and the American College of Chest Physicians diagnostic CT categories of fibrotic hypersensitivity pneumonia on high-resolution CT

HRCT Pattern	Typical HP	Compatible with HP	Indeterminate for HP
ATS/JRS/ALAT	Fibrosis: • Predominant coarse reticulation/irregular linear opacities *AND* ≥1 feature of small airway disease: • Ill-defined centrilobular nodules and/or GGO • Mosaicism, three-density sign and/or air trapping *AND* Distribution possibilities: • Diffuse (Axial, craniocaudal planes) • Mid-lung predominant • Basilar sparing	Fibrosis: • UIP pattern • Subtle fibrosis and extensive GGO *AND* ≥1 feature of small airway disease: • Ill-defined centrilobular nodules • Three-density sign and/or air trapping *AND* Distribution possibilities: • Craniocaudal: upper lung predominant • Axial: peribronchovascular, subpleural	Fibrosis without compelling features of HP • Indeterminate, probable, typical UIP • Fibrotic NSIP • Organizing pneumonia • Indeterminate
ACCP	Fibrosis *AND* • Profuse and diffuse ill-defined centrilobular ground-glass nodules *OR* • Mosaicism with three-density sign *AND* • Lack of features to support an alternative diagnosis	Fibrosis *AND* • Non-profuse ill-defined centrilobular *OR* • Mosaicism and air trapping not meeting criteria for typical HP *OR* • Patchy or diffuse GGO *AND* • Lack of features to support an alternative diagnosis	Fibrosis without other features of HP

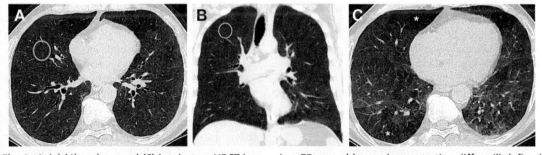

Fig. 1. Axial (*A*) and coronal (*B*) inspiratory HRCT images in a 75-year-old man demonstrating diffuse ill-defined centrilobular nodularity of ground-glass attenuation (*circle, A* and *B*). Axial expiratory (*C*) HRCT image demonstrating persistent regions of hypoattenuation reflective of air trapping (*asterisk, C*) in corresponding regions of inspiratory mosaicism (*A*). Findings were consistent with a typical non-fibrotic HP pattern per the ACCP and ATS/JRS/ALAT guidelines. Clinical interrogation revealed recurrent exposure to chemical solvents applied during woodworking. The patient regularly performed woodwork in a poorly ventilated space without mask protection.

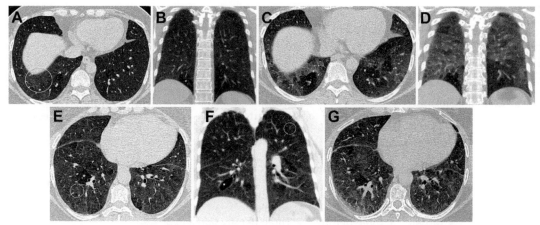

Fig. 2. Axial (*A*) and coronal (*B*) inspiratory HRCT images in a 54-year-old woman demonstrating diffuse faint ground-glass attenuation and centrilobular nodularity (*circle, A*) adjacent to lobular regions of hypoattenuation (*asterix, A* and *B*) reflective of mosaicism. Axial (*C*) and coronal (*D*) expiratory HRCT images demonstrating persistent lobular hypoattenuation reflective of air trapping. Similarly, axial (*E*) and coronal (*F*) inspiratory HRCT images in a 58-year-old woman demonstrating diffuse ill-defined centrilobular ground-glass nodularity (*circle, E* and *F*) and mosaicism (*asterix, E* and *F*). Axial (*G*) expiratory HRCT image demonstrating persistent lobular hypoattenuation reflective of air trapping in the regions of corresponding inspiratory mosaicism. Findings were consistent with a typical non-fibrotic HP pattern as per the ACCP and ATS/JRS/ALAT guidelines in both patients. Clinical interrogation revealed continuous exposure to bird antigens and hay in the first patient and recurrent hot tub exposure in the second patient.

axially. In addition to SAD manifestations described in non-fibrotic HP, the three-density sign is added to both typical and compatible fibrotic HP patterns (**Figs. 4** and **5**). The three-density sign has been shown to be highly specific for fibrotic HP.[25] The involvement of at least five lobules in a minimum of three lobes was also shown to be specific in distinguishing HP from UIP/IPF, although grading of mosaicism remains in large part subjective in clinical practice.[25] The ACCP categorization scheme differs in that detailed descriptions of fibrotic patterns are not provided, and distribution is not emphasized (see **Fig. 5**). HRCT is considered typical for HP when fibrosis is associated with diffusely distributed ground-glass CLNs or with mosaicism and the three-density sign. In HRCTs compatible with HP, fibrosis may be coupled with a lesser degree of CLNs, patchy or diffuse GGO or mosaicism and air trapping. In both categorization schemes, an indeterminate HRCT pattern for HP includes patterns suggestive of alternate diagnoses in the absence of compelling HP findings (**Fig. 6**).

Histopathologic evaluation

Lung biopsy should be avoided when a high level of diagnostic confidence can be achieved at MDD on a review of available exposure history, HRCT and BAL data. When a confident diagnosis cannot be made from available information, lung biopsy should be considered following an

assessment of patients' risks and benefits.[6,7] Histopathology is a powerful tool in the diagnostic workup of HP. Similar to HRCT, an initial determination to include or exclude the presence of fibrosis is crucial. Under the ATS/JRS/ALAT guidelines, both fibrotic and non-fibrotic forms of HP can be categorized at histopathology as typical, probable, or indeterminate. As per the ATS/JRS/ALAT guidelines, a typical HP pattern at histopathology allows, at a minimum, a high-confidence diagnosis (80% to 89%) when HRCT is indeterminate and an exposure cannot be identified. In all other scenarios, a typical HP pattern at histopathology allows a definite HP diagnosis ($\geq$90%) regardless of exposure history or HRCT confidence level.[7] Although these guidelines suggest pathologic categorization of HP as typical, probable, or indeterminate, the practical use of this categorization has faced criticism within the pathology community and poses several challenges. First, for ILD, pathologists provide a histologic diagnosis based on the microscopic findings without use of the terms typical, probable, or indeterminate. Second, the strict nature of the criteria makes its practical application challenging for interpretation of the typical case. For example, any case may have a single focus suggestive of aspirated material; however, under the ATS/JRS/ALAT criteria, any such case is functionally excluded from evaluation as this meets exclusionary criteria for all categories. Finally, the

Table 3
Basic high-resolution CT descriptors of use in hypersensitivity pneumonia relevant to parenchymal infiltration and small airway disease

Key disease characteristics	Term	Definition	Example
Parenchymal infiltration	Ground-glass opacity (GGO)	Patchy regions of increased parenchymal attenuation	
	Mosaicism	Juxtaposed regions of varying attenuation on inspiratory CT may reflect the presence of GGO	
Small airway disease	Centrilobular nodules	Ill-defined ground-glass nodules ≤ 5 mm at the center of secondary pulmonary lobules	

(continued on next page)

Table 3
(continued)

Key disease characteristics	Term	Definition	Example
	Air trapping	Geographic/lobular regions of relative low-attenuation on expiratory CT reflecting trapped air distal to small airway obstruction	
	Three-density pattern	Juxtaposed regions of low attenuation (air trapping), intermediate attenuation (unaffected lung), and high attenuation (infiltration)	

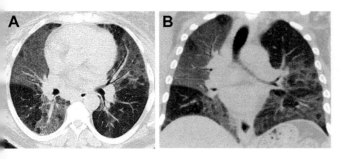

Fig. 3. Axial (*A*) and coronal (*B*) inspiratory HRCT images in a 48-year-old woman demonstrating randomly distributed bilateral ground-glass opacity and mosaicism indicating parenchymal infiltration. The absence of an expiratory phase of imaging precluded the assessment for air trapping and centrilobular nodularity was not present. Findings were therefore compatible with a nonfibrotic HP pattern as per the ACCP and ATS/JRS/ALAT.

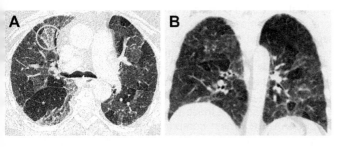

Fig. 4. Axial (*A*) inspiratory HRCT images in a 76-year-old woman demonstrating axially diffuse multifocal coarse reticulation and the three-density sign. The three-density sign corresponds to the combination of geographic hypoattenuation due to air trapping (*asterisk, A*), ground-glass opacity due to parenchymal infiltration (*circle, A*), and intervening intermediate density reflecting spared lung (*arrow, A*). Coronal HRCT image (*B*) demonstrates the diffuse distribution of abnormality in the craniocaudal plane. Findings were consistent with a typical fibrotic HP pattern as per the ACCP and ATS/JRS/ALAT guidelines.

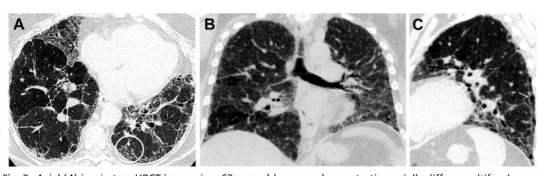

Fig. 5. Axial (*A*) inspiratory HRCT images in a 62-year-old woman demonstrating axially diffuse multifocal coarse reticulation and the three-density sign. Geographic hypoattenuation due to air trapping in the right lung (*asterisk, A*) is interposed between ground-glass opacity due to parenchymal infiltration anteriorly and intermediate density reflecting spared lung posteriorly. Left lower lobe predominant subpleural honeycomb cysts are seen (*circle, A*) (*arrow, C*). Coronal (*B*) and sagittal (*C*) HRCT images demonstrate the lower lobe predominance of abnormality in the craniocaudal plane. Findings were consistent with fibrotic HP as per the ACCP guidelines, although compatible with fibrotic HP as per the ATS/JRS/ALAT guidelines given the lower lobe involvement. The HP panel was notable for the presence of anti-*Micropolyspora faeni* IgGs. The patient had a known bird exposure for 20 years.

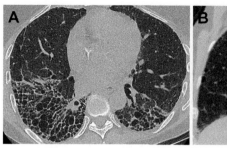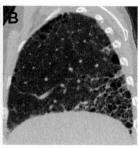

Fig. 6. Axial (*A*) inspiratory and sagittal (*B*) HRCT images in a 74-year-old woman demonstrating lower lobe predominant exuberant honeycombing. The pattern is highly suggestive of connective tissue-ILD, and the pattern therefore deemed indeterminate for HP as per the ACCP and ATS/JRS/ALAT guidelines.

guidelines discourage a differential diagnosis as the focus is placed entirely on the presence or absence of features of HP. These categories are best reserved for MDD.[26]

Non-fibrotic HP: Major features of non-fibrotic HP at histopathology include a lymphocytic predominant airway-centered cellular interstitial pneumonia resembling cellular nonspecific interstitial pneumonia (**Fig. 7**), a lymphocytic predominant cellular bronchiolitis (**Fig. 8**), and the presence of poorly formed non-necrotizing granulomas (**Fig. 9**).[5,7] The loose appearance, small size, and absence of surrounding hyaline fibrosis are helpful features in distinguishing these from sarcoid-type granulomas. After discussion at MDD, the pathologic diagnosis can be categorized into typical, probable, or indeterminate patterns. A typical pattern implies the presence of all three findings in at least one biopsy site. A probable HP pattern is present if granulomas are not found but the remaining two cardinal findings are present concurrently on a specimen. When either interstitial or peribronchiolar lymphocytic inflammation is present, the pattern is considered indeterminate.

Fibrotic HP: Major features of fibrotic HP at histopathology include airway-centered fibrosis, chronic fibrosing interstitial pneumonia, and the presence of poorly formed non-necrotizing granulomas (**Figs. 10 and 11**). After discussion at MDD, the pathologic diagnosis can similarly be categorized into typical, probable, or indeterminate patterns. A typical pattern implies the presence of all three findings in at least one biopsy site. A probable HP pattern implies the absence of granulomas and the identification of airway-centered and interstitial fibrosis concurrently on a specimen. If only interstitial fibrosis is seen, the pattern is considered indeterminate.[7] Airway-centered fibrosis in HP is characterized by peribronchiolar metaplasia (**Fig. 12**) and bridging fibrosis. Although these findings are more pronounced in HP when compared with UIP/IPF, substantial overlap exists.[12,27] Interstitial fibrosis may be reminiscent of a UIP pattern with the presence of fibroblastic foci and subpleural honeycombing, as it may resemble fibrotic NSIP. Fibrotic features may be superimposed on the chronic interstitial and airway-centered inflammation seen in non-fibrotic HP.[7,12] Additional findings that may be encountered in both fibrotic and non-fibrotic HP forms include Masson bodies of organizing pneumonia and scattered multinucleated giant cells containing cytoplasmic inclusions.[5,28] In both

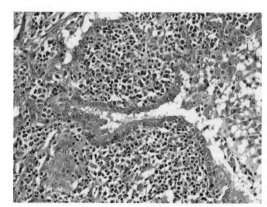

Fig. 7. Hematoxylin and eosin (H&E) stain showing airway-centered (*arrowhead*) mild interstitial chronic inflammation focally associated with reactive pneumocytes (NSIP-like pattern).

Fig. 8. H&E stain showing chronic bronchiolitis with submucosal lymphocytes and plasma cells.

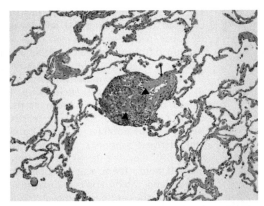

Fig. 9. H&E stain showing an interstitial non-necrotizing granuloma and multinucleated giant cells (*arrowheads*) adjacent to a pulmonary arteriole (*arrow*).

disease forms, features suggestive of an alternative diagnosis should be absent such as plasmacytic predominance, necrotizing or sarcoid-type granulomas, or aspirated material.[7]

CLINICAL OUTCOMES

Several prognostic factors have been identified in HP. Imaging and histopathologic evidence of fibrosis has been consistently shown to adversely impact outcomes, particularly when a UIP pattern of fibrosis is identified.[14,17,29] This underlines the role of radiology and pathology in portending prognosis. Patients with fibrotic HP are also more likely to be older, have an unidentified exposure, lack typical BAL findings of lymphocytosis, and present with greater functional impairment; all factors independently associated with worse survival.[12,17] Smoking-related changes on radiologic–pathologic specimens also infer a

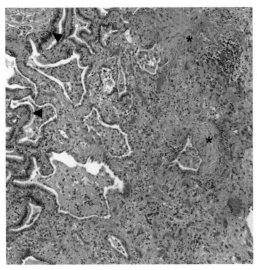

Fig. 11. H&E stain showing fibrotic HP with fibroblastic foci (*asterisks*) (suggestive of a UIP-pattern) and interstitial fibrosis with bronchiolar metaplasia (*arrowheads*).

worse prognosis as smoking is associated with a higher likelihood of delayed diagnosis and adverse outcomes.[18] Beyond the identification of prognostic factors, imaging may impact disease course by assisting in timely diagnosis and prompting a search for the culprit antigen. Removal of exposure and appropriate management may prevent progression and allow recovery, even in fibrotic disease (**Fig. 13**)[11,14][PMID: 35236720]. In addition, categorizing patients as having fibrotic HP could prompt evaluation for underlying genetic factors such as short telomere lengths that carry prognostic value and can potentially impact decisions on immunosuppressive therapy [PMID: 33122338].

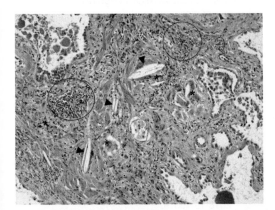

Fig. 10. H&E showing fibrotic HP with poorly defined granulomas (*asterisks*) adjacent to airways, some which contain cholesterol clefts (*arrowhead*) and a lymphoplasmocytic infiltrate (*circles*).

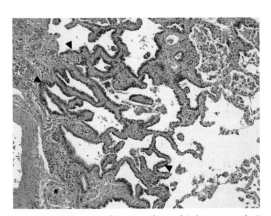

Fig. 12. H&E stain showing bronchiolar metaplasia (*arrowheads*) with a small non-necrotizing granuloma (*asterisk*).

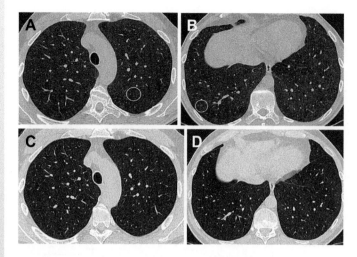

Fig. 13. Axial inspiratory HRCT images centered on the upper (*A*) and lower (*B*) lobes in a 47-year-old man demonstrating diffuse ill-defined centrilobular nodularity of ground-glass attenuation (*circle, A* and *B*) and mosaicism (*asterisk, B*). Findings were consistent with a typical non-fibrotic HP pattern as per the ACCP and ATS/JRS/ALAT guidelines. HP panel was notable for positivity of mold-derived antigens. Home tests confirmed elevated levels of environmental mold. There was a significant clinical and radiographic improvement following the antigen removal. Axial inspiratory HRCT images at comparable upper (*C*) and lower (*D*) lobe sections 17 months following initial CT demonstrating resolution of the findings.

SUMMARY

In summary, HP is a heterogeneous subgroup of ILDs resulting from the immune-mediated reaction to an airborne antigen in a sensitized host. Diagnosis is made challenging by the breadth of possible inciting exposures and the great variability in disease epidemiology and presentations. A thorough investigation of possible exposures is crucial. Because of the significant overlap between HP and other types of ILD, notably IPF, HP should be suspected in any patient presenting with ILD until a definite diagnostic determination is made. HRCT is key in the diagnostic workup and assisted by bronchoscopic and histopathologic specimens when required. Radiologic–pathologic assessment is valuable to distinguish fibrotic and non-fibrotic forms of the disease, as fibrosis portends a worse prognosis. MDD is central in establishing a confident HP diagnosis by incorporating available clinical, radiologic, and pathologic information.

CLINICS CARE POINTS

- Hypersensitivity pneumonia (HP) should be suspected in any patient presenting with interstitial lung disease.

- The absence of an identifiable causative antigen does not exclude HP.

- There is a significant overlap in the clinical presentation and radiologic appearance of fibrotic HP and UIP/idiopathic pulmonary fibrosis.

- Fibrotic HP carries a worse prognosis when compared with non-fibrotic HP.

REFERENCES

1. Ramazzini B. Diseases of Workers. Translated from the Latin Text De Morbis Artificum of 1713 by Wilmer Cave Wright, with an Introduction by George Rosen. New York, London: Hafner, 1964.

2. Towey JW, Sweany HC, Huron WH. Severe bronchial asthma apparently due to fungus spores found in maple bark. J Am Med Assoc 1932;99:453–9.

3. Bourke SJ, Dalphin JC, Boyd G, et al. Hypersensitivity pneumonitis: current concepts. Eur Respir J Suppl 2001;32:81s–92s.

4. Vasakova M, Selman M, Morell F, et al. Hypersensitivity pneumonitis: current concepts of pathogenesis and potential targets for treatment. Am J Respir Crit Care Med 2019;200:301–8.

5. Hirschmann JV, Pipavath SN, Godwin JD. Hypersensitivity pneumonitis: a historical, clinical, and radiologic review. Radiographics 2009;29:1921–38.

6. Fernandez Perez ER, Travis WD, Lynch DA, et al. Diagnosis and evaluation of hypersensitivity pneumonitis: CHEST guideline and expert panel report. Chest 2021;160:e97–156.

7. Raghu G, Remy-Jardin M, Ryerson CJ, et al. Diagnosis of hypersensitivity pneumonitis in adults. An Official ATS/JRS/ALAT clinical practice guideline. Am J Respir Crit Care Med 2020;202:e36–69.

8. Thomeer MJ, Costabe U, Rizzato G, et al. Comparison of registries of interstitial lung diseases in three European countries. Eur Respir J Suppl 2001;32:114s–8s.

9. Fernandez Perez ER, Kong AM, Raimundo K, et al. Epidemiology of hypersensitivity pneumonitis among an insured population in the United States: a claims-based cohort analysis. Ann Am Thorac Soc 2018;15:460–9.

10. Kaul B, Cottin V, Collard HR, et al. Variability in global prevalence of interstitial lung disease. Front Med (Lausanne) 2021;8:751181.

11. Fernandez Perez ER, Swigris JJ, Forssen AV, et al. Identifying an inciting antigen is associated with improved survival in patients with chronic hypersensitivity pneumonitis. Chest 2013;144:1644–51.

12. Hamblin M, Prosch H, Vasakova M. Diagnosis, course and management of hypersensitivity pneumonitis. Eur Respir Rev 2022;31:210169.

13. Baldwin CI, Todd A, Bourke SJ, et al. Pigeon fanciers' lung: identification of disease-associated carbohydrate epitopes on pigeon intestinal mucin. Clin Exp Immunol 1999;117:230–6.

14. De Sadeleer LJ, Hermans F, De Dycker E, et al. Effects of corticosteroid treatment and antigen avoidance in a large hypersensitivity pneumonitis cohort: a single-centre cohort study. J Clin Med 2018;8.

15. Depierre A, Dalphin JC, Pernet D, et al. Epidemiological study of farmer's lung in five districts of the French Doubs province. Thorax 1988;43:429–35.

16. Blanchet MR, Israel-Assayag E, Cormier Y. Inhibitory effect of nicotine on experimental hypersensitivity pneumonitis in vivo and in vitro. Am J Respir Crit Care Med 2004;169:903–9.

17. Creamer AW, Barratt SL. Prognostic factors in chronic hypersensitivity pneumonitis. Eur Respir Rev 2020;29.

18. Dangman KH, Storey E, Schenck P, et al. Effects of cigarette smoking on diagnostic tests for work-related hypersensitivity pneumonitis: data from an outbreak of lung disease in metalworkers. Am J Ind Med 2004;45:455–67.

19. Allen DH, Basten A, Williams GV, et al. Familial hypersensitivity pneumonitis. Am J Med 1975;59: 505–14.

20. Lacasse Y, Selman M, Costabel U, et al. Clinical diagnosis of hypersensitivity pneumonitis. Am J Respir Crit Care Med 2003;168:952–8.

21. Woge MJ, Ryu JH, Moua T. Diagnostic implications of positive avian serology in suspected hypersensitivity pneumonitis. Respir Med 2017;129:173–8.

22. Burrell R, Rylander R. A critical review of the role of precipitins in hypersensitivity pneumonitis. Eur J Respir Dis 1981;62:332–43.

23. Vasakova M, Morell F, Walsh S, et al. Hypersensitivity pneumonitis: perspectives in diagnosis and management. Am J Respir Crit Care Med 2017;196: 680–9.

24. Lacasse Y, Cormier Y. Hypersensitivity pneumonitis. Orphanet J Rare Dis 2006;1:25.

25. Barnett J, Molyneaux PL, Rawal B, et al. Variable utility of mosaic attenuation to distinguish fibrotic hypersensitivity pneumonitis from idiopathic pulmonary fibrosis. Eur Respir J 2019;54.

26. Churg A. Hypersensitivity pneumonitis: new concepts and classifications. Mod Pathol 2022;35: 15–27.

27. Akashi T, Takemura T, Ando N, et al. Histopathologic analysis of sixteen autopsy cases of chronic hypersensitivity pneumonitis and comparison with idiopathic pulmonary fibrosis/usual interstitial pneumonia. Am J Clin Pathol 2009;131:405–15.

28. Castonguay MC, Ryu JH, Yi ES, et al. Granulomas and giant cells in hypersensitivity pneumonitis. Hum Pathol 2015;46:607–13.

29. Mooney JJ, Elicker BM, Urbania TH, et al. Radiographic fibrosis score predicts survival in hypersensitivity pneumonitis. Chest 2013;144:586–92.

Imaging of Pulmonary Manifestations of Connective Tissue Disease

Kimberly Kallianos, MD

KEYWORDS

- Connective tissue disease • Interstitial lung disease • Nonspecific interstitial pneumonia
- Organizing pneumonia • Lymphoid interstitial pneumonia • Usual interstitial pneumonia
- Interstitial pneumonia with autoimmune features

KEY POINTS

- The diagnosis of connective tissue disease-related interstitial lung disease is a multidisciplinary process, integrating clinical findings, serologic data, and imaging patterns.
- Although connective tissue disease-associated interstitial lung disease connective tissue disease-related usual interstitial pneumonia (CTD-ILD) can present with any pattern, the most commonly seen patterns are nonspecific interstitial pneumonia (NSIP), organizing pneumonia (OP), NSIP/OP overlap, and lymphoid interstitial pneumonia. CTD-UIP is also seen, most commonly in patients with rheumatoid arthritis.
- Multicompartmental disease, when seen, supports a diagnosis of CTD-ILD. These features include airways disease, pleural/pericardial effusions, and pulmonary hypertension.

CLINICAL DIAGNOSIS OF CONNECTIVE TISSUES DISEASE

The majority of connective tissue diseases (CTDs) are multisystem disorders that are often heterogeneous in their presentation and do not have a single laboratory, histologic, or radiologic feature that is defined as the gold standard to support a specific diagnosis.[1] Given this challenging situation, the diagnosis of CTD is a process that requires the synthesis of multidisciplinary data which may include patient clinical symptoms, serologic evaluation, laboratory testing, histology from tissue biopsy, and imaging (**Table 1**).[2–6]

Thus, the goals of a radiologist in the workup of a patient with suspected CTD are several. Image interpretation and identification of pulmonary and extrapulmonary manifestations that would suggest an underlying CTD is a primary goal; however, the radiologist also must be comfortable with the multidisciplinary data supplied by the other arms of the patient's workup so as to place the imaging findings in the appropriate clinical context. In fact, a radiologist with broad knowledge of the features and presentation of CTD is a great asset in the diagnosis of CTD patients, as imaging findings are not infrequently the initial presenting symptom. In a series of 114 patients evaluated in an interstitial lung disease program, 34 (30%) satisfied criteria American College of Rheumatology criteria for a CTD, 17 (15%) of which were newly diagnosed with CTD as a direct result of their evaluation by the interstitial lung disease program.[7] In addition, a subset of patients with presumed idiopathic interstitial pneumonia such as idiopathic pulmonary fibrosis followed longitudinally will subsequently be diagnosed with a CTD at follow-up. In one series of 68 patients diagnosed with idiopathic interstitial lung disease, 13 patients (19%) developed a CTD over the 1 to 11 year follow-up period.[8]

The author has nothing to disclose.
Department of Radiology and Biomedical Imaging, UCSF, 505 Parnassus Avenue, M391, San Francisco, CA 94143, USA
E-mail address: Kimberly.Kallianos@ucsf.edu

Table 1
Classification criteria for connective tissue diseases

Lupus	Scleroderma	Rheumatoid Arthritis	Myositis	Sjogren
Skin rash/ photosensitivity	Sclerodactyly	Joint symptoms	Proximal muscle weakness	Ocular symptoms
Oral ulcers	Fingertip lesions	Duration > 6 wk	Dysphagia	Oral symptoms
Arthritis	Telangiectasia	Rheumatoid nodules	Muscle biopsy	Salivary gland biopsy
Serositis	Pulmonary hypertension and/or interstitial lung disease	Rheumatoid factor	Elevated skeletal muscle enzymes	Sjogren-related autoantibodies
Systemic disorders—renal, neurologic, hematologic, immunologic	Raynaud phenomenon	Radiographic erosions	EMG findings	
Antinuclear antibody	SSc-related autoantibodies		Skin rash	

SEROLOGIC ANALYSIS

Evaluation for the presence of autoantibodies is a key feature in the workup of patients with presumed CTD. Although a comprehensive understanding of the breath of autoantibodies evaluated in the practice of rheumatology is beyond the scope of practice for radiologists, a general familiarity with the common autoantibodies associated with CTDs allows radiologists involved in the diagnosis of patients with interstitial lung disease to engage fully in the multidisciplinary conversation that takes place to distinguish patients with idiopathic ILD from those with an underlying connective tissue disorder. Multidisciplinary assessment of patients with interstitial lung disease has been shown in the literature to improve dialogistic certainty, resulting in a change in diagnosis from IPF to CTD-ILD in 28% of patients.[9]

The ATS/ERS/JRS/ALAT Clinical Practice Guidelines for patients with newly diagnosed interstitial lung disease who are clinically suspected of having IPF recommend serologic testing to aid in the exclusion CTD as a cause of the patient's lung disease.[10,11] Guidelines recommend testing for antinuclear antibody (ANA), anti-cyclic citrullinated peptide (anti-CCP), and rheumatoid factor (RF) in all patients with suspected ILD. More focused antibody tests such as Scl70, SSA/Ro, SSB/La, RNP, and myositis–related antibodies can be performed in specific cases, as discussed below.

ANA titers are very commonly tested in patients with presumed CTD. Low-level titers (for example 1:40 dilution) can be seen in up to 32% of normal individuals, and thus a higher cut-off of 1:160 or 1:320 dilution improves the identification of a clinically significant positive ANA result.[12] Positive ANA is sensitive for the diagnosis of lupus (93%) and scleroderma (85%); however, it can be less helpful in the diagnosis of other connective tissue disorders. For example, myositis or anti-synthetase syndrome is classically ANA negative.[13] In addition to the presence of a positive ANA, the pattern of staining is also a relevant feature—with options including nuclear, nucleolar, and centromeric patterns. Anti-centromeric pattern is strongly associated with scleroderma.[14]

Rheumatoid factor positivity has a high sensitivity and specificity for the diagnosis of rheumatoid arthritis (both near 70%), whereas anti-CCP has an even higher specificity (95%–99%).[12] Anti-topoisomerase I, also known as anti-Scl70 has a very high specificity for scleroderma (90%–100%). Other highly specific autoantibodies for a defined CTD include anti-ds-DNA and anti-Smith antibodies which have a specificity for SLE of 97% and 96% respectively. A positive anti-RNP in isolation is both highly sensitive and specific for mixed CTD. The combination of positive anti-SSA/Ro and anti-SSB/La antibodies is suggestive of Sjogren's disease, although positive SSA in isolation can also be seen with a variety of other CTDs, particularly scleroderma.[15] Finally, a variety of autoantibodies can be detected in patients with myositis (either polymyositis or dermatomyositis) and are associated with an increased risk of interstitial lung disease. Anti-tRNA synthetase antibodies (Jo-1, PL-7, PL-12, EJ, OJ, KS, Ha, Zo) are specific for the diagnosis of myositis, of which anti Jo-1 is the most common (seen in 20%–30%), followed by anti PL-7 and PL-12 (seen in 3%–4%).[15] Anti-Jo1 antibody positivity is seen in 30% to 75% of myositis patients with ILD.[16]

CT FINDINGS IN CONNECTIVE TISSUE DISEASE PATIENTS

Nearly all patterns of interstitial lung disease can be seen in patients with CTD, although the four most common patterns of interstitial lung disease seen in patients with CTD are nonspecific interstitial pneumonia (NSIP), organizing pneumonia (OP), NSIP/OP overlap, and lymphoid interstitial pneumonia (LIP). Surgical biopsy to confirm a particular pattern of interstitial lung disease is rarely performed, and therefore high-resolution computed tomography (CT) is very frequently used to determine the primary pattern of lung pathology.

The most common pattern of interstitial lung disease seen in patients with CTD is NSIP (**Fig. 1**). CT findings in NSIP include (1) symmetric bilateral ground-glass opacity, (2) irregular reticulation, and (3) traction bronchiectasis.[17] The combination of ground-glass opacity with reticulation and relatively minimal honeycombing has a 96% sensitivity for NSIP versus UIP; however, only a moderate specificity (41%).[18] Histologically, these findings correspond to varying degrees of fibrosis and interstitial inflammation uniformly involving the peripheral and basilar lung.[19] Relative subpleural sparing, although not a sensitive finding, is highly specific for distinguishing NSIP from UIP pattern (96%).[20]

Organizing pneumonia seen in patients with CTD has a similar CT appearance to organizing pneumonia due to other causes (**Fig. 2**). Common findings include symmetric, peripheral, or peribronchovascular ground-glass opacity and consolidation.[21] The atoll or reverse halo sign characterized by rounded or crescentic regions of consolidation with central clearing or ground-glass opacity may also be seen in 20% of patients with OP.[22] Combined features of NSIP and OP, also called "NSIP/OP overlap", include the greater extent of consolidation and greater frequency of combined peripheral plus peribronchovascular distribution than is seen in patients with isolated NSIP pattern[23] (**Fig. 3**).

LIP/follicular bronchiolitis is characterized by interstitial infiltration by lymphocytes and plasma cells; however, these are polyclonal in origin, which helps to distinguish from these findings from low-grade lymphoma. The major CT findings corresponding to this histology include ground-glass opacity, small ill-defined nodules, and perivascular cysts[24] (**Fig. 4**).

Usual interstitial pneumonia (UIP) pattern is also seen in patients with CTD. CTD-UIP patients tend to be younger and more likely to be female compared with patients with UIP pattern due to idiopathic pulmonary fibrosis (IPF).[25] UIP pattern is defined by basilar and peripheral predominate fibrosis with reticulation, traction bronchiectasis, and honeycombing[11] (**Fig. 5**). Several CT findings have been reported as useful in distinguishing UIP pattern due to CTD versus UIP pattern in patients with IPF. These include the "anterior upper

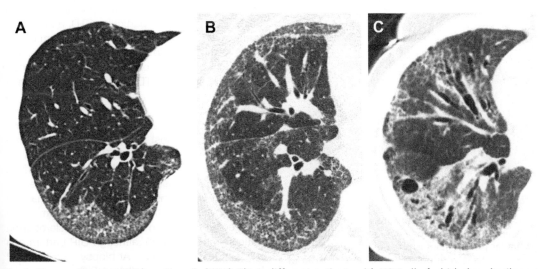

Fig. 1. Nonspecific interstitial pneumonia (NSIP). Three different patients with NSIP, all of which show basilar predominant findings with subpleural sparing. The spectrum of findings seen in NSIP include ground-glass opacity (*A*), irregular reticulation (*B*), and traction bronchiectasis (*C*).

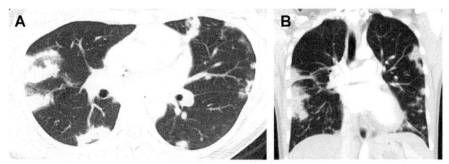

Fig. 2. Organizing pneumonia. Axial (*A*) and coronal reformatted (*B*) images show typical findings of organizing pneumonia in a patient with systemic lupus erythematosus. Patchy basilar predominant subpleural and peribronchovascular regions of consolidation with the reversed halo sign are typical findings.

lobe sign", with concentration of fibrosis in the anterior lung and relative sparing of other regions; the "straight edge sign", with a sharp line of demarcation in the craniocaudal plane between normal lung and regions involved by fibrosis; and the "exuberant honeycombing sign", with exuberant honeycomb cysts occupying 70% of the fibrotic involvement of the lung. The specificities of each of these signs alone exceed 87% for CTD-UIP, and the presence of two of the three signs has a sensitivity for CTD-UIP of 95%.[26] It is important to acknowledge that CT findings may evolve over time. Over 3 years of longitudinal follow-up in a series of 48 patients with biopsy-proven NSIP, 28% of patients with NSIP pattern on initial CT progressed to findings of UIP pattern[27] (**Fig. 6**).

In addition to pulmonary parenchymal involvement by interstitial lung disease, there are associated "multicompartmental" findings which also support a diagnosis of connective tissue-related

ILD. These include intrinsic airway disease (such as bronchiolitis obliterans as manifested by mosaic perfusion on inspiratory imaging and air trapping on expiratory imaging), pleural or pericardial effusions, and pulmonary vascular disease such as pulmonary hypertension[28] (**Fig. 7**).

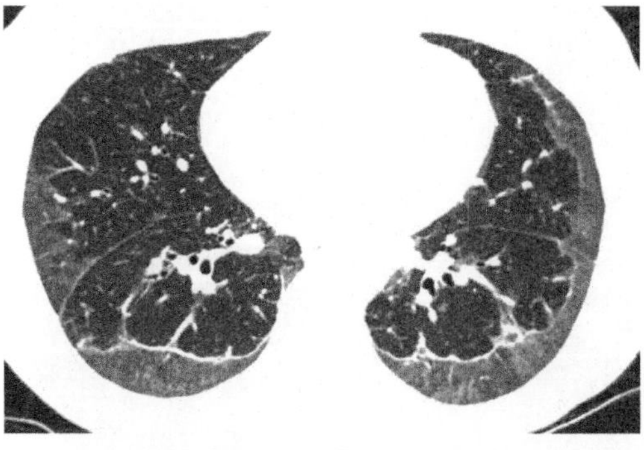

Pulmonary hypertension is defined as elevated pulmonary artery pressures greater than 25 mm Hg at rest of greater than 30 mm Hg during exercise. A variety of size thresholds of the pulmonary artery have been described in the literature; however, pulmonary artery size has only moderate sensitivity (range 47%–87%) and specificity (range 41%–100%) for the detection of pulmonary hypertension. Pulmonary artery to aorta ratio greater than 1 is a stronger predictor for pulmonary hypertension than pulmonary artery diameter alone, with a positive predictive value of 92% to 95%.[29,30]

SPECIFIC CONNECTIVE TISSUE DISEASES

There is no one pattern of interstitial lung disease that is diagnostic of a particular CTD, and all patterns have been seen across the spectrum of patients with CTD. However, certain patterns are seen more commonly or are more strongly associated with particular CTD diagnoses. These trends are summarized in **Table 2** and discussed in further detail below.

Scleroderma (**Figs. 8** and **9**)—Interstitial lung disease occurs most commonly in scleroderma compared with the other CTDs, occurring in up to 90% of patients with both limited and diffuse forms of the disease. Interstitial lung disease and pulmonary hypertension contribute to the majority (60%) of deaths in this patient population.[31] The most common pattern of ILD seen in scleroderma patients is NSIP (77%), although UIP pattern can be seen less commonly. At biopsy, fibrotic NSIP is more common than cellular NSIP.[32]

Rheumatoid arthritis (**Fig. 10**)—Interstitial lung disease is reported in up to 40% of patients with

Fig. 3. Overlap of nonspecific interstitial pneumonia (NSIP) and organizing pneumonia (OP). Subpleural and basilar predominant ground-glass opacity is present in a patient with polymyositis. Note the rim of consolidation at the interface between the ground glass opacity and normal lung. This appearance is typical of an overlap of NSIP and OP.

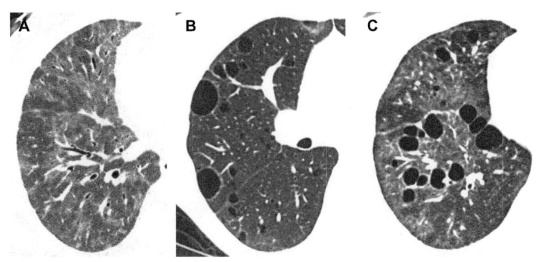

Fig. 4. Lymphoid interstitial pneumonia. Three separate patients with connective tissue disease and lymphoid interstitial pneumonia. Typical findings include ground-glass opacity (*A*), isolated cysts (*B*), and a combination of ground glass and cysts (*C*).

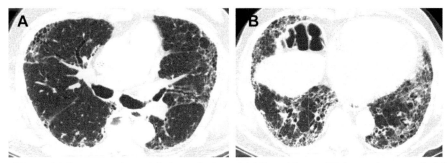

Fig. 5. Usual interstitial pneumonia. Axial through the mid (*A*) and lower (*B*) lungs shows typical findings of fibrosis and honeycombing (*arrow*) with a patchy subpleural and basilar predominance.

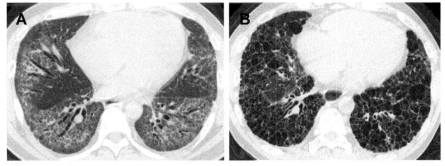

Fig. 6. Nonspecific interstitial pneumonia, evolution over time. Baseline CT (*A*) shows typical findings of nonspecific interstitial pneumonia with basilar predominant reticulation and traction bronchiectasis with subpleural sparing. Six years later (*B*), the same patient shows findings typical of usual interstitial pneumonia with extensive honeycombing.

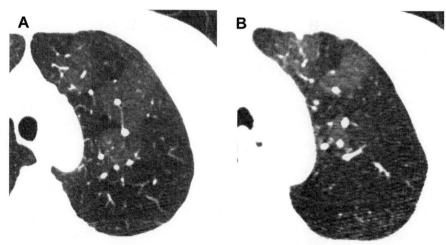

Fig. 7. Airways disease. Inspiratory (*A*) and expiratory (*B*) CT images in a patient with constrictive bronchiolitis showing mosaic perfusion, geographic regions of decreased lung density, and corresponding air trapping on the expiratory phase.

rheumatoid arthritis. Although both UIP and NSIP patterns are seen in this population, with UIP pattern reported more frequently (41%–56% vs 30%–33%).[33,34] The presence of UIP pattern in patients with RA-ILD is also associated with more rapid disease progression and increased mortality compared with NSIP pattern, although there is mixed data regarding the prognosis of patients with UIP in the setting of RA-ILD versus IPF.[35] Rheumatoid arthritis is also associated with airways disease such as bronchiolitis obliterans as well as organizing pneumonia.[36]

Myositis (**Fig. 11**)—Anti-synthetase syndrome occurs in a subset of patients with inflammatory myositis (dermatomyositis/polymyositis) who have myositis-related antibodies, including antibodies to the aminoacyl-tRNA synthetase enzymes. A substantial proportion of patients with the anti-synthetase syndrome (70%–90%) have interstitial lung disease, with the most common CT patterns in this patient population including NSIP (45%), OP (21%), or NSIP/OP overlap (24%).[37] The natural history of ILD in this patient population is a decrease of resolution of

consolidation over time in the majority of patients following treatment with corticosteroids and immunosuppression; however, fibrosis develops in a subset (38%), and the minority of patients evolve to UIP pattern of fibrosis.[38] Patients with anti-synthetase syndrome and anti-MDA-5 antibodies may also present with fulminant respiratory failure and diffuse alveolar damage, with a particularly high risk of mortality (84%).[39]

Sjogren syndrome (**Fig. 12**)—LIP is the most common interstitial lung disease seen in patients with Sjogren syndrome, seen in 50%. Airways diseases such as follicular bronchiolitis, bronchiolitis, and bronchiectasis less commonly occur.[40]

Systemic lupus erythematosus (**Fig. 13**)—The most common CT abnormality seen in up to 50% to 60% of patients with lupus is serositis including pleuritis and pleural/pericardial effusions, with lung parenchymal involvement such as pulmonary hemorrhage, pulmonary edema, and lupus pneumonitis/diffuse alveolar damage occurring in a smaller subset (3%–7%).[41,42] Pulmonary fibrosis is seen much less commonly in lupus patients than in those with other CTDs.[36]

Table 2					
Common and less common manifestations of connective tissue diseases by diagnosis					
	Scleroderma	**Rheumatoid Arthritis**	**Myositis**	**Sjogrens**	**Lupus**
Common	NSIP PAH	UIP NSIP	NSIP OP	LIP	Edema Hemorrhage DAD
Less common	UIP	Airways disease OP	DAD	Airways disease	Fibrosis

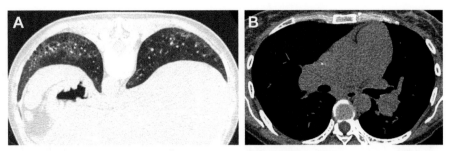

Fig. 8. Scleroderma, interstitial lung disease and pulmonary hypertension. Lung windows at the bases (A) show mild ground-glass opacity with subpleural sparing compatible with early nonspecific interstitial pneumonia in a patient with marked dyspnea. Soft tissue windows (see B) shows a markedly enlarged pulmonary artery, measuring 4.1 cm, compatible with pulmonary hypertension.

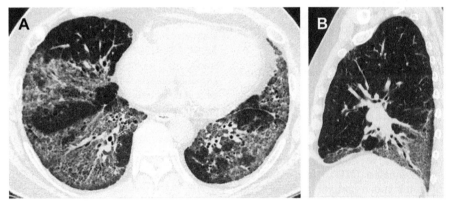

Fig. 9. Scleroderma. Axial (A) and sagittal reformatted (B) images show basilar predominant reticulation and traction bronchiectasis with subpleural sparing. Nonspecific interstitial pneumonia is the most common pattern seen in scleroderma patients.

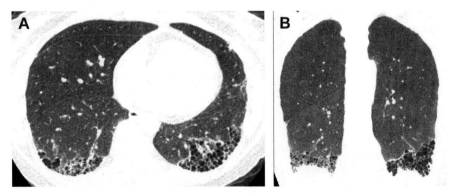

Fig. 10. Rheumatoid arthritis. Axial (A) and coronal reformatted (B) images show typical findings of usual interstitial pneumonia with peripheral and basilar fibrosis with honeycombing. In the setting of connective tissue disease, usual interstitial pneumonia is most closely associated with rheumatoid arthritis.

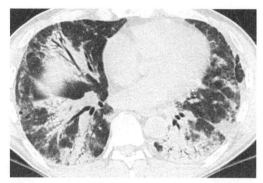

Fig. 11. Antisynthetase syndrome. A subpleural and basilar predominance of consolidation is typical of an overlap of nonspecific interstitial pneumonia and organizing pneumonia. This pattern is often seen with myositis and antisynthetase syndrome.

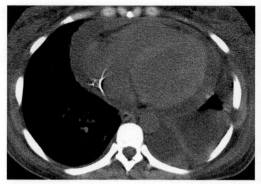

Fig. 13. Systemic lupus erythematosus (SLE). Serositis is a common finding in patients with SLE. In this patient with SLE, pericardial effusion/thickening and left-sided pleural effusion is indicative of a serositis.

Mixed Connective Tissue Disease (MCTD)—The CT features of mixed connective tissue disease (MCTD) most closely mimic those of scleroderma (NSIP) and myositis (OP), as well as an overlap of these features.[43]

Idiopathic Pneumonia with Autoimmune Features—Patients with clinical features suggesting a diagnosis of CTD but not meeting established criteria for any disorder may present with interstitial lung disease. Several different terms have been used to describe these patients including "idiopathic pneumonia with autoimmune features (IPAF)", "undifferentiated CTD", "lung-dominant CTD", and "autoimmune-featured diffuse lung disease".

To establish a diagnosis of IPAF, patients must (1) have an interstitial pneumonia by HRCT or lung biopsy, (2) not meet diagnostic criteria for a defined CTD, (3) not have another explanation for their lung disease, and (4) meet at least one feature

from two of three domains—clinical, serologic, and morphologic.[44]

Imaging findings fall under the morphologic domain, with suggestive HRCT patterns including NSIP, OP, NSIP/OP overlap, and LIP or the presence of multicompartment involvement (as described above) in addition to ILD. Other patterns of ILD have been described in patients diagnosed with IPAF (for example UIP); however, this pattern of ILD does not fulfill one of the necessary domains, and as such, features from two other domains such as clinical and serologic must also be present.[45-47]

EXACERBATION OF INTERSTITIAL LUNG DISEASE

In addition to the utility of imaging for the diagnosis of CTD, CT is also useful for the evaluation of acute symptoms in CTD patients, which may be due to worsening/exacerbation of ILD versus infection. Exacerbation of interstitial lung disease manifests with worsening fibrosis, organizing pneumonia, and/or diffuse alveolar damage—which will appear as increased diffuse ground glass and/or consolidation. Overall prognosis of ILD exacerbation is poor, with a 66% mortality rate in one series of 24 biopsy-proven ILD patients, which included patients with CTD-NSIP (3/24) and CTD-UIP (8/24).[48]

SUMMARY

Although any pattern of interstitial lung disease can be seen in patients with CTD, NSIP, OP, NSIP/OP overlap, LIP, and less commonly UIP are classically associated with CTD as described above. Familiarity with these common imaging patterns, as well as the clinical and serologic manifestations of CTD, will allow the radiologist to

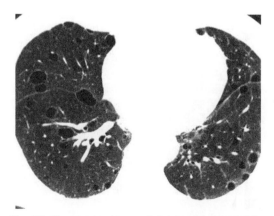

Fig. 12. Sjogren syndrome. Axial image shows thin-walled pulmonary cysts and mild ground-glass opacity in a patient with Sjogren syndrome.

contribute fully in the multidisciplinary diagnosis of patients with CTD.

CLINICS CARE POINTS

- Common CT patterns in CTD-ILD include NSIP, OP, NSIP/OP overlap, LIP, and UIP
- Multicompartmental disease including pulmonary hypertension and airways disease also support a diagnosis of CTD-ILD

REFERENCES

1. Aggarwal R, Ringold S, Khanna D, et al. Distinctions between diagnostic and classification criteria? Arthritis Care Res 2015;67(7):891–7.
2. van den Hoogen F, Khanna D, Fransen J, et al. 2013 classification criteria for systemic sclerosis: an American college of rheumatology/European league against rheumatism collaborative initiative. Ann Rheum Dis 2013;72(11):1747–55.
3. Vitali C, Bombardieri S, Jonsson R, et al. Classification criteria for Sjögren's syndrome: a revised version of the European criteria proposed by the American-European Consensus Group. Ann Rheum Dis 2002;61(6):554–8.
4. Arnett FC, Edworthy SM, Bloch DA, et al. The American Rheumatism Association 1987 revised criteria for the classification of rheumatoid arthritis. Arthritis Rheum 1988;31(3):315–24.
5. Dalakas MC, Hohlfeld R. Polymyositis and dermatomyositis. Lancet 2003;362(9388):971–82.
6. Tan EM, Cohen AS, Fries JF, et al. The 1982 revised criteria for the classification of systemic lupus erythematosus. Arthritis Rheum 1982;25(11):1271–7.
7. Mittoo S, Gelber AC, Christopher-Stine L, et al. Ascertainment of collagen vascular disease in patients presenting with interstitial lung disease. Respir Med 2009;103(8):1152–8.
8. Homma Y, Ohtsuka Y, Tanimura K, et al. Can interstitial pneumonia as the sole presentation of collagen vascular diseases be differentiated from idiopathic interstitial pneumonia? Respiration 1995;62(5):248–51.
9. Castelino FV, Goldberg H, Dellaripa PF. The impact of rheumatological evaluation in the management of patients with interstitial lung disease. Rheumatology 2010;50(3):489–93.
10. Raghu G, Rochwerg B, Zhang Y, et al. An Official ATS/ERS/JRS/ALAT Clinical Practice Guideline: Treatment of Idiopathic Pulmonary Fibrosis. An Update of the 2011 Clinical Practice Guideline. Am J Respir Crit Care Med 2015;192(2):e3–19.
11. Raghu G, Remy-Jardin M, Myers JL, et al. Diagnosis of Idiopathic Pulmonary Fibrosis. An Official ATS/ERS/JRS/ALAT Clinical Practice Guideline. Am J Respir Crit Care Med 2018;198(5):e44–68.
12. Satoh M, Vázquez-Del Mercado M, Chan EKL. Clinical interpretation of antinuclear antibody tests in systemic rheumatic diseases. Mod Rheumatol 2009;19(3):219–28.
13. Solomon DH, Kavanaugh AJ, Schur PH. Evidence-based guidelines for the use of immunologic tests: antinuclear antibody testing. Arthritis Rheum 2002;47(4):434–44.
14. Ho KT, Reveille JD. The clinical relevance of autoantibodies in scleroderma. Arthritis Res Ther 2003;5(2):80–93.
15. Jee AS, Adelstein S, Bleasel J, et al. Role of autoantibodies in the diagnosis of connective-tissue disease ILD (CTD-ILD) and interstitial pneumonia with autoimmune features (IPAF). J Clin Med 2017;6(5):51.
16. Fischer A, Swigris JJ, du Bois RM, et al. Anti-synthetase syndrome in ANA and anti-Jo-1 negative patients presenting with idiopathic interstitial pneumonia. Respir Med 2009;103(11):1719–24.
17. Travis WD, Costabel U, Hansell DM, et al. An official American Thoracic Society/European Respiratory Society statement: Update of the international multidisciplinary classification of the idiopathic interstitial pneumonias. Am J Respir Crit Care Med 2013;188(6):733–48.
18. Elliot TL, Lynch DA, Newell JD Jr, et al. High-resolution computed tomography features of nonspecific interstitial pneumonia and usual interstitial pneumonia. J Comput Assist Tomogr 2005;29(3):339–45.
19. Johkoh T, Müller NL, Colby TV, et al. Nonspecific interstitial pneumonia: correlation between thin-section CT findings and pathologic subgroups in 55 patients. Radiology 2002;225(1):199–204.
20. Silva CIS, Müller NL, Lynch DA, et al. Chronic hypersensitivity pneumonitis: differentiation from idiopathic pulmonary fibrosis and nonspecific interstitial pneumonia by using thin-section CT. Radiology 2008;246(1):288–97.
21. Zare Mehrjardi M, Kahkouee S, Pourabdollah M. Radio-pathological correlation of organizing pneumonia (OP): a pictorial review. Br J Radiol 2017;90(1071):20160723.
22. Kim SJ, Lee KS, Ryu YH, et al. Reversed halo sign on high-resolution CT of cryptogenic organizing pneumonia: diagnostic implications. AJR Am J Roentgenol 2003;180(5):1251–4.
23. Enomoto N, Sumikawa H, Sugiura H, et al. Clinical, radiological, and pathological evaluation of "NSIP with OP overlap" pattern compared with NSIP in patients with idiopathic interstitial pneumonias. Respir Med 2020;174:106201.
24. Lynch DA, Travis WD, Müller NL, et al. Idiopathic interstitial pneumonias: CT features. Radiology 2005;236(1):10–21.

25. Park JH, Kim DS, Park IN, et al. Prognosis of fibrotic interstitial pneumonia: idiopathic versus collagen vascular disease-related subtypes. Am J Respir Crit Care Med 2007;175(7):705–11.

26. Chung JH, Cox CW, Montner SM, et al. CT features of the usual interstitial pneumonia pattern: differentiating connective tissue disease-associated interstitial lung disease from idiopathic pulmonary fibrosis. AJR Am J Roentgenol 2018;210(2):307–13.

27. Silva CI, Müller NL, Hansell DM, et al. Nonspecific interstitial pneumonia and idiopathic pulmonary fibrosis: changes in pattern and distribution of disease over time. Radiology 2008;247(1):251–9.

28. Oldham JM, Adegunsoye A, Valenzi E, et al. Characterisation of patients with interstitial pneumonia with autoimmune features. Eur Respir J 2016;47(6): 1767–75.

29. Peña E, Dennie C, Veinot J, et al. Pulmonary hypertension: how the radiologist can help. Radiographics 2012;32(1):9–32.

30. Mohamed Hoesein FA, Besselink T, Pompe E, et al. Accuracy of CT Pulmonary Artery Diameter for Pulmonary Hypertension in End-Stage COPD. Lung 2016;194(5):813–9.

31. Solomon JJ, Olson AL, Fischer A, et al. Scleroderma lung disease. Eur Respir Rev 2013;22(127):6–19.

32. Bouros D, Wells AU, Nicholson AG, et al. Histopathologic subsets of fibrosing alveolitis in patients with systemic sclerosis and their relationship to outcome. Am J Respir Crit Care Med 2002;165(12):1581–6.

33. Lee HK, Kim DS, Yoo B, et al. Histopathologic pattern and clinical features of rheumatoid arthritis-associated interstitial lung disease. Chest 2005; 127(6):2019–27.

34. Tanaka N, Kim JS, Newell JD, et al. Rheumatoid arthritis-related lung diseases: CT findings. Radiology 2004;232(1):81–91.

35. Kim EJ, Collard HR, King TE Jr. Rheumatoid arthritis-associated interstitial lung disease: the relevance of histopathologic and radiographic pattern. Chest 2009;136(5):1397–405.

36. Mayberry JP, Primack SL, Müller NL. Thoracic Manifestations of Systemic Autoimmune Diseases: Radiographic and High-Resolution CT Findings. RadioGraphics 2000;20(6):1623–35.

37. Debray MP, Borie R, Revel MP, et al. Interstitial lung disease in anti-synthetase syndrome: initial and follow-up CT findings. Eur J Radiol 2015;84(3): 516–23.

38. Tillie-Leblond I, Wislez M, Valeyre D, et al. Interstitial lung disease and anti-Jo-1 antibodies: difference between acute and gradual onset. Thorax 2008; 63(1):53–9.

39. Vuillard C, Pineton de Chambrun M, de Prost N, et al. Clinical features and outcome of patients with acute respiratory failure revealing anti-synthetase or anti-MDA-5 dermato-pulmonary syndrome: a French multicenter retrospective study. Ann Intensive Care 2018;8(1):87.

40. Kim EA, Lee KS, Johkoh T, et al. Interstitial Lung Diseases Associated with Collagen Vascular Diseases: Radiologic and Histopathologic Findings. RadioGraphics 2002;22(suppl_1):S151–65.

41. Murin S, Wiedemann HP, Matthay RA. Pulmonary manifestations of systemic lupus erythematosus. Clin Chest Med 1998;19(4):641–65, viii.

42. Cervera R, Khamashta MA, Font J, et al. Systemic lupus erythematosus: clinical and immunologic patterns of disease expression in a cohort of 1,000 patients. Eur Working Party Systemic Lupus Erythematosus. Med (Baltimore) 1993;72(2):113–24.

43. Yamanaka Y, Baba T, Hagiwara E, et al. Radiological images of interstitial pneumonia in mixed connective tissue disease compared with scleroderma and polymyositis/dermatomyositis. Eur J Radiol 2018; 107:26–32.

44. Fischer A, Antoniou KM, Brown KK, et al. An official European Respiratory Society/American Thoracic Society research statement: interstitial pneumonia with autoimmune features. Eur Respir J 2015;46(4): 976–87.

45. Fischer A, Collard HR, Cottin V. Interstitial pneumonia with autoimmune features: the new consensus-based definition for this cohort of patients should be broadened. Eur Respir J 2016; 47(4):1295.

46. Dai J, Wang L, Yan X, et al. Clinical features, risk factors, and outcomes of patients with interstitial pneumonia with autoimmune features: a population-based study. Clin Rheumatol 2018;37(8):2125–32.

47. Ahmad K, Barba T, Gamondes D, et al. Interstitial pneumonia with autoimmune features: Clinical, radiologic, and histological characteristics and outcome in a series of 57 patients. Respir Med 2017;123:56–62.

48. Silva CIS, Müller NL, Fujimoto K, et al. Acute exacerbation of chronic interstitial pneumonia: high-resolution computed tomography and pathologic findings. J Thorac Imaging 2007;22(3):221–9.

Pathogenesis, Imaging, and Evolution of Acute Lung Injury

Seth Kligerman, MD

KEYWORDS

• Organizing pneumonia • Diffuse alveolar damage • CT • Fibrosis

KEY POINTS

- Acute lung injury exists on a continuum ranging from organizing pneumonia to diffuse alveolar damage.
- The site of injury in all forms of ALI is at the level of the type I alveolar epithelial cell, capillary endothelial cell, and intervening basement membrane.
- Imaging manifestations in diffuse alveolar damage (DAD), acute fibrinous and organizing pneumonia (AFOP), and organizing pneumonia (OP) share numerous patterns likely related to the same site of initial injury.
- Once the injury occurs, repair depends on the presence of type II pneumocytes and integrity of the basement membrane.
- Although the lung can repair itself in cases of ALI, in many cases permanent fibrosis occurs, which can be severe.

INTRODUCTION

There are numerous etiologies of acute lung injury (ALI) with the insult causing disruption of the framework of the lung with damage centered on capillary endothelium and alveolar epithelium and the intervening shared basement membrane.[1] This damage leads to cell death, exudation of proteinaceous and cellular material into the alveoli and interstitium, subsequent organization with alveolar collapse, and attempts at repair. ALI exists on a clinical, radiologic, and pathologic spectrum ranging from the milder organizing pneumonia (OP) pattern of injury to the extremely severe diffuse alveolar damage (DAD) pattern of injury. Acute fibrinous and OP (AFOP) is a pathologic finding highlighted by the exudation of fibrin and exists somewhere along the spectrum between OP and DAD. ALI remains a significant cause of patient morbidity and mortality, a fact highlighted by the SARS-CoV-2 (COVID-19) pandemic. Even if a patient survives the ALI, resultant pulmonary fibrosis can lead to chronic debilitation. This article discusses the clinical, radiologic, and pathologic findings of ALI, focusing on the stages of injury and pathways to repair or fibrosis.

DIFFUSE ALVEOLAR DAMAGE
Causes and Exudative Phase

DAD is the pathologic finding corresponding to a severe lung injury of which there are numerous causes including inhalation lung injury, drug toxicity, shock, and sepsis.[2] However, the most common cause of DAD is infection, which was true even before the dramatic increase in ALI seen during the COVID-19 pandemic.[3] In addition, DAD is a common pathologic process seen in acute exacerbations of underlying fibrotic lung disease.[4] In instances where the underlying cause of DAD is unknown, it is termed acute interstitial pneumonia. Although these various etiologies may seem distinct clinically, the underlying pathologic process remains constant. During the first week of injury, termed the acute exudative phase,

University of California, San Diego, 200 West Arbor Drive, San Diego, CA 92103, USA
E-mail address: skligerman@health.ucsd.edu

Radiol Clin N Am 60 (2022) 925–939
https://doi.org/10.1016/j.rcl.2022.06.005
0033-8389/22/© 2022 Elsevier Inc. All rights reserved.

there is diffuse damage to the alveolar epithelial cells, capillary endothelial cells, and intervening basement membranes with subsequent cell death and denudation of the alveolar walls.[5–10] Because of the increased capillary permeability, fluid, proteinaceous material, fibrin, and neutrophils flow into the alveoli.[6,11,12] In severe cases, damage to the blood-oxygen interface leads to leakage of red blood cells into the alveoli.[13] Hyaline membranes, eosinophilic structures composed of cellular debris, plasma proteins, and surfactant from pneumocyte death, line the alveolar walls and are the hallmark of the acute stage of DAD.[2,5]

The alveoli and alveolar septa also become infiltrated with myofibroblasts and fibroblasts as part of the normal healing process. Myofibroblasts are beneficial to closing open wounds, whereas the extracellular matrix proteins, cytokines, and growth factors released by fibroblasts are essential for wound healing.[14] However, if these cells are not removed in a timely manner, they can lead to permanent fibrosis, which can begin in less than a week after injury.[1] Myofibroblast contracture in the lungs can create distortion of the alveolar and bronchial architecture and promotes, in conjunction with the lack of surfactant because of pneumocyte death, alveolar collapse.[15,16] In addition, persistent fibroblastic activation, leading to the continued deposition of collagen in the alveoli and interstitium, can lead to permanent lung fibrosis.

On computed tomography (CT), the exudative phase of DAD is manifest as basilar predominant, but often diffuse ground-glass opacity (GGO) with areas of consolidation that are often dependent but are patchy or nodular (Fig. 1). Sparing of the anterior portions of the lungs is common. Septal thickening, caused by a combination of edema, interstitial inflammation, and alveolar collapse, is often most pronounced in the posterior aspects of the lungs because of their dependent nature.[17,18] Focal areas of spared, normal attenuated secondary lobules, termed lobular sparing, or more confluent subpleural sparing are common throughout the spectrum of ALI.[8,19,20] Bronchial dilation and volume loss are often mild in this phase.[20] The injury is essentially always bilateral and usually symmetric, although asymmetric injury can occur (Fig. 2).

Organizing Phase of Diffuse Alveolar Damage

Although there is overlap between phases because of the varying severity and distribution of injury, typically 1 week after the acute phase of DAD the organizing phase begins, eventually becoming the predominant finding by 3 weeks

postinjury.[21] Although there are many components to the organizing phase, it is most denoted by two processes: extensive volume loss caused by alveolar collapse; and organization of the exudative material filling the alveoli, alveolar ducts, and interstitium into whorls or plugs of fibroblasts and activated myofibroblasts embedded in connective tissue matrix.[22–25] These organizing plugs are similar if not identical to those seen in OP and AFOP. However, compared with OP, in DAD there is more severe architectural destruction and alveolar collapse, which can become permanent in some cases.[5,9,24,26] Nonetheless, in some instances, a pathologists may have difficulty in differentiating a severe case of OP and DAD on biopsy.[1,15] This organizing phase of DAD is also commonly referred to as the proliferative phase denoting the proliferation of epithelial and connective tissue cells in an attempt to repair the damage and re-expand the collapsed alveoli.

CT findings mirror the pathologic organization and volume loss. Although the injury may still be lower lobe–predominant with anterior sparing, in some cases the injury is so widespread that no zonal distribution can be elucidated. GGO and consolidation remain the predominant finding, although the extent of consolidation often increases (see Figs. 1 and 2). There is more extensive volume loss compared with the exudative phase, secondary to a combination of alveolar collapse and possible early fibrosis. During this stage of injury, reticulation and airway dilation can develop rapidly[8,19,27,28] and are associated with a decreased likelihood of survival.[2,28–30] It should be noted that the airway dilation seen in DAD, AFOP, or OP may not be permanent and can resolve with lung repair and alveolar re-expansion (see Fig. 2; Fig. 3). Therefore, because bronchiectasis is often used to define a permanent airway dilation,[31] the term of traction bronchiectasis, although still widely used to describe this often transitory finding, may not be technically correct. Distended and distorted subpleural secondary lobules, which can mimic cicatricial emphysema, may also form but can also abate after lung repair likely related to increased lung volumes (see Fig. 3).

Lung Repair and Fibrosis in Diffuse Alveolar Damage

Mechanisms of lung repair after DAD are extremely complex and rely on the presence of type II pneumocytes, a repairable basement membrane, and a fibrinolytic system to remove the OP plugs. Because type I pneumocytes cannot themselves regenerate, lung repair in any form of ALI

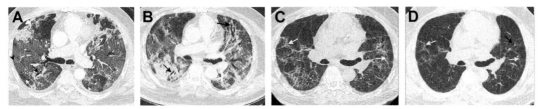

Fig. 1. (*A–D*) Diffuse alveolar damage caused by COVID in a 61-year-old man. (*A*) Axial image from a CT scan shows diffuse GGO with associated septal thickening (*black arrowhead*) and scattered areas of consolidation. Areas of subpleural (*white arrows*) and lobular (*white arrowhead*) sparing are present. There is minimal bronchial dilation (*black arrow*) and only mild volume loss. (*B*) Axial CT imaging at the same level 10 days later demonstrates increasing peribronchiolar consolidation with persistent lobular and subpleural sparing. There is associated increased volume loss with increased dilation of many airways (*black arrows*) despite being on a ventilator with high positive end pressures. (*C*) Axial CT image 5 months later shows areas of peribronchiolar GGO with architectural distortion (*white arrow*). Areas of bronchial dilation are improved but persist in some areas concerning for permanent bronchiectasis. Lung volumes are improved. (*D*) Axial CT image 12 months after the initial injury shows continued improvement of GGO and architectural distortion. However, persistent linear bands of subpleural and peribronchiolar GGO persist (*white arrows*) and represent permanent fibrosis and the residual dilated airways represent permanent traction bronchiectasis (*black arrow*). Overall, the degree of fibrosis is mild given the severity of lung injury. Importantly, the lung continued to heal even 5 months after the initial injury, so be wary of calling fibrosis early after a lung injury. (*Courtesy of* S Kligerman, MD, San Diego, California.)

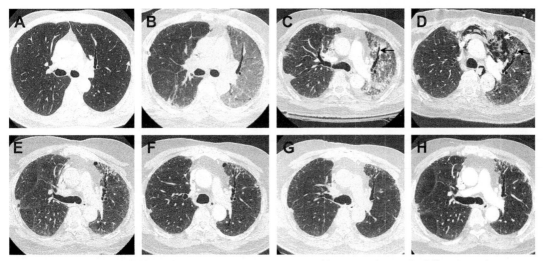

Fig. 2. (*A–H*) Asymmetric diffuse alveolar damage in a 64-year-old man with poorly differentiated pancreatic adenocarcinoma status post right lung wedge resection for an isolated pulmonary metastasis. He underwent Whipple procedure in January 2017. His course was complicated by pancreatic leak, severe sepsis, and acute kidney injury. (*A*) Baseline scan from 2016 at the level of the left upper lobe bronchus shows minimal scattered subpleural reticulation (*white arrows*) but otherwise no evidence of significant fibrosis. (*B*) Four days after Whipple procedure, on February 1st, the patient developed acute respiratory distress syndrome with diffuse left lung GGO with mild areas of opacity on the right. There is no significant airway dilation or volume loss. Although the injury is asymmetric, findings are consistent with the exudative phase of DAD (*C*). Two weeks later, finding of the organizing phase of DAD is seen with increased consolidation and volume loss with increasing bronchial dilation (*arrow*). (*D*) In mid-March, GGO and consolidation have improved but there is persistent dilation of the anterior segment left upper lobe bronchus (*black arrow*). Pneumomediastinum (*white arrow*) is present and is a common complication during prolonged ventilation in patients with DAD. (*E*) CT image at the same level in late May shows improved lung aeration with continued decrease in GGO but persistent airway dilation and subpleural reticulation concerning for permanent fibrosis. (*F–H*) CT images at the same level from 10 months (*F*), 1 year (*G*), and 4 years (*H*) post-DAD show stable findings with asymmetric anterior predominant fibrosis with traction bronchiectasis involving the left upper lobe anterior segmental bronchus and subpleural reticulation. The fibrosis has not progressed because no additional episodes of lung injury had occurred after the initial injury in February 2017. (*Courtesy of* S Kligerman, MD, San Diego, California.)

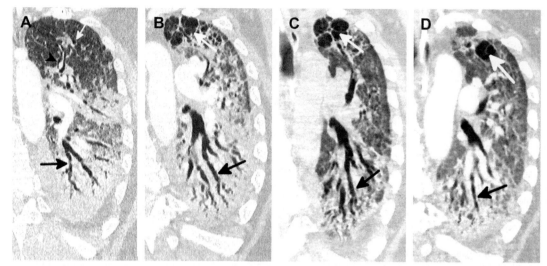

Fig. 3. Rapid development of cystic change in a nonsmoking patient with diffuse alveolar damage caused by dermatomyositis. (*A*) Coronal oblique CT image through the left lung shows lower lobe–predominant consolidation with areas of ground-glass opacity and bronchial dilation (*black arrow*). A few areas of pulmonary interstitial emphysema are present (*black arrowhead*). There are a few areas of lucency in the lungs (*white arrow*). (*B*) Coronal oblique CT image 1 week later shows increasing diffuse consolidation with increasing bronchial dilation (*black arrow*). There has been development of upper lobe parenchymal cystic change (*white arrow*) with an appearance suggesting of secondary lobules that have been pulled apart secondary to the extensive volume loss, suggestive of cicatricial emphysema. (*C*) Coronal oblique CT image 8 days later shows decreasing consolidation with slight improvement in lung volumes. Bronchial dilation (*black arrow*) and cystic change with an appearance of distended pulmonary lobules (*white arrow*) are seen but slightly improved. (*D*) Coronal oblique CT image 1 month later shows decreasing airway dilation (*black arrow*) as the injury begins to heal and lung volumes improve. Additionally, the subpleural cystic change has significantly improved (*white arrow*), likely related to decreased tension on the apical lobules as the lung volumes have increased. (*Courtesy of* S Kligerman, MD, San Diego, California.)

relies on the presence of type II pneumocytes to proliferate and then differentiate into type I pneumocytes, which then re-epithelialize over the denuded, and ideally repaired, basement membrane.[1] Additionally, type II pneumocytes secrete surfactant, which decreases the surface tension at the air/liquid interface of the lung.[32] This allows for some degree of lung repair and alveolar re-expansion.[15] Absence of type II pneumocytes would lead to permanent alveolar collapse. In addition, in areas with extensive basement membrane infoldings because of the initial injury, granular pneumocytes attempting to repair and re-epithelialize the denuded basal lamina can proliferate over apposed septa, thereby fusing the partial or completely collapsed alveoli into a single thickened septum leading to permanent alveolar volume loss.[9] Lastly, if the OP plugs are not removed by fibrinolysis,[15] two possible outcomes may occur. If the plugs remain in the alveoli, there is often epithelization and incorporation of these interalveolar buds into the interstitium.[6,8,9] This fibrosis by accretion is an important mechanism of lung remodeling not only in ALI but also seen in usual interstitial pneumonia (UIP) and

nonspecific interstitial pneumonia (NSIP).[1,2,6,8,9,15] The organizing plugs of fibroblastic tissue may also remain in the alveolar lumens and form large swaths of concretions, completely obliterating whole areas of lung in a process sometimes referred to as obliterative fibrosis.[15]

If the patient survives the exudative and organizing phase of DAD, consolidation and GGO slowly improve. Although findings on CT may return to normal in a small percentage of patients,[33] most patients have some degree of residual fibrosis because of mechanisms described previously.[1] In most cases the fibrosis often involves less than 25% of the lung (see **Figs. 1** and **2**).[33–35] The limited degree of fibrosis in comparison with the extensive parenchymal involvement seen earlier in the injury suggests that a healing response has occurred with reorganization of the damaged epithelial basement membranes and aeration of previously collapsed alveoli. However, in some patients the degree of permanent injury is so extensive that lung transplant is performed; 7% of lung transplants in the United States performed from August 1, 2020 to September 30,

2021 were performed secondary to COVID-19-related DAD.[36] Another question commonly posed is when the findings seen on CT during lung repair of ALI represent permanent fibrosis versus continued healing. Although there is no set time point as to when imaging findings demarcate fibrosis, in the author's experience, lung injury can continue to improve up to 6 months after the initial injury so the word fibrosis should be used sparingly before that time (see **Fig. 1**).

The distribution of post-DAD-related fibrosis is variable, although areas of reticulation, bronchiectasis, and cystic spaces are often present. Although the fibrosis is classically described as being most pronounced in the anterior, nondependent portions of the lung, fibrosis can occur in numerous patterns (see **Figs. 1** and **2**), and in some instances the pattern could be classified as UIP (**Fig. 4**).[17,19,28,33] The fibrosis seen with DAD should not progress unless subsequent episodes of lung injury occur.

Association of Diffuse Alveolar Damage with Usual Interstitial Pneumonia

An association between organizing lung injury and UIP was described in 1973 and has been confirmed in many studies.[37,38] This association is documented in the setting of an acute exacerbation, or accelerated phase, of UIP where imaging and histologic findings of DAD, or less commonly of OP, are superimposed on underlying UIP pattern of fibrosis (**Fig. 5**). This acute injury often leads to rapid clinical deterioration and even death.[4,39–42] In 2016, the definition of acute exacerbation was changed and importantly does not exclude infection as an underlying trigger to the lung injury (**Table 1**).[39,43] The imaging and histology often coincide findings of DAD superimposed on an underlying UIP pattern, which can, on occasion, be difficult to recognize given the superimposed lung injury. If the patient survives, much of the ALI can resolve, although worsening fibrosis is often seen.[1] Basement membrane damage is a

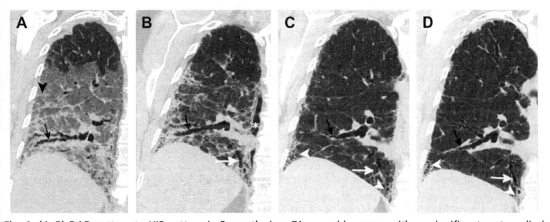

Fig. 4. (*A–D*) DAD pattern to UIP pattern in 3 months in a 71-year-old woman with no significant past medical history. (*A*) A few days after admission for shortness of breath, coronal CT image shows mid and lower lung–predominant GGO with septal thickening (*black arrowhead*) with mild volume loss and airway dilation. (*B*) Coronal CT image at the same level 2 weeks later shows normal evolution of DAD with decreasing GGO and increasing areas of subpleural and peribronchovascular consolidation. There is increased volume loss with increasing airway dilation (*black arrow, white arrow*). Pneumomediastinum (*asterisk*) has developed because of barotrauma from ventilation. Extensive work-up revealed no underlying cause and the patient was diagnosed with acute interstitial pneumonia. (*C*) Coronal CT image 3 months after initial injury shows what would be described as a probable UIP pattern with lower lobe subpleural reticulation (*white arrowheads*) and airway dilation most conspicuous in the posterior segment of the right lower lobe (*white arrow*). The dilation of the lateral segmental bronchus (*black arrow*) is significantly improved because of surrounding alveolar re-expansion from healing. (*D*) Coronal CT image 18 months after initial injury shows no change in what would be classified as a probable UIP pattern with permanent subpleural reticulation (*white arrowheads*) and traction bronchiectasis (*white arrow*). The lateral segmental bronchus (*black arrow*), which was significantly dilated during the acute injury, shows mild irregularities but tapers normally. Although a UIP pattern is commonly associated with progression, this fibrosis, secondary to DAD, has remained stable for more than 3 years because it represented sequela of a single severe lung injury and not repeated episodes of injury. (*Courtesy of* S Kligerman, MD, San Diego, California.)

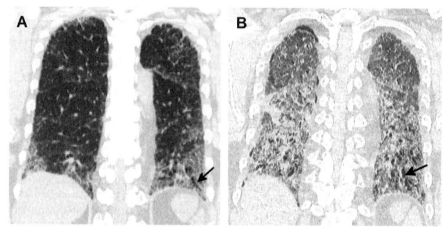

Fig. 5. (*A, B*) Acute exacerbation in 60-year-old man with UIP. (*A*) Baseline CT shows UIP pattern of fibrosis with lower lobe subpleural reticulation and traction bronchiectasis (*arrow*). Mild honeycombing, not seen in this image, was present. (*B*) Four months later, the patient was admitted to the hospital for rapidly developing shortness of breath. Coronal CT at the same level shows interval development of a DAD pattern of lung injury with diffuse but lower lobe–predominant ground-glass opacity and consolidation with increasing bronchial dilation (*arrow*). Given the baseline UIP pattern, this was termed an acute exacerbation. The patient received a lung transplant while in the hospital, which pathologically confirmed findings of DAD with underlying UIP pattern of fibrosis. (*Courtesy of* S Kligerman, MD, San Diego, California.)

common finding at electron microscopy in patients with UIP even in the absence of an acute exacerbation.[9,38,44] The relationship between UIP and the organization that occurs in response to acute or subacute lung injury is not entirely understood. However, the common histologic findings suggest that repeated episodes of lung injury and subsequent abnormal lung repair are partially responsible.

Table 1
Comparison between 2016 and 2007 criteria for acute exacerbation of idiopathic pulmonary fibrosis

	2016 Criteria[43]	2007 Criteria[39]
Definition	An acute, clinically significant respiratory deterioration characterized by evidence of new widespread alveolar abnormality	An acute, clinically significant, respiratory deterioration of unidentifiable cause
Underlying diagnosis	Previous or concurrent diagnosis of IPF	Previous or concurrent diagnosis of IPF
Clinical presentation	Acute worsening or development of dyspnea typically within 1 mo duration	Unexplained worsening or development of dyspnea within 30 d
CT findings	New bilateral ground-glass opacity and/or consolidation superimposed on a background pattern consistent with usual interstitial pneumonia pattern	New bilateral ground-glass abnormality and/or consolidation superimposed on a background of reticular or honeycomb pattern consistent with usual interstitial pneumonia pattern
Exclusion	Deterioration not fully explained by cardiac failure or fluid overload	No evidence of pulmonary infection by endotracheal aspirate or bronchoalveolar lavage Exclusion of alterative causes including left heart failure, pulmonary embolism, or any identifiable cause of acute lung injury

Abbreviation: IPF, idiopathic pulmonary fibrosis.

ACUTE FIBRINOUS ORGANIZING PNEUMONIA

AFOP is a histologic pattern of ALI that lies along a continuum somewhere between that of OP and DAD. The main histologic difference in AFOP is the presence of reddish fibrin "balls" within the alveoli intermixed with areas of OP.[29] However, hyaline membranes associated with DAD are absent. The underlying etiologies of AFOP mirror that of DAD and OP and include, but are not limited to, infection, autoimmune disease, drug toxicity, and toxic inhalation, such as e-cigarette/vaping-associated ALI.[45–49] The imaging findings and outcomes are variable depending on the study. For instance, in one study of 17 patients with AFOP, nine patients had a severe lung injury with imaging findings like those with DAD (Fig. 6) and demonstrated rapid progression to death.[29] The remaining patients had a subclinical course with imaging and recovery like that of OP.[24] In a more recent paper with 34 cases, the imaging findings had an OP pattern in 85% of cases and only two patients with a more severe pattern of injury akin to DAD on imaging died.[50] AFOP, like DAD and OP, can lead to pulmonary fibrosis.[1] Given the lack of ability to differentiate AFOP from either OP or DAD or imaging, this finding should remain a pathologic diagnosis and not an imaging one.

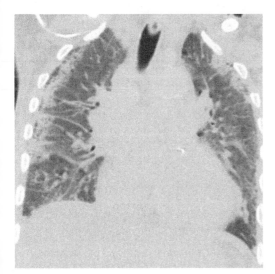

Fig. 6. AFOP in a 69-year-old man. Coronal CT image shows diffuse ground-glass opacity with areas of subpleural consolidation and septal thickening. Given the severity of lung injury, the patient was thought to have DAD. However, biopsy revealed AFOP, which is a pathologic pattern of lung injury where there is extensive deposition of fibrin in the airspaces alongside plugs of organizing pneumonia. The pattern of injury on imaging can range from a mild organizing pneumonia pattern to a severe DAD pattern. (*Courtesy of* S Kligerman, MD, San Diego, California.)

ORGANIZING PNEUMONIA
Etiology

The pathologic response of OP was first recognized during the turn of the nineteenth century in patients with "unresolved" pneumococcal pneumonias. OP was recognized as a distinct pathologic response to pulmonary infection where intra-alveolar exudates were transformed into connective tissue and is associated with the development of or occurs in conjunction with pulmonary fibrosis.[51]

OP is a nonspecific response to lung injury with the initial injury being the same as that seen with AFOP and DAD.[1] Like DAD, infection is the leading cause of OP, although numerous other etiologies include, but are not limited to, toxic inhalation, drug reaction, radiation, aspiration, and the sequela of a systemic inflammatory condition, such as that seen with certain collagen vascular diseases. In some, an inciting cause of the OP is never discovered, and the clinical entity is labeled cryptogenic OP. The underlying cause of OP, just like that of DAD and AFOP, is difficult to elucidate without contributory clinical and laboratory data because the imaging and pathologic findings are often identical to one another.[52]

Focal Imaging Patterns

On CT, numerous imaging patterns are associated with OP. These findings are most often diffuse, but focal abnormalities do occur. OP can present as a solitary pulmonary nodule or as a focal area of consolidation and/or GGO in 10% to 38% of patients.[35,53–55] Focal OP can have various appearances, which can range from benign-appearing areas of consolidation to nodules with spiculation or internal air bronchograms, which can mimic lung cancer or lymphoma, respectively. Architectural distortion, fibrosis, and marginal irregularities within and surrounding these nodules are correlated with alveolar collapse, interstitial inflammation, and fibrosis. A surrounding desmoplastic reaction similar to that seen with lung adenocarcinomas can also occur.[56,57] In many instances, focal OP is preceded by recent infection.[58] Additionally, with focal OP that is more consolidative than mass-like, the distribution is often peribronchovascular or subpleural (Fig. 7). Lobular or subpleural sparing, like that seen with diffuse forms, can occur. Unfortunately, in cases where the imaging does overlap with malignancy, lung biopsy may still be necessary if no prior imaging is available and there are no clinical findings to suggest OP. In rare instances where malignancy is still highly suspected, surgical excision is still sometimes necessary even if a biopsy shows OP

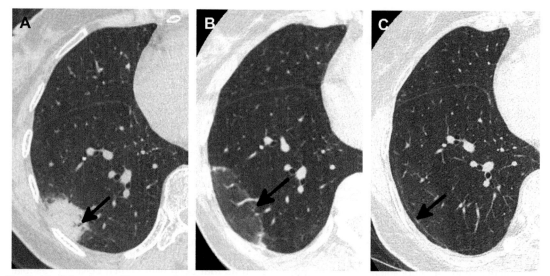

Fig. 7. (*A–C*) Focal mass-like areas of OP in a 44-year-old man with chest pain and abnormal chest radiograph. (*A*) Axial image shows a 3.8-cm subpleural right lower lobe mass with internal air bronchograms (*arrow*). The anterior edge of the mass shows mild ground-glass opacity. Although this was believed to represent an infection, the possibility of malignancy, including pulmonary lymphoma, was raised. The patient underwent biopsy, which showed OP. Subsequent *Coccidioides* titers were positive. (*B*) A few weeks after starting antifungals, axial CT image shows the lesion has expanded outward with near complete resolution of the consolidative portion, which has been replaced by nearly all ground-glass opacity (*arrow*). A remaining band of linear consolidation is along the periphery of the lesion consistent with a reverse halo sign. (*C*) Six months later, there is only a thin linear band of subpleural scarring (*arrow*) in the site of prior infection. (*Courtesy of* S Kligerman, MD, San Diego, California.)

because this pathologic finding can occur adjacent to a lung malignancy.[59]

Diffuse Imaging Patterns

Idiopathic and secondary causes of OP can present with various patterns of diffuse lung disease on imaging. Although some patterns are suggestive of a diagnosis of OP, in many instances the findings are nonspecific. The dominant finding in OP, which itself is completely nonspecific, is bilateral consolidation and/or GGO, occurring in 80% to 95% of cases.[19,60,61] However, it is the distribution of the opacities that helps to suggest the diagnosis of OP. These include subpleural or peribronchovascular predominant consolidation often with areas of lobular or subpleural sparing (Fig. 8).[62–64] In some instances, the subpleural consolidation forms linear bands that can parallel the underlying pleural surface. The peribronchovascular distribution may be related to the extensive epithelial damage involving peribronchiolar alveolar septa on pathology.[65] The areas of lobular sparing relate to the zonal distribution of injury where one lobular is filled with OP and the adjacent lobular is spared.[1] The cause of the subpleural sparing is unclear but may be related to clearance mechanisms via the subpleural lymphatics. Septal thickening is also a common finding and may be

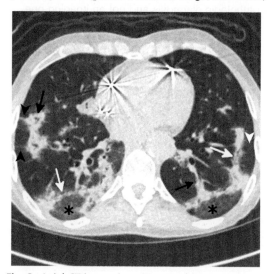

Fig. 8. Axial CT image in a 67-year-old woman being treated with nivolumab for metastatic non–small cell lung cancer shows classic imaging findings of organizing pneumonia including peribronchovascular (*black arrows*) and subpleural (*white arrows*) consolidation with areas of septal thickening (*black arrowheads*). The subpleural consolidation forms linear bands that run parallel to the pleural surface often with intervening subpleural sparing (*white arrowhead*). Additionally, ground-glass opacity is seen between the subpleural consolidation and the pleural surface creating a reverse halo sign (*asterisks*). (*Courtesy of* S Kligerman, MD, San Diego, California.)

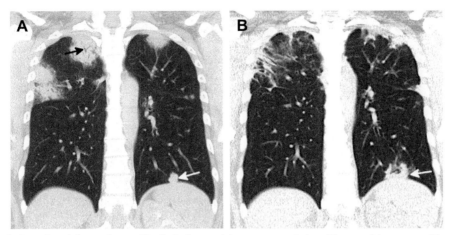

Fig. 9. Evolution of nodular and mass-like foci of organizing pneumonia in a 38-year-old woman with mixed connective tissue disease. (*A*) Coronal CT image shows numerous subpleural round subpleural masses (*black arrow*) and nodules (*white arrow*). (*B*) 16 days after the initiation of steroids, the areas of consolidation have improved with residual areas of subpleural and peribronchovascular consolidation. The lower lobe nodule now demonstrates a "reverse-halo" sign (*white arrow*). (*Courtesy of* S Kligerman, MD, San Diego, California.)

related to septal edema in acute injury, which can progress to septal fibrosis if the injury does not resolve.[1]

The "reverse halo" or "atoll" sign is a CT finding defined as a focal area of GGO surrounded by a ring, or halo, of consolidation (see **Figs. 7** and **8**; **Fig. 9**). It can occur with a unilateral or bilateral injury and is often preceded by a focus of nodular or mass-like consolidation. Over time, the nodule or mass expands outward with decreasing attenuation centrally creating this imaging finding (see **Figs. 7** and **9**). Why this occurs is unclear, but it may represent a healing response. Although initially thought to be a sign diagnostic of OP, it is seen with a variety of infections, infarction, noninfectious granulomatous abnormalities, and even adenocarcinoma in situ.[66,67]

In focal and diffuse forms, OP can appear as airway-centered or peribronchiolar nodules. These nodules are variable in size but are often subpleural and may demonstrate internal air bronchograms when large.[68] The distribution of nodules suggests that the initial site of injury involves the airway.[65] In many instances, these nodules coexist with additional parenchymal manifestations of OP, as discussed previously. This may help to differentiate these nodules from other pathologic processes that can have a similar appearance, such as parenchymal lymphoma, septic emboli, or granulomatosis with polyangiitis. In certain instances, diffuse tree-in-bud nodularity can represent OP on pathology (**Fig. 10**). This has been seen with inhalational injuries caused by synthetic marijuana and e-cigarette/vaping-associated ALI.[69,70]

Treatment of OP centers around removing known inciting factors and corticosteroids treatment, either alone or in conjunction with cytotoxic agents.[23,62,71] How steroids cause the plugs of OP to resolve in still unclear. Prognosis is usually good, and many cases demonstrate complete or near complete resolution with only minimal areas of scarring (**Fig. 11**). In most, the extent of lung

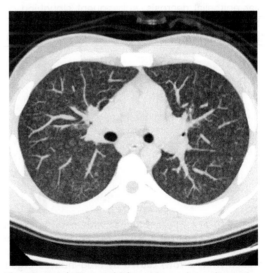

Fig. 10. Axial 10-mm-thick maximum intensity projection image shows diffuse ill-defined ground-glass centrilobular nodules in a 20-year-old man diagnosed with e-cigarette/vaping-associated acute lung injury. Biopsy was performed, which showed organizing pneumonia centered around the respiratory bronchioles caused by the toxic inhalation injury. (*Courtesy of* S Kligerman, MD, San Diego, California.)

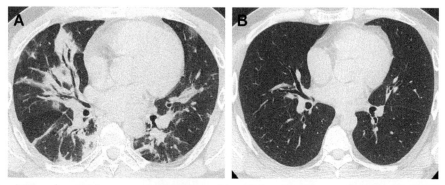

Fig. 11. Resolution of organizing pneumonia pattern of lung injury in a 45-year-old man with COVID-19-related pneumonia. (*A*) Axial image during admission shows peribronchovascular and subpleural consolidation. (*B*) Axial image 6 months later shows a complete resolution of lung injury on CT. (*Courtesy of* S Kligerman, MD, San Diego, California.)

injury is mild, and the lung repairs itself without permanent injury.[7,65,72–74] However, in certain instances, the degree of injury is severe leading to permanent damage and interstitial fibrosis.

Organization as a Pathway to Fibrosis

The pathways of injury in OP, AFOP, and DAD are essentially identical and exist along a continuum. The initial insult leads to injury of the alveolar and capillary epithelium with subsequent proteinaceous exudates filling the airspaces and distal airways.[8,65,72,75,76] Although the degree of injury is more severe in DAD than OP, both lead to alveolar epithelial necrosis, subsequent sloughing of the dead pneumocytes, and associated denudation of the alveolar basal lamina.[9,65,76] The basal

lamina is an integral part in normal lung repair by providing an underlying scaffolding for the lung and aid in lung repair.[77,78] New parenchymal cells migrate from adjacent healthy alveoli, repopulate alveolar epithelial cells, and help unfold the pleated basal lamina.[9,65,78] Similar to that seen with DAD, infolding of the basal lamina can lead to permanent epithelial damage with alveolar collapse as repopulating epithelial cells epithelialize over the deformed and infolded basal lamina causing permanent apposition.[65,72] Additionally, intraluminal plugs of organizing fibrotic tissue are epithelialized by proliferating type II pneumocytes with subsequent incorporation into the interstitium.[8,9,65,72,76] Once in the interstitium, they share morphologic characteristics of and look identical to fibroblastic foci seen in UIP.[7,8]

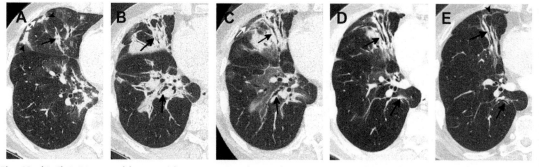

Fig. 12. (*A–E*) A 71-year-old man with metastatic colorectal cancer on an immune checkpoint inhibitor develops shortness of breath and cough. (*A*) Axial image during time of emergency department visit shows peribronchovascular (*black arrow*) and subpleural (*black arrowheads*) consolidation with areas of subpleural sparing (*double-headed white arrow*) caused by drug-induced organizing pneumonia. (*B*) Four days later, there is increasing peribronchovascular consolidation (*black arrows*) with persistent areas of subpleural sparing. (*C*) Ten days after initial injury and 4 days after initiation of steroids, consolidation has decreased with increased GGO in the previous areas of consolidation. Bronchial dilation (*black arrows*) in seen in certain regions. Conspicuous subpleural sparing (*white arrow*) is present. (*D*) Axial CT image 1 month after injury shows continued decrease in consolidation and decrease in GGO. Persistent airway dilation is present in the right middle lobe (*black arrows*). (*E*) Axial CT image 2 years after injury shows right middle lobe greater than right lower lobe peribronchiolar fibrosis (*black arrows*) with linear subpleural bands of scarring (*black arrowhead*). Overall, the degree of fibrosis is mild given the extent of lung injury. (*Courtesy of* S Kligerman, MD, San Diego, California.)

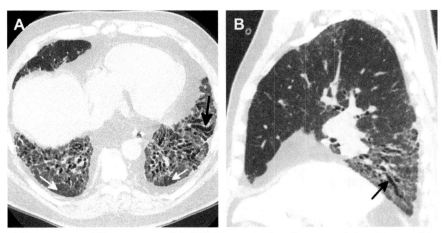

Fig. 13. (*A, B*) NSIP pattern of fibrosis 14 months after COVID-19-related pneumonia in a 54-year-old man with no past medical history. Axial (*A*) and sagittal (*B*) images show lower lobe–predominant fibrosis with ground-glass opacity, traction bronchiectasis (*black arrows*), and areas of subpleural and lobular sparing (*white arrows*) sugges-tive of an NSIP pattern of fibrosis. This pattern can occur after a single episode of acute lung injury. (*Courtesy of* S Kligerman, MD, San Diego, California.)

Given that the initial insult to the basal lamina is more severe in DAD than in OP, it is of little surprise that DAD can lead to fibrosis, as discussed previ-ously. The development of fibrosis secondary to

OP is less commonly reported in the radiology literature. In these cases, the distribution of fibrosis often mirrors the distribution of the initial injury and often shows peribronchiolar or

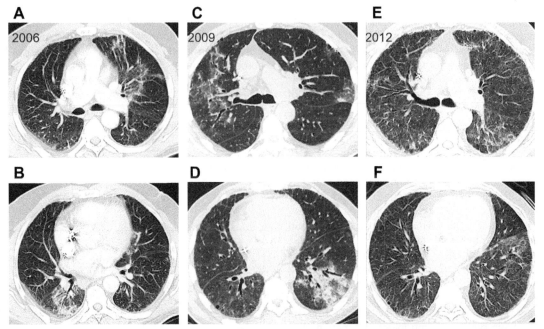

Fig. 14. (*A–F*) A 62-year-old man with reactive arthritis with numerous repeated episodes of OP caused by medical noncompliance. Axial images through the carina (*A*) and through the lower lobes (*B*) in 2006 show patchy areas of peribronchovascular consolidation and GGO, which was shown to be OP on biopsy. The abnormality resolved after steroid treatment. Axial images through the carina (*C*) and lower lobes (*D*) in 2009 show new areas of peri-bronchovascular consolidation and GGO because of OP. Mild areas of fibrosis are present in the right lower lobe and left upper lobe because of prior insult. Axial images through the carina (*E*) and through the lower lobes (*F*) in 2012 show more diffuse hazy peribronchovascular and subpleural GGO. Although some of this represents acute injury, many areas represented permanent fibrosis as demonstrated on continued follow-up imaging (not shown). Repeated episodes of lung injury can lead to worsening fibrosis after each insult. (*Courtesy of* S Kliger-man, MD, San Diego, California.)

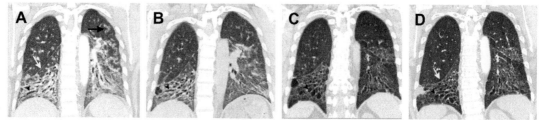

Fig. 15. Progression of OP with areas of NSIP to NSIP in a 39-year-old woman with scleroderma. (*A*) Coronal image shows extensive peribronchovascular GGO and consolidation (*black arrow*) with dilated airways (*black arrowhead*) and inferior displacement of the right major fissure (*white arrow*). Open lung biopsy showed predominantly OP with scattered areas of NSIP pattern of fibrosis. (*B*) After steroid treatment coronal CT scan shows decreasing GGO and near complete resolution of consolidation. Airway dilation *(black arrowhead)*, persists. It is unclear if the residual GGO represents areas of OP or fine fibrosis. Coronal CT images 12 months (*C*) and 18 months (*D*) after the initial CT show near complete resolution of GGO. There is extensive lower lobe–predominant fibrosis with lower lobe volume loss, manifest with inferior displacement of the major fissure (*white arrow*) and associated traction bronchiectasis *(black arrowhead)*. Conspicuous subpleural sparing is present. Bilateral lung transplant showed NSIP pattern of fibrosis with only a few plugs of OP. Although the author believes that OP is the pattern of injury that leads to an NSIP pattern of fibrosis, the concept remains controversial. (*Courtesy of* S Kligerman, MD, San Diego, California.)

subpleural bands of fibrosis with GGO, tractional bronchiectasis, and architectural distortion (**Fig. 12**). In other instances, diffuse OP can heal with a pattern identical to that of NSIP, which is reported to occur in up to 45% of patients (**Fig. 13**).[79] Fibrosis that occurs with OP secondary to a single event, such as a severe pneumonia, should not lead to progressive fibrosis. However, OP relapses are common, being seen 13% to 58% of patients.[23,53,60,62] With each repeated episode of insult, areas of fibrosis can develop (**Fig. 14**).

Lastly, OP is commonly associated with other pathologic forms of interstitial pulmonary fibrosis, most notably NSIP and less frequently UIP.[38,80] The relationship between NSIP and OP is controversial. However, OP is commonly seen in cases of NSIP, and in the American Thoracic Society study on NSIP, OP was seen in 52% of biopsy specimens[81] with similar findings seen in numerous additional studies.[82–84] Additionally, the presence of OP in patients with NSIP is associated with more rapid disease progression and a worse prognosis.[80] Given this clear relationship and evolution from OP to NSIP on imaging in many patients, the author believes that OP is the pathologic pattern of lung injury that may lead to an NSIP pattern of fibrosis in many cases (**Fig. 15**). However, this remains a controversial topic.

SUMMARY

ALI exists on a spectrum. Although there is a tendency to divide injuries into distinct entities, the primary site of injury in all remains the same with injury to the shared basement membrane between the capillary endothelium and type I pneumocyte, which leads to exudation, organization, and attempts at repair. The radiologic findings in ALI depend on the degree of injury and the subsequent healing response. Although ALI can heal without permanent injury, the development of fibrosis after injury is not uncommon and may be debilitating. When ALI does lead to fibrosis, other histologic and imaging patterns, such as those seen with NSIP, can occur, suggesting that the injury associated with organization may be the underlying cause.

CLINICS CARE POINTS

- The pathologic manifestations of acute lung injury exist on a spectrum including organizing pneumonia, acute fibrinous and organizing pneumonia, and diffuse alveolar damage.

- Given that acute lung injury exists on a spectrum, imaging and pathologic findings can overlap.

- Acute fibrinous and organizing pneumonia (AFOP) is a pathologic diagnosis. Imaging findings overlap with both organizing pneumonia and diffuse alveolar damage. There is no way to suggest the diagnosis of AFOP based on imaging alone.

- Organizing pneumonia, acute fibrinous and organizing pneumonia, and diffuse alveolar damage represent nonspecific patterns of lung injury with numerous causes. A radiologist can diagnose ALI but the clincan needs to find the underlying cause.

- No lung injury is truly idiopathicl; it is just that the underlying cause has not been elucidated.

DISCLOSURE

The author has nothing to disclose.

REFERENCES

1. Kligerman SJ, Franks TJ, Galvin JR. From the radiologic pathology archives: organization and fibrosis as a response to lung injury in diffuse alveolar damage, organizing pneumonia, and acute fibrinous and organizing pneumonia. Radiographics 2013;33(7): 1951–75.

2. Castro CY. ARDS and diffuse alveolar damage: a pathologist's perspective. Semin Thorac Cardiovasc Surg 2006;18(1):13–9.

3. Parambil JG, Myers JL, Aubry MC, et al. Causes and prognosis of diffuse alveolar damage diagnosed on surgical lung biopsy. Chest 2007;132(1):50–7.

4. Silva CIS, Muller NL, Fujimoto K, et al. Acute exacerbation of chronic interstitial pneumonia: high-resolution computed tomography and pathologic findings. J Thorac Imaging 2007;22(3):221–9.

5. Fukuda Y, Ishizaki M, Masuda Y, et al. The role of intraalveolar fibrosis in the process of pulmonary structural remodeling in patients with diffuse alveolar damage. Am J Pathol 1987;126(1):171–82.

6. Tomashefski JF Jr. Pulmonary pathology of acute respiratory distress syndrome. Clin Chest Med 2000;21(3):435–66.

7. Cordier JF. Cryptogenic organising pneumonia. Eur Respir J 2006;28(2):422–46.

8. Galvin JR, Frazier AA, Franks TJ. Collaborative radiologic and histopathologic assessment of fibrotic lung disease. Radiology 2010;255(3):692–706.

9. Katzenstein AL. Pathogenesis of "fibrosis" in interstitial pneumonia: an electron microscopic study. Hum Pathol 1985;16(10):1015–24.

10. Vassiliou AG, Kotanidou A, Dimopoulou I, et al. Endothelial damage in acute respiratory distress syndrome. Int J Mol Sci 2020;21(22):8793.

11. Pierrakos C, Karanikolas M, Scolletta S, et al. Acute respiratory distress syndrome: pathophysiology and therapeutic options. J Clin Med Res 2011;4(1):7–16.

12. Idell S. Coagulation, fibrinolysis, and fibrin deposition in acute lung injury. Crit Care Med 2003;31(4 Suppl):S213–20.

13. Matthay MA, Zemans RL. The acute respiratory distress syndrome: pathogenesis and treatment. Annu Rev Pathol 2011;6:147–63.

14. Quesnel C, Nardelli L, Piednoir P, et al. Alveolar fibroblasts in acute lung injury: biological behaviour and clinical relevance. Eur Respir J 2010;35(6): 1312–21.

15. Corrin B, Nicholson AG. Acute alveolar injury and repair. Pathol Lungs 2011;135–53.

16. Gunther A, Ruppert C, Schmidt R, et al. Surfactant alteration and replacement in acute respiratory distress syndrome. Respir Res 2001;2(6):353–64.

17. Ferguson EC, Berkowitz EA, Lung CT. Part 2, The interstitial pneumonias: clinical, histologic, and CT manifestations. AJR Am J Roentgenol 2011;199(4): W464–76.

18. Rouby J-J, Puybasset L, Nieszkowska A, et al. Acute respiratory distress syndrome: lessons from computed tomography of the whole lung. Crit Care Med 2003;31(4 Suppl):S285–95.

19. Lynch DA, Travis WD, Muller NL, et al. Idiopathic interstitial pneumonias: CT features. Radiology 2005;236(1):10–21.

20. Ichikado K, Suga M, Gushima Y, et al. Hyperoxia-induced diffuse alveolar damage in pigs: correlation between thin-section CT and histopathologic findings. Radiology 2000;216(2):531–8.

21. Thille AW, Esteban A, Fernandez-Segoviano P, et al. Chronology of histological lesions in acute respiratory distress syndrome with diffuse alveolar damage: a prospective cohort study of clinical autopsies. Lancet Respir Med 2013;1(5):395–401.

22. Savici D, Katzenstein AL. Diffuse alveolar damage and recurrent respiratory failure: report of 6 cases. Hum Pathol 2001;32(12):1398–402.

23. Cordier JF. Organising pneumonia. Thorax 2000; 55(4):318–28.

24. Chapman HA. Epithelial-mesenchymal interactions in pulmonary fibrosis. Annu Rev Physiol 2011;73: 413–35.

25. Izykowski N, Kuehnel M, Hussein K, et al. Organizing pneumonia in mice and men. J Transl Med 2016;14(1):169.

26. Burkhardt A. Alveolitis and collapse in the pathogenesis of pulmonary fibrosis. Am Rev Respir Dis 1989; 140(2):513–24.

27. Desai SR, Wells AU, Rubens MB, et al. Acute respiratory distress syndrome: CT abnormalities at long-term follow-up. Radiology 1999;210(1):29–35.

28. Ichikado K, Suga M, Muller NL, et al. Acute interstitial pneumonia: comparison of high-resolution computed tomography findings between survivors and nonsurvivors. Am J Respir Crit Care Med 2002;165(11):1551–6.

29. Beasley MB, Franks TJ, Galvin JR, et al. Acute fibrinous and organizing pneumonia: a histological pattern of lung injury and possible variant of diffuse

alveolar damage. Arch Pathol Lab Med 2002;126(9):1064–70.

30. Ichikado K, Suga M, Muranaka H, et al. Prediction of prognosis for acute respiratory distress syndrome with thin-section CT: validation in 44 cases. Radiology 2006;238(1):321–9.

31. Hansell DM, Bankier AA, MacMahon H, et al. Fleischner Society: glossary of terms for thoracic imaging. Radiology 2008;246(3):697–722.

32. Veldhuizen EJ, Haagsman HP. Role of pulmonary surfactant components in surface film formation and dynamics. Biochim Biophys Acta 2000;1467(2):255–70.

33. Masclans JR, Roca O, Munoz X, et al. Quality of life, pulmonary function, and tomographic scan abnormalities after ARDS. Chest 2011;139(6):1340–6.

34. Joynt GM, Antonio GE, Lam P, et al. Late-stage adult respiratory distress syndrome caused by severe acute respiratory syndrome: abnormal findings at thin-section CT. Radiology 2004;230(2):339–46.

35. Drakopanagiotakis F, Polychronopoulos V, Judson MA. Organizing pneumonia. Am J Med Sci 2008;335(1):34–9.

36.. Roach A, Chikwe J, Catarino P, et al. Lung transplantation for Covid-19–related respiratory failure in the United States. N Engl J Med 2022;386(12):1187–8.

37. Gosink BB, Friedman PJ, Liebow AA. Bronchiolitis obliterans. Roentgenologic-pathologic correlation. Am J Roentgenol Radium Ther Nucl Med 1973;117(4):816–32.

38. Katzenstein A-LA, Zisman DA, Litzky LA, et al. Usual interstitial pneumonia: histologic study of biopsy and explant specimens. Am J Surg Pathol 2002;26(12):1567–77.

39. Collard HR, Moore BB, Flaherty KR, et al. Acute exacerbations of idiopathic pulmonary fibrosis. Am J Respir Crit Care Med 2007;176(7):636–43.

40. Kim DS, Park JH, Park BK, et al. Acute exacerbation of idiopathic pulmonary fibrosis: frequency and clinical features. Eur Respir J 2006;27(1):143–50.

41. Kondoh Y, Taniguchi H, Kawabata Y, et al. Acute exacerbation in idiopathic pulmonary fibrosis. Analysis of clinical and pathologic findings in three cases. Chest 1993;103(6):1808–12.

42. Parambil JG, Myers JL, Ryu JH. Histopathologic features and outcome of patients with acute exacerbation of idiopathic pulmonary fibrosis undergoing surgical lung biopsy. Chest 2005;128(5):3310–5.

43. Collard HR, Ryerson CJ, Corte TJ, et al. Acute exacerbation of idiopathic pulmonary fibrosis. An International Working Group Report. Am J Respir Crit Care Med 2016;194(3):265–75.

44. Strieter RM. What differentiates normal lung repair and fibrosis? Inflammation, resolution of repair, and fibrosis. Proc Am Thorac Soc 2008;5(3):305–10.

45. Hwang DM, Chamberlain DW, Poutanen SM, et al. Pulmonary pathology of severe acute respiratory syndrome in Toronto. Mod Pathol 2005;18(1):1–10.

46. Lee SM, Park J-J, Sung SH, et al. Acute fibrinous and organizing pneumonia following hematopoietic stem cell transplantation. Korean J Intern Med 2009;24(2):156–9.

47. Papiris SA, Triantafillidou C, Kolilekas L, et al. Amiodarone: review of pulmonary effects and toxicity. Drug Saf 2010;33(7):539–58.

48. Valim V, Rocha RH, Couto RB, et al. Acute fibrinous and organizing pneumonia and undifferentiated connective tissue disease: a case report. Case Rep Rheumatol 2012;2012:549298.

49. Butt YM, Smith ML, Tazelaar HD, et al. Pathology of vaping-associated lung injury. N Engl J Med 2019;381(18):1780–1.

50. Onishi Y, Kawamura T, Higashino T, et al. Clinical features of acute fibrinous and organizing pneumonia: an early histologic pattern of various acute inflammatory lung diseases. PLoS One 2021;16(4):e0249300.

51. Symmers D, Hoffman AM. The increased incidence of organizing pneumonia: preliminary communication. J Am Med Assoc 1923;81(4):297–8.

52. Pardo J, Panizo A, Sola I, et al. Prognostic value of clinical, morphologic, and immunohistochemical factors in patients with bronchiolitis obliterans-organizing pneumonia. Hum Pathol 2013;44(5):718–24.

53. Lohr RH, Boland BJ, Douglas WW, et al. Organizing pneumonia. Features and prognosis of cryptogenic, secondary, and focal variants. Arch Intern Med 1997;157(12):1323–9.

54. Cazzato S, Zompatori M, Baruzzi G, et al. Bronchiolitis obliterans-organizing pneumonia: an Italian experience. Respir Med 2000;94(7):702–8.

55. Oymak FS, Demirbas HM, Mavili E, et al. Bronchiolitis obliterans organizing pneumonia. Clinical and roentgenological features in 26 cases. Respiration 2005;72(3):254–62.

56. Yang PS, Lee KS, Han J, et al. Focal organizing pneumonia: CT and pathologic findings. J Korean Med Sci 2001;16(5):573–8.

57. Aoki T, Tomoda Y, Watanabe H, et al. Peripheral lung adenocarcinoma: correlation of thin-section CT findings with histologic prognostic factors and survival. Radiology 2001;220(3):803–9.

58. Melloni G, Cremona G, Bandiera A, et al. Localized organizing pneumonia: report of 21 cases. Ann Thorac Surg 2007;83(6):1946–51.

59. Romero S, Barroso E, Rodriguez-Paniagua M, et al. Organizing pneumonia adjacent to lung cancer: frequency and clinico-pathologic features. Lung Cancer 2002;35(2):195–201.

60. Vasu TS, Cavallazzi R, Hirani A, et al. Clinical and radiologic distinctions between secondary bronchiolitis obliterans organizing pneumonia and

cryptogenic organizing pneumonia. Respir Care 2009;54(8):1028–32.

61. Ujita M, Renzoni EA, Veeraraghavan S, et al. Organizing pneumonia: perilobular pattern at thin-section CT. Radiology 2004;232(3):757–61.

62. Drakopanagiotakis F, Paschalaki K, Abu-Hijleh M, et al. Cryptogenic and secondary organizing pneumonia: clinical presentation, radiographic findings, treatment response, and prognosis. Chest 2011;139(4):893–900.

63. Epler GR. Bronchiolitis obliterans organizing pneumonia. Arch Intern Med 2001;161(2):158–64.

64. Roberton BJ, Hansell DM. Organizing pneumonia: a kaleidoscope of concepts and morphologies. Eur Radiol 2011;21(11):2244–54.

65. Myers JL, Katzenstein AL. Ultrastructural evidence of alveolar epithelial injury in idiopathic bronchiolitis obliterans-organizing pneumonia. Am J Pathol 1988;132(1):102–9.

66. Marchiori E, Zanetti G, Meirelles GSP, et al. The reversed halo sign on high-resolution CT in infectious and noninfectious pulmonary diseases. AJR Am J Roentgenol 2011;197(1):W69–75.

67. Kim SJ, Lee KS, Ryu YH, et al. Reversed halo sign on high-resolution CT of cryptogenic organizing pneumonia: diagnostic implications. AJR Am J Roentgenol 2003;180(5):1251–4.

68. Akira M, Yamamoto S, Sakatani M. Bronchiolitis obliterans organizing pneumonia manifesting as multiple large nodules or masses. AJR Am J Roentgenol 1998;170(2):291–5.

69. Kligerman SJ, Kay FU, Raptis CA, et al. CT findings and patterns of e-cigarette or vaping product use-associated lung injury: a multicenter cohort of 160 cases. Chest 2021;160(4):1492–511.

70. Berkowitz EA, Henry TS, Veeraraghavan S, et al. Pulmonary effects of synthetic marijuana: chest radiography and CT findings. AJR Am J Roentgenol 2015; 204(4):750–7.

71. Yoo J-W, Song JW, Jang SJ, et al. Comparison between cryptogenic organizing pneumonia and connective tissue disease-related organizing pneumonia. Rheumatology (Oxford) 2010;50(5): 932–8.

72. Basset F, Ferrans VJ, Soler P, et al. Intraluminal fibrosis in interstitial lung disorders. Am J Pathol 1986;122(3):443–61.

73. Davison AG, Heard BE, McAllister WA, et al. Cryptogenic organizing pneumonitis. Q J Med 1983; 52(207):382–94.

74. Epler GR, Colby TV, McLoud TC, et al. Bronchiolitis obliterans organizing pneumonia. N Engl J Med 1985;312(3):152–8.

75. Nagai S, Izumi T. Bronchiolitis obliterans with organizing pneumonia. Curr Opin Pulm Med 1996;2(5): 419–23.

76. Peyrol S, Cordier JF, Grimaud JA. Intra-alveolar fibrosis of idiopathic bronchiolitis obliterans-organizing pneumonia. Cell-matrix patterns. Am J Pathol 1990;137(1):155–70.

77. Rennard SI, Bitterman PB, Crystal RG. Response of the lower respiratory tract to injury. Mechanisms of repair of the parenchymal cells of the alveolar wall. Chest 1983;84(6):735–9.

78. Vracko R. Basal lamina scaffold-anatomy and significance for maintenance of orderly tissue structure. Am J Pathol 1974;77(2):314–46.

79. Lee JW, Lee KS, Lee HY, et al. Cryptogenic organizing pneumonia: serial high-resolution CT findings in 22 patients. AJR Am J Roentgenol 2010;195(4): 916–22.

80. Todd NW, Marciniak ET, Sachdeva A, et al. Organizing pneumonia/non-specific interstitial pneumonia overlap is associated with unfavorable lung disease progression. Respir Med 2015;109(11): 1460–8.

81. Travis WD, Hunninghake G, King TE Jr, et al. Idiopathic nonspecific interstitial pneumonia: report of an American Thoracic Society project. Am J Respir Crit Care Med 2008;177(12):1338–47.

82. Cottin V, Donsbeck AV, Revel D, et al. Nonspecific interstitial pneumonia. Individualization of a clinico-pathologic entity in a series of 12 patients. Am J Respir Crit Care Med 1998;158(4):1286–93.

83. Katzenstein AL, Fiorelli RF. Nonspecific interstitial pneumonia/fibrosis. Histologic features and clinical significance. Am J Surg Pathol 1994;18(2):136–47.

84. Nagai S, Kitaichi M, Itoh H, et al. Idiopathic nonspecific interstitial pneumonia/fibrosis: comparison with idiopathic pulmonary fibrosis and BOOP. Eur Respir J 1998;12(5):1010–9.

Imaging of Smoking and Vaping Related Diffuse Lung Injury

Katherine A. Cheng, MD[a],*, Holly Nichols, MD[a], H. Page McAdams, MD[a], Travis S. Henry, MD[a], Lacey Washington, MD[a]

KEYWORDS

- Smoking-related lung injury • EVALI • Crack lung • Respiratory bronchiolitis
- Langerhans cell histiocytosis

KEY POINTS

- Smoking-related lung injury demonstrates a range of clinical presentations and radiologic findings.
- Variable imaging findings reflect a variety of possible substances inhaled and pathologic mechanisms for lung injury.
- Radiologists should be familiar with acute and subacute patterns of smoking-related lung disease and EVALI to ensure timely diagnosis and treatment.

INTRODUCTION

Smoking, whether of tobacco or other substances, is one of the most common causes of lung injury. Multiple mechanisms are responsible for smoking-related lung injury, including direct and indirect effects of toxins. Particle size, chemical makeup and solubility, inhaled volume, and presence of contaminants also play a substantial role in determining the effects of the exposure.[1] Given these factors, it is not surprising that the findings of smoking-related lung injury may overlap. The timeline of the patient's initial symptoms and presentation can play an essential role in diagnosis and management. Therefore, this review organizes the patterns of lung injury from inhaled toxins based on acuity of presentation: the acute category consisting of acute eosinophilic pneumonia, synthetic marijuana, e-cigarette or vaping product use–associated lung injury (EVALI), and illicit drug use; the subacute category comprising Langerhans cell histiocytosis (LCH) and the respiratory bronchiolitis (RB) and desquamative interstitial pneumonitis (DIP) disease spectrum; and lastly the chronic category including smoking-related fibrosis and emphysema.

WHEN TO SUSPECT SMOKING-RELATED LUNG INJURY

An accurate and comprehensive patient history is a powerful resource for the clinician and radiologist, helping narrow the differential diagnosis to smoking-related and other inhalational lung diseases, particularly in the acute setting. Thus the radiologist should consider lung injury from an inhaled toxin when acute clinical decompensation occurs in the absence of infection and cardiac dysfunction. In this setting, imaging features are often nonspecific. For example, acute lung injury may present with diffuse centrilobular nodules that might otherwise be suggestive of infection. Lung injury may also mimic pulmonary edema with central ground-glass opacities, interlobular septal thickening, and pleural effusions.

[a] Department of Radiology, Duke University, Duke University Medical Center, 2301 Erwin Road, Box 3808, Durham, NC 27710, USA

* Corresponding author.

E-mail address: katherine.cheng@duke.edu

Radiol Clin N Am 60 (2022) 941–950

https://doi.org/10.1016/j.rcl.2022.06.004

0033-8389/22/Published by Elsevier Inc.

ACUTE PRESENTATIONS
Acute Eosinophilic Pneumonia

Patient presentation
Acute eosinophilic pneumonia is caused by multiple etiologies, including infections, drug reactions, and inhalation of illicit drugs. However, there remains to be a close association of acute eosinophilic pneumonia with cigarette smoking, particularly when there is an increase in smoking habits. Patients with smoking-related acute eosinophilic pneumonia are most commonly young men in their 20s to 40s, presenting with acute febrile illness and impaired respiratory function that may mimic acute respiratory distress syndrome (ARDS).[2]

Pathophysiology
Although the mechanisms of lung injury for acute eosinophilic pneumonia have yet to be fully determined, the pathology stems from the recruitment of eosinophils and their degranulation of proteins that promote inflammation and lung injury. Although peripheral eosinophils remain within the normal range, pulmonary eosinophilia greater than 25% is seen on bronchioloalveolar lavage (BAL), distinguishing this entity from ARDS in which neutrophilia is seen on BAL.[2]

Imaging
Diagnosis of acute eosinophilic pneumonia is guided by the Philit criteria, which include acute respiratory symptoms of less than 1 month, pulmonary opacities on thoracic imaging, pulmonary eosinophilia (>25% eosinophils on BAL), and absence of other pulmonary eosinophilic diseases.[2] Thoracic imaging reveals multifocal or diffuse ground-glass opacities, sometimes with superimposed consolidation and interlobular septal thickening as seen in **Fig. 1**. Small to moderate pleural effusions may also be present.[3] Although the radiographic findings may mimic ARDS or pulmonary edema, accurate diagnosis for acute eosinophilic pneumonia is imperative. Rapid response to corticosteroid treatment is a hallmark of the disease; the clinical course can result in death without timely treatment.[2]

Synthetic Marijuana

Patient presentation
Developed to simulate the cannabis effect, synthetic cannabinoids are mood-altering chemicals that were initially sprayed onto dry plant material, which could then be smoked. Lung injury related to this practice may be considered in adolescents and young adults who present with compromised respiratory function and altered mental status.[4] These substances are now also used in electronic cigarette and vaping devices, and the findings in that setting are described with other vaping-related lung diseases.

Pathophysiology
Although the exact mechanism is unknown, injury to the endothelium of the airway most likely precipitates an immune response that triggers inflammation, damaging surrounding normal lung tissue. Histology from patients who smoked synthetic cannabinoids demonstrated plugs of granulation tissue centered around the bronchioles (organizing pneumonia) and foci of acute lung injury.[4,5]

Imaging
Although the pulmonary manifestations of synthetic marijuana have not been fully investigated, case reports have demonstrated diffuse centrilobular nodules and tree-in-bud opacities, which parallel the histology of an airway-centered injury as seen in **Fig. 2**. In addition, patterns of organizing pneumonia, including areas of superimposed patchy consolidation, have also been observed. Synthetic marijuana use may also result in cardiac dysfunction, and as such the imaging manifestations of pulmonary edema may also be present.[4]

E-Cigarette or Vaping Product Use–Associated Lung Injury

Patient presentation
EVALI has emerged as a deadly trend, particularly among young patients in whom cigarette smoking is being supplanted by the use of vaping products. Like other inhalational injuries, EVALI is a diagnosis of exclusion. Patients are often young and present not only with respiratory symptoms and chest pain, but also with nonspecific signs including gastrointestinal symptoms. Most cases of EVALI are attributable to inhalation of nicotine or marijuana/THC derivatives. This customization is an alluring but deadly feature of electronic cigarettes. Severe cases may result in intensive care unit level care and a minority of patients have died of EVALI.[6]

Pathophysiology
As with any inhaled toxin, the body's response to electronic cigarettes creates a cascade of immune responses that ultimately culminates in inflammation and leads to lung injury. Histology has demonstrated airway-centered lung injury. However, the exact mechanism of injury is poorly understood, possibly because of the wide variety of contents seen in electronic cigarettes.[6] Everything regarding electronic cigarettes can be personalized, from the type of compound that is vaporized, particle size, inhaled quantity and duration, and so

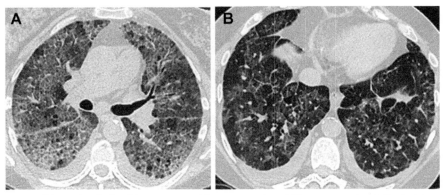

Fig. 1. A 57-year-old previously healthy woman with acute eosinophilic pneumonia attributed to smoking to-bacco. She was admitted for acute respiratory failure and underwent computed tomography (CT), which shows bilateral ground-glass opacitiesand small pleural effusions as seen in Panel A. Imaging also included smooth interlobular septal thickening, best illustrated in Panel B. The diagnosis was confirmed at surgical lung biopsy and the patient quickly improved after initiation of corticosteroid treatment.

forth. The most common findings of EVALI at pathology include organizing pneumonia and diffuse alveolar damage. Acute eosinophilic pneumonia and diffuse alveolar hemorrhage may also be seen.[6]

Imaging
The inherent variability of exposures with these devices results in a wide range of mechanisms that can lead to lung injury and thus variability in imaging presentation. Although organizing pneumonia can demonstrate a wide variety of imaging presentations, the pattern seen in the setting of EVALI tends to be somewhat less variable. Patients often present with bilateral symmetric ground-glass opacities with associated septal thickening, often resulting in a crazy paving pattern. Subpleural sparing is commonly present. There may also be sparing along the peribronchovascular interstitium.[6,7]

Patients with a diffuse alveolar damage pattern of injury may present with a more severe clinical and imaging presentation, including lower lobe–predominant consolidation and volume loss as seen in **Fig. 3**B. Findings may overlap with those of organizing pneumonia with peribronchovascular ground-glass opacities, for example please refer to **Fig. 3**C. Patients may also demonstrate a crazy paving pattern as seen in **Fig. 3**A.[6,7] Less commonly, patients with EVALI may also present with diffuse centrilobular nodules as depicted in **Fig** 3D. This pattern likely reflects airway-centered organizing pneumonia (similar to synthetic marijuana). Pulmonary hemorrhage is a rare manifestation with bilateral ground-glass opacities or consolidation.

Cocaine

Patient presentation
Crack cocaine is the highly addictive precipitant solid form of cocaine that is evaporated at high temperatures and smoked, causing neurologic and cardiovascular symptoms and throat

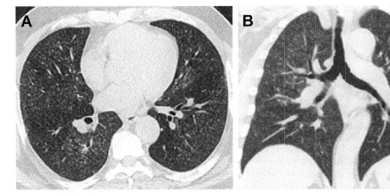

Fig. 2. (A, B) Diffuse bilateral centrilobular nodules in a patient with history of smoking synthetic marijuana.

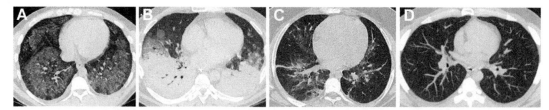

Fig. 3. Spectrum of imaging findings from four different patients with EVALI. (*A*) Bilateral ground-glass opacities and crazy paving. (*B*) Dependent consolidation from lung injury. (*C*) Mild peribronchovascular ground-glass opacities and linear consolidation consistent with organizing pneumonia. (*D*) Axial maximum intensity projection image showing diffuse centrilobular nodules in a 40-year-old man who vaped THC.

tightness or pain, chest pain, dyspnea, hemoptysis, and cough with black sputum.[8] Specifically, "crack lung" is used to describe an acute respiratory compromise that manifests within 48 hours of use and associated with ancillary symptoms, such as fever and hemoptysis.[9]

Pathophysiology

"Crack lung" comprises diffuse alveolar damage and alveolar hemorrhage. Pulmonary hemorrhage can occur at the level of the airways with bleeding of the bronchial and tracheal vessels or from destruction of the capillary alveolar interface.[8] In a histologic review of 52 autopsies from patients that tested positive for cocaine, 58% showed acute pulmonary hemorrhage (**Fig. 4**) and 40% showed chronic pulmonary hemorrhage with hemosiderin-laden macrophages.[10]

Imaging

Although the mechanism for damage to the capillary alveolar membrane in crack lung is not fully characterized, the resulting increase in permeability leads to increased edema fluid in the alveolar spaces, which was seen in 77% patients in the previously mentioned histologic review.[10] Although the increased permeability can account for the noncardiogenic pulmonary edema,

impaired cardiac function from cocaine-induced myocardial ischemia can also result in cardiogenic pulmonary edema. The radiologic findings of pulmonary edema include interlobular septal thickening, perihilar opacities, effusions, and parenchymal consolidation or ground-glass opacities with possible subpleural sparring as seen in **Fig. 5**. Ground-glass opacities with subpleural sparing is a common feature in "crack lung."[11] Images in patients with diffuse alveolar hemorrhage demonstrate diffuse opacities without geographic predilection, predominantly ground-glass in attenuation with or without superimposed areas of consolidation, and occasionally with superimposed interlobular septal thickening giving rise to a "crazy paving" appearance.

Other radiologic abnormalities that may be seen in association with inhaled cocaine include pneumothorax or pneumomediastinum from barotrauma, findings of organizing pneumonia, bronchiolitis obliterans, and pulmonary eosinophilia.[8]

Heroin

Patient presentation

Although typically injected intravenously, heroin can also be inhaled or smoked, often in conjunction with cannabis. At an inpatient rehabilitation center, a

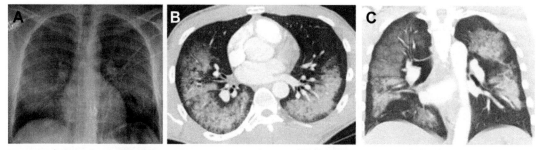

Fig. 4. (*A*) Bilateral central opacities in a patient presenting for acute shortness of breath after smoking crack cocaine. (*B, C*) CT finding of that same patient; central ground-glass opacities with subpleural sparing and superimposed confluent areas of consolidation and interlobular septal thickening. Findings compatible with significant pulmonary edema.

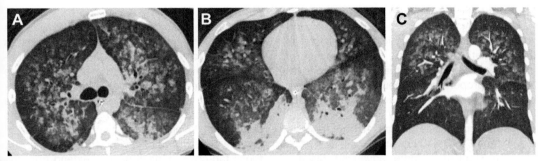

Fig. 5. (*A, B*) A 33-year-old homeless man who presented with respiratory failure bloody secretions. He was a regular cocaine user and admitted to recently smoking heroin before admission. CT images show symmetric ground-glass opacities, dependent consolidation, and smooth interlobular septal thickening. These findings were believed to represent a combination of permeability edema and hemorrhage in the context of bloody secretions. (*C*) A 24-year-old man who presented with lung injury from smoking the gel out of a fentanyl patch. He was hypoxic to 89% on room air and coughing up blood at the time of presentation. CT was negative for pulmonary embolism but showed symmetric bilateral ground-glass opacities attributable to smoking fentanyl. Patient's symptoms improved and he was discharged the following day.

sample of 300 heroin users were assessed and 70.3% of them were smokers of heroin laced with cannabis.[12] Patients often mistakenly believe that smoking heroin rather than administering it intravenously removes the addictive and destructive nature of heroin. Reports of patients smoking fentanyl have also been described.[13] Clinical signs include mental status change and euphoria, nausea, vomiting, dyspnea, cough, fevers, and depressed respiratory function. Compromised respiratory status often occurs acutely.[14]

Pathophysiology
Similar to cocaine, heroin is associated with damage to the capillary alveolar interface, resulting in increased permeability. In addition, the neurologic response to heroin itself may also provoke neurologic pulmonary edema. Regardless of the pathophysiology, noncardiogenic pulmonary edema is a common manifestation of heroin and opioid use, whether through inhalation or intravenous injection.[1] Heroin is also a stimulator of mast cells, which release histamine and trigger bronchospasm.[14]

Imaging
Imaging in patients with heroin or other opiate inhalation may demonstrate classic findings of pulmonary edema and lung injury. Other histologic manifestations that may be seen in these patients include eosinophilic pneumonia and, rarely, alveolar proteinosis, which have been reported in case reports.[15]

SUBACUTE PRESENTATIONS
Pulmonary Langerhans Cell Histiocytosis

Clinical presentation
Pulmonary LCH is highly associated with smokers and more commonly seen in young adults ranging

from 20 to 40 years of age. Although nearly all patients with pulmonary LCH have a personal history of smoking or prolonged exposure to secondhand smoke, only a minority of patients with smoking history actually develop pulmonary LCH, implying a possible genetic predisposition.[16,17] In a review of 20 lobectomy specimens from patients with a smoking history, only one patient had the histologic findings of LCH. This contrasts with the 18 patients who had RB, which is described in the following section.[18]

There is a broad clinical presentation and course for LCH; patients may be asymptomatic, present with vague symptoms of dyspnea and cough, or succumb to severe respiratory compromise. Pneumothorax is a classic complication and can prompt the initial clinical presentation. Patients with more advanced disease and symptoms may require steroid therapy or even lung transplantation.[16]

Pathophysiology
LCH is the abnormal proliferation and accumulation of Langerhans cells, a subset of dendritic cells that are identified through their characteristic Birbeck granules or X-bodies. These cells are the immune protectors of the respiratory tract; therefore, they are predictably increased in smokers, reflecting an immune-mediated inflammatory response.[17]

Imaging
Biopsy is used for definitive diagnosis but can often be avoided in patients who demonstrate "classic" imaging findings and mild symptoms that are managed with smoking cessation. Therefore, it is imperative that the radiologist be familiar with the imaging patterns of LCH. The recruitment and accumulation of the dendritic cells along the

airways manifest as airway-centered nodules, which develop central lucencies that may expand and evolve into irregular, thick-walled cysts as the inflammation progresses.[17] The presence of cysts that may rupture into the pleural spaces results in the propensity for pneumothorax. Sparing of the costophrenic angles is the radiologic hallmark of this disease. In early phases of the disease, small nodules less than 10 mm tend to predominate (**Fig. 6**A). Cysts are seen in all phases but often suggest a more advanced disease state.[16] Extensive cystic parenchmymal destruction can create a "burnt out" appearance as seen in Fig. 6B and 6C. LCH may also be observed in conjunction with other smoking-related lung diseases.

Respiratory Bronchiolitis and Desquamative Interstitial Pneumonia

Clinical presentation
Respiratory Bronchiolitis (RB), respiratory bronchiolitis with interstitial lung disease (RB-ILD), and desquamative interstitial pneumonia (DIP) represent a spectrum of disease, seen in the same patient population and representing different distributions of similar macrophages. These histologic patterns are typically seen in smokers and management primarily consists of smoking cessation. RB is characterized by the accumulation of airway-centered macrophages without clinical symptoms. When patients exhibit clinical manifestations, such as abnormal pulmonary function tests, shortness of breath, or cough, the term RB-ILD is applied.[19] In a cohort of 109 surgically confirmed cases of RB, 98% were smokers. Smoking cessation can potentially alleviate the symptoms and reverse the lung injury in most cases. In that same cohort, RB remained in one-third of patients after 5 years of smoking cessation.[20] DIP is associated with alveolar accumulation of macrophages. Its clinical manifestations include cough, clubbing of the fingers, and shortness of breath with a slight male preponderance.[21]

Pathophysiology
The pathophysiology of RB and DIP involves the accumulation and migration of macrophages as a response to the inflammation incited by the inhalation of smoking toxins. These macrophages engulf and remove the toxins, turning their cytoplasm into a tan color hue, earning the nickname "smokers' macrophages." In RB and RB-ILD, the studding of the airways with these colored macrophages gives rise to centrilobular nodules. In DIP, those tan-colored macrophages extend from the airways and fill the alveolar spaces. Alveolar wall fibrosis and concurrent inflammation may be present in both pathologies. Because DIP is merely an extension of RB and both diseases stem from smoking, it is common for both pathologies to coexist with histologic and radiographic overlap.[17]

Imaging
Like other smoking-related lung injury patterns, RB presents radiographically as ill-defined, centrilobular nodules with an upper lobe–predominance (**Fig. 7**). The upper lung–predominant distribution may be attributed to the more robust lymphatic drainage system in the lower lungs, allowing for better clearance of the particles.[17] For reasons unknown, these centrilobular nodules do not cavitate or progress into cysts, a distinguishing feature from LCH. As in other small airway diseases, mosaic attenuation may be seen.

Because DIP involves the accumulation of smokers' macrophages in the alveolar spaces, this radiographically translates into the nonspecific pattern of symmetric ground-glass opacities interposed with normal areas of lung parenchyma. However, despite the aforementioned robust lower lung lymphatic system, these ground-glass opacities tend to be basilar predominant (**Fig. 8**). Cystic changes and emphysema may also be seen; however, honeycombing is unusual. The fibrosis pattern in DIP consists of symmetric wall thickening of the alveoli without destruction of the lung architecture, mirroring the nonspecific interstitial pneumonia pattern in histology.[19]

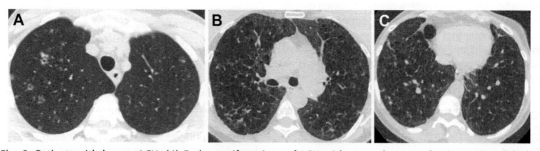

Fig. 6. Patients with known LCH. (*A*) Early manifestations of LCH with upper lung–predominant centrilobular nodules, some of which show cavitations. (*B, C*) Patient with advanced or "burnt out" LCH with extensive cystic parenchymal destruction.

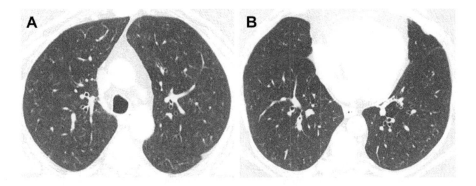

Fig. 7. (*A, B*) Diffuse centrilobular nodules in a patient with a long-standing history of smoking and suspected RB-ILD.

CHRONIC LUNG DISEASE
Smoking-Related Interstitial Fibrosis

Patient presentation
The importance of diagnosing smoking-related interstitial lung fibrosis (SRIF), also referred to as airspace enlargement with fibrosis or RB with fibrosis, lies in its different prognosis from that of other forms of fibrosis, specifically idiopathic pulmonary fibrosis (IPF).[22] It is therefore important to distinguish these entities, although the distinction is challenging for the clinician, radiologist, and pathologist. In contrast to IPF, there have been no reports of significant clinical impairment related to SRIF. In fact, studies have described SRIF (**Fig. 9**) in patients without clinical suspicion for ILD.[18]

Pathophysiology
Although it is not surprising that the toxic effects of cigarette smoking can cause fibrosis, the pathophysiology of SRIF is poorly understood but probably multifactorial. Cigarette toxins promote inflammation, recruit and accumulate immune cells, and cause the release of cytokines and growth factors. Specifically, nicotine is a suspected culprit because it can induce cell damage, incite inflammation, and initiate collagen production. These combined effects likely play a role in the pathogenesis of SRIF.[21] Histologically, SRIF consists of alveolar wall thickening with increased collagen accumulation. In contrast to IPF, SRIF is distinguished by overall preserved lung architecture and lack of temporal variability.[18]

Imaging
Even in the presence of the histologic findings of fibrosis, patients may have normal imaging on high-resolution computed tomography. In patients with abnormal imaging, findings typically include a background centrilobular nodules and

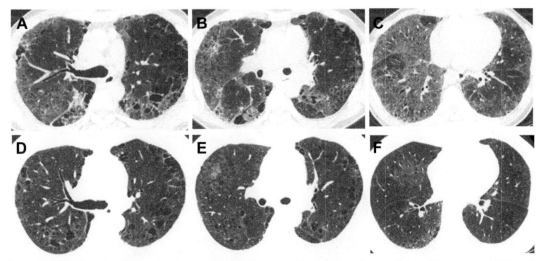

Fig. 8. (*A–C*) Diffuse basilar-predominant ground-glass opacities are seen in a patient with suspected DIP in the setting of emphysema. After smoking cessation and short-term treatment of steroids, there is significant decrease in the ground-glass opacities (*D–F*), which is expected in DIP.

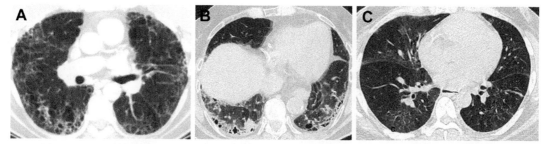

Fig. 9. (A) Findings of SRIF with reticulation and ground-glass opacities on a background of emphysema and respiratory bronchiolitis. Pathology showed bronchiolocentric fibrosis suggestive of SRIF. (B) Patient with ground-glass opacities, reticulation, and cystic changes found to be distal lobular airspace enlargement on histology. (C) Separate patient that also had histology suggestive of SRIF with ground-glass opacities as the predominant findings.

ground-glass opacities (reflecting RB spectrum disease) and upper lung–predominant emphysema with concurrent reticulation.[21] Although SRIF and usual interstitial pneumonia differ in their clinical presentation, progression, and management, distinguishing between the two pathologies is challenging, especially because they can share radiologic features, such as honeycombing, and both are seen in conjunction with emphysema. Chae and colleagues[23] advocated for the location of emphysema and honeycombing and their relationship with respect to each other as helpful tools for the radiologist; honeycombing bordering to emphysema, uneven areas of honeycombing, and absence of honeycombing in the upper lungs all favor SRIF over usual interstitial pneumonia.

Emphysema

Clinical presentation

Emphysema is a ubiquitous disease among smokers causing significant clinical impairment and respiratory compromise. Patients present with cough, dyspnea on exertion, and abnormal pulmonary function tests including increased total lung capacity and decreased forced expiratory volume in 1 second.[24]

Pathophysiology

Smoking causes airway-centered injury that progresses to alveolar destruction through a cascade of inflammatory pathways that lead to cellular destruction and remodeling mediated by immune cells, cytokines, oxidative stress, and extracellular matrix proteolysis. Emphysema related to smoking is predominantly centrilobular in distribution, although paraseptal emphysema (Fig. 10) may also be seen. On histologic review, there is destruction of the alveolar walls with enlargement of the airspaces.[25]

Imaging

Focal areas of lucency without perceptible walls are the hallmark imaging findings of emphysema. In smokers, these focal lucencies are usually centered around the airways, otherwise described as centrilobular in location. These lucencies can merge as the disease process progresses and form bullae. Alternatively, these lucencies may be located in the periphery near the pleural spaces, giving rise to paraseptal emphysema.[25] The pulmonary vessels are diminutive in the areas of emphysema further decreasing the attenuation of the affected areas, because the lung directs blood flow away from areas of hypoxia to areas of preserved ventilation to promote effective vascular gas exchange.

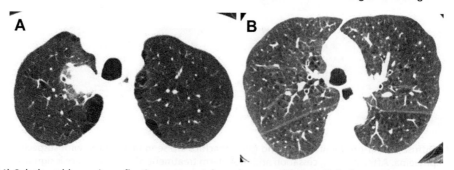

Fig. 10. (A) Subpleural lucencies reflecting paraseptal emphysema. (B) Centrilobular emphysema.

Table 1
Summary table

Presentation	Disease Entity	Mechanism of Injury	Common Imaging Findings
Acute	Acute eosinophilic pneumonia	Recruitment of eosinophils and release of degranulation proteins	Multifocal or diffuse ground-glass opacities, ± superimposed consolidation or ground-glass opacities.
	Synthetic marijuana use	Airway-centered injury, organizing pneumonia	Apical-predominant centrilobular nodules. Patchy consolidation, crazy paving.
	EVALI	Variable: organizing pneumonia, diffuse alveolar damage, acute eosinophilic pneumonia, diffuse alveolar hemorrhage	Ground-glass opacities with septal thickening (crazy paving), subpleural sparing. May demonstrate lower lobe–predominant consolidation.
	Crack lung	Diffuse alveolar damage, alveolar hemorrhage	Diffuse ground-glass opacities, ± superimposed consolidation, occasional crazy paving.
	Heroin inhalation	Damage to the capillary alveolar interface	Findings of pulmonary edema: ground-glass opacities with interlobular septal thickening. ± pleural effusions.
Subacute	LCH	Langerhans cell proliferation and associated inflammatory response	Irregular centrilobular nodules. Thick-walled, irregular cysts. Sparing of the costophrenic angles.
	RB	Macrophage accumulation along the airways	Ill-defined apical-predominant centrilobular micronodules.
	DIP	Macrophage accumulation in the alveolar spaces	Bilateral lower lung–predominant ground-glass opacities.
Chronic	Emphysema	Inflammatory cascade resulting in alveolar destruction	Lucencies without perceptible walls, which may be centrilobular or paraseptal in distribution.
	SRIF	Poorly understood mechanism resulting in alveolar wall thickening and collagen accumulation	Basal- and peripheral-predominant septal thickening. May demonstrate ground-glass opacities. With or without imaging findings of other smoking-related lung disease.

SUMMARY

Smoking-related lung injury comprises a broad spectrum of pathologies that can share overlapping imaging features, making diagnosis challenging to the radiologist and clinician. Furthermore, the category of smoking-related lung injury has also evolved to include pathologies that extend beyond nicotine cigarette smoking to include inhalation of illicit drugs and electronic cigarettes. Despite these challenges, imaging remains a powerful clinical tool that can aid in diagnosis and prognosis by expediting appropriate treatment. By categorizing smoking-related lung injury based on the timeline and acuity of the patient's symptoms, we hope to improve the radiologist's understanding of the pathophysiology and imaging features of smoking-related lung injury (Table 1).

CLINICS CARE POINTS

- Acute presentations are uncommon with cigarette smoking and more common with related inhalational injuries.
- Centrilobular nodules and ground-glass opacities are nonspecific findings that may be seen in the acute setting but are also commonly seen in subacute smoking-related lung diseases.
- Chronic smoking-related lung injury tends to have an insidious clinical presentation.

DISCLOSURE

The authors have nothing to disclose.

REFERENCES

1. Mégarbane B, Chevillard L. The large spectrum of pulmonary complications following illicit drug use: features and mechanisms. Chem Biol Interact 2013;206(3):444–51.
2. De Giacomi F, Vassallo R, Yi ES, et al. Acute eosinophilic pneumonia. Causes, diagnosis, and management. Am J Respir Crit Care Med 2018;197(6): 728–36.
3. Jeong YJ, Kim K-I, Seo IJ, et al. Eosinophilic lung diseases: a clinical, radiologic, and pathologic overview. RadioGraphics 2007;27(3):617–37.
4. Berkowitz EA, Henry TS, Veeraraghavan S, et al. Pulmonary effects of synthetic marijuana: chest radiography and CT findings. AJR Am J Roentgenol 2015; 204(4):750–7.
5. Kourouni I, Mourad B, Khouli H, et al. Critical illness secondary to synthetic cannabinoid ingestion. JAMA Netw Open 2020;3(7):e208516.
6. Kligerman S, Raptis C, Larsen B, et al. Radiologic, pathologic, clinical, and physiologic findings of electronic cigarette or vaping product use-associated lung injury (EVALI): evolving knowledge and remaining questions. Radiology 2020;294(3): 491–505.
7. Kligerman SJ, Kay FU, Raptis CA, et al. CT findings and patterns of e-cigarette or vaping product use-associated lung injury: a multicenter cohort of 160 cases. Chest 2021;160(4):1492–511.
8. Restrepo CS, Carrillo JA, Martínez S, et al. Pulmonary complications from cocaine and cocaine-based substances: imaging manifestations. Radiographics 2007;27(4):941–56.
9. Giacomi FD, Srivali N. Cocaine use and crack lung syndrome. QJM 2019;112(2):125–6.
10. Bailey ME, Fraire AE, Greenberg SD, et al. Pulmonary histopathology in cocaine abusers. Hum Pathol 1994;25(2):203–7.
11. Chong WH, Saha BK, Austin A, et al. The significance of subpleural sparing in CT chest: a state-of-the-art review. Am J Med Sci 2021;361(4): 427–35.
12. Morgan N, Daniels W, Subramaney U. Smoking heroin with cannabis versus injecting heroin: unexpected impact on treatment outcomes. Harm Reduct J 2019;16(1):65.
13. Tambe V, Desai P, Kondapi D, et al. 1156: Inhaled fentanyl leading to diffuse alveolar hemorrhage. Crit Care Med 2019;47(1):555.
14. Radke JB, Owen KP, Sutter ME, et al. The effects of opioids on the lung. Clin Rev Allergy Immunol 2014; 46(1):54–64.
15. Chapman E, Leipsic J, Satkunam N, et al. Pulmonary alveolar proteinosis as a reaction to fentanyl patch smoke. Chest 2012;141(5):1321–3.
16. Suri HS, Yi ES, Nowakowski GS, et al. Pulmonary Langerhans cell histiocytosis. Orphanet J Rare Dis 2012;7:16.
17. Kligerman S, Franks TJ, Galvin JR. Clinical-radiologic-pathologic correlation of smoking-related diffuse parenchymal lung disease. Radiol Clin North Am 2016;54(6):1047–63.
18. Katzenstein AL, Mukhopadhyay S, Zanardi C, et al. Clinically occult interstitial fibrosis in smokers: classification and significance of a surprisingly common finding in lobectomy specimens. Hum Pathol 2010; 41(3):316–25.
19. Elicker BM, Kallianos KG, Jones KD, et al. Smoking-related lung disease. Semin Ultrasound CT MR 2019;40(3):229–38.
20. Fraig M, Shreesha U, Savici D, et al. Respiratory bronchiolitis: a clinicopathologic study in current smokers, ex-smokers, and never-smokers. Am J Surg Pathol 2002;26(5):647–53.
21. Margaritopoulos GA, Harari S, Caminati A, et al. Smoking-related idiopathic interstitial pneumonia: a review. Respirology 2016;21(1):57–64.
22. Watanabe Y, Kawabata Y, Kanauchi T, et al. Multiple, thin-walled cysts are one of the HRCT features of airspace enlargement with fibrosis. Eur J Radiol 2015;84(5):986–92.
23. Chae KJ, Jin GY, Jung HN, et al. Differentiating smoking-related interstitial fibrosis (SRIF) from usual interstitial pneumonia (UIP) with emphysema using CT features based on pathologically proven cases. PLoS One 2016;11(9):e0162231.
24. Newell JD Jr. CT of emphysema. Radiol Clin North Am 2002;40(1):31–42, vii.
25. Yoshida T, Tuder RM. Pathobiology of cigarette smoke-induced chronic obstructive pulmonary disease. Physiol Rev 2007;87(3):1047–82.

Imaging of Cystic Lung Disease

Cato Chan, MD[a,b], Christopher Lee, MD[a,b],*

KEYWORDS

- Cystic lung disease • Lymphangioleiomyomatosis • Pulmonary cysts
- High-resolution computed tomography

KEY POINTS

- Diffuse cystic lung disease refers to multiple rounded lucencies or low-attenuating areas with well-defined interfaces with normal lung.
- Other parenchymal lucencies, such as cavitary disease, bronchiectasis, honeycombing, and emphysema, may mimic cystic lung disease.
- Cystic lung disease generally has a nonspecific presentation and can be found incidentally. Recurrent pneumothorax is a complication that can be seen with multiple cystic lung diseases.
- Cystic lung disease can present in isolation or with ancillary imaging features, such as ground-glass opacities or nodules. Clinical features, such as connective tissue disease, cancer, and gender, can further assist in narrowing the differential diagnosis.
- In cases with indeterminate imaging and clinical features, open lung biopsy should be considered.

INTRODUCTION

Diffuse cystic lung disease (DCLD) encompasses a group of diverse pathophysiological processes presenting as multiple air-filled spaces in the pulmonary parenchyma. They can represent a significant diagnostic challenge, especially in patients without pathognomonic computed tomographic (CT) findings and nonspecific clinical presentation. Delayed diagnosis can lead to adverse events, such as recurrent pneumothoraces or progression of cancer. High-resolution computed tomography (HRCT), in conjunction with clinical and pathologic data, is key to establishing a diagnosis.

PATHOPHYSIOLOGY

The pathophysiology of cyst formation (Table 1) in DCLD varies and depends on the underlying condition. Many cystic lung diseases develop via the ball-valve effect. This occurs when peribronchiolar infiltration obstructs the proximal bronchiole, preventing egress of air on expiration but allowing air to pass through on inspiration, which results in cystic dilation of the distal parenchyma. Interstitial fibrosis can also give rise to cysts through retraction of the parenchyma, causing traction bronchiolectasis or alveolar ectasia. Finally, alveolar dissolution from ischemia or alveolar rupture can also result in cyst formation.[1]

IMAGING TECHNIQUE/PROTOCOLS

As with most diffuse lung diseases, HRCT (Table 2) is the optimal method for evaluating cystic lung disease. A standard HRCT protocol consists of noncontrast end-inspiratory images in the supine position, end-expiratory images in the supine position, and end-inspiratory images in the prone position. Volumetric single breath-hold acquisition with thin-section reconstruction using a high-spatial frequency algorithm is recommended. Using contiguous thin-section imaging in the setting of cystic lung disease can help evaluate the cysts for any evidence of mural nodularity or wall thickening. Volumetric acquisitions also allow for the

a Cedars Sinai Imaging, Cedars Sinai Medical Center, 8700 Beverly Boulevard, Suite M-335, Los Angeles, CA 90048, USA; b 8705 Gracie Allen Drive, Suite M-335, Los Angeles, CA 90048, USA
* Corresponding author. 8705 Gracie Allen Drive, Suite M-335, Los Angeles, CA 90048.
E-mail address: christopher.lee3@cshs.org

Radiol Clin N Am 60 (2022) 951–962
https://doi.org/10.1016/j.rcl.2022.06.006

Table 1
Mechanisms for cyst formation and common cystic lung disease

Mechanisms for Cyst Formation	Cystic Lung Disease
Ball-valve effect owing to proximal obstruction by peribronchiolar infiltration/mass effect	LAM, LIP, PLCH, DIP, neoplasm
Traction bronchiolectasis or alveolar ectasia owing to interstitial fibrosis and parenchymal retraction	HP, PLCH
Alveolar dissolution or rupture ± confluence of air spaces	BHD, amyloidosis

creation of multiplanar reformats and maximum/minimum intensity projections, which can be helpful in evaluating the distribution of cysts in the craniocaudal plane. The expiratory and prone series can be acquired with axial (step-and-shoot) technique for radiation dose reduction, in which axial images are obtained at 10- to 20-mm intervals. Expiratory images can identify small airways-related air-trapping as seen in hypersensitivity pneumonitis (HP). Prone images can confirm honeycombing, a mimicker of cystic lung disease.[2]

CLASSIFICATION OF CYSTIC LUNG DISEASE

Pulmonary cysts are round parenchymal lucencies or low-attenuating areas with well-defined interfaces with normal lung. The walls of the cysts vary in thickness but typically measure less than 2 mm.[3] Incidental pulmonary cysts are typically few (<5), are lower lobe in distribution, and are seen in 7.6% of patients older than 40 years of age.[4] Unfortunately, cyst features have significant overlap with other hypodense parenchymal lesions, and no standardized classification exists to distinguish cysts from these other hypodense lesions (**Table 3**).

ISOLATED CYSTIC LUNG DISEASE
Lymphangioleiomyomatosis

Lymphangioleiomyomatosis (LAM) is a rare multisystem disease involving abnormal smooth musclelike cells with loss-of-function mutations in tumor suppressor genes TSC-1 (hamartin protein) and TSC-2 (tuberin). It can occur sporadically or as a manifestation of tuberous sclerosis complex.[5] There is a strong predilection for women of childbearing age. Patients often present with recurrent pneumothoraces or progressive dyspnea, or less commonly with chylous pleural effusion, hemoptysis, or retroperitoneal hemorrhage from a renal angiomyolipoma. Obstruction of lymphatic channels by LAM cells may be the mechanism for chylous effusions. Bronchiolar obstruction by LAM cells produces pulmonary cysts via the ball-valve effect. The production of matrix metalloproteinases and cathepsin-K by LAM cells can degrade the pulmonary interstitium, also leading to cyst formation.[6] Patients with tuberous sclerosis complex may also exhibit hamartomas and benign neoplasms, such as giant cell astrocytomas, cortical tubers, renal angiomyolipomas, and cardiac rhabdomyomas.[7]

LAM can be treated with sirolimus, which stabilizes lung function, reduces symptoms, and improves quality of life.[8] Recurrent pneumothoraces are typically treated with pleurodesis.[9]

Table 2
High-resolution computed tomography protocol

Position	Supine		Prone
Respiration	Inspiratory	Expiratory	Inspiratory
Slice thickness	0.625–1.5 mm		
Gantry rotation	<1 s		
Acquisition	Helical (volumetric)	Helical or axial	
Reformats/reconstruction	High-spatial-frequency algorithm Thin sections MIP/minIP		
Field-of-view	Apex to costophrenic sulcus		

Table 3
Classification of cystic structures within the lungs

	Fleischner Society Description	Wall Thickness	Comments
Cyst	Round parenchymal lucency or low-attenuating area with a well-defined interface with normal lung	<2 mm	
Cavity	Gas-filled space within a pulmonary consolidation, mass, or nodule	>3 mm	
Bleb	Small gas-containing space within the visceral pleura or subpleural lung	<1 mm	
Emphysema	Enlarged airspaces with alveolar wall destruction, appearing as areas of low attenuation without visible walls	Not seen	Associated with tobacco exposure
Bulla	Thin-walled airspace measuring more than 1 cm in diameter, usually accompanied by emphysema	<1 mm	Associated with tobacco exposure
Pneumatocele	Thin-walled gas-filled space within the lung	<1 mm	Most frequently owing to acute pneumonia, trauma, or aspiration of hydrocarbon fluid
Honeycombing	Fibrotic lung tissue containing clustered, thick-walled, cystic airspaces within the subpleural lung	1–3 mm	Represents end-stage fibrotic lung disease, classically usual interstitial pneumonia
Cystic bronchiectasis	Saccular appearance of irreversible bronchial dilation	1–3 mm	

On CT, LAM manifests as diffusely distributed, air-filled, thin-walled cysts of varying size but uniform shape (**Fig. 1**). The intervening lung parenchyma between the cysts is typically normal. Ill-defined areas of increased attenuation may be secondary to hemorrhage or edema. Air-trapping is rarely seen.[10]

A definitive diagnosis of LAM can be achieved with a characteristic clinical history and CT appearance, as well as other specific features, such as serum vascular endothelial growth factor-D levels. Histopathologic confirmation is usually not required.[9]

Birt-Hogg-Dubé Syndrome

Birt-Hogg-Dubé (BHD) syndrome, also known as *Hornstein-Knickenberg* syndrome, is an autosomal dominant systemic multiorgan disorder that classically presents with cutaneous lesions (fibrofolliculomas, trichodiscoma, acrochordons), renal tumors (oncocytomas, renal cell carcinoma), and spontaneous recurrent pneumothoraces from cystic lung disease.[11] BHD syndrome occurs owing to autosomal dominant loss-of-function germline mutations in the folliculin gene (FLCN) on chromosome 17. It is hypothesized that folliculin has key interactions with cell-cell adhesion mechanisms. With repeated stretching from respirations, alveolar spaces expand at "anchor points" to the pleura, leading to cyst formation.[12]

CT of BHD syndrome demonstrates a lower lung predominant distribution of cysts, with characteristically greater than 2 elliptical paramediastinal cysts or disproportionate paramediastinal cysts (**Fig. 2**).[13] Cysts are thin walled, and the intervening lung parenchyma is normal.

Diagnostic criteria suggestive of BHD syndrome includes the presence of characteristic cutaneous

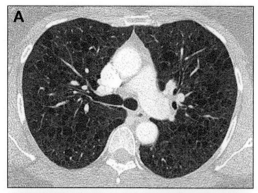

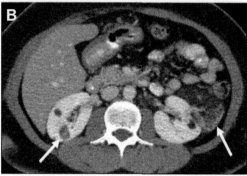

Fig. 1. CT scan in a patient with sporadic LAM. Axial image through the lungs (*A*) demonstrates innumerable round thin-walled cysts evenly distributed throughout the lungs. There is normal intervening parenchyma without nodules or ground-glass opacities. Axial image through the upper abdomen (*B*) shows multiple fat-containing lesions within both kidneys consistent with angiomyolipomas (*arrows*). Angiomyolipomas may be present in both LAM associated with tuberous sclerosis and sporadic LAM.

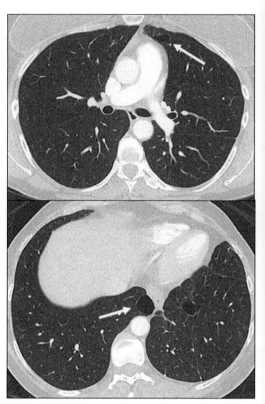

Fig. 2. Axial CT images in a patient with BHD syndrome demonstrate bilateral cysts, including prominent paramediastinal cysts (*arrows*). A disproportionate number of elliptical paramediastinal cysts is characteristic of this disease.

lesions, family history, renal tumors, and/or pulmonary cysts. A genetic test positive for germline FLCN mutation is considered confirmatory of BHD syndrome.[14]

CYSTIC LUNG DISEASE ASSOCIATED WITH GROUND-GLASS OPACITIES
Lymphocytic Interstitial Pneumonia

Lymphocytic interstitial pneumonia (LIP) is a benign lymphoproliferative disorder with diffuse interstitial proliferation of polyclonal lymphocytes and plasma cells. It is commonly associated with immune-related abnormalities, such as Sjögren syndrome, AIDS, autoimmune thyroid disease, and Castleman disease, but can also be idiopathic. Peribronchiolar infiltration causing partial bronchiolar obstruction via the ball-valve effect is thought to result in cyst formation.[15] Nonspecific pulmonary symptoms include progressive

dyspnea and dry cough. Systemic symptoms are less common. Therapy usually involves corticosteroids and treatment of the underlying disease.[16]

CT findings of LIP include diffuse centrilobular ground-glass opacities, poorly defined centrilobular nodules, thickening of bronchovascular bundles, interlobular septal thickening, and mediastinal/hilar lymphadenopathy (Fig. 3). Cysts are seen in up to 68% of patients.[17] Characteristically, the cysts are small (1–30 mm), few in number (<10% of the lung), and random in distribution.[15,18] LIP can present as isolated cystic lung disease and have been described as "perivascular" in some reports. On follow-up CT, ground-glass opacities and nodules may regress, whereas the cysts persist.[19] The presence of small nodules and cysts can help differentiate LIP from lymphoma, a common mimicker.[20]

Desquamative Interstitial Pneumonia

Desquamative interstitial pneumonia (DIP) is an uncommon form of interstitial lung disease

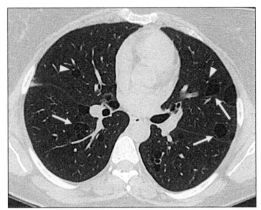

Fig. 3. Axial CT image in a patient with LIP demonstrates scattered cysts in a perivascular distribution (*arrows*). Note the vessels (*arrowheads*) along the cyst walls. LIP may occasionally present as isolated cystic lung disease.

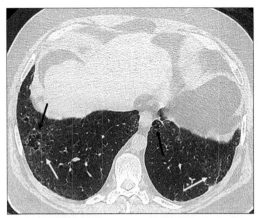

Fig. 4. Axial CT image in a patient with a significant smoking history and DIP demonstrates peripheral lower-lobe predominant ground-glass opacities (*white arrows*) with superimposed cystic lesions (*black arrows*).

typically affecting male smokers in their fourth or fifth decades. Significant overlap between the CT findings of respiratory bronchiolitis-interstitial lung disease and DIP suggests that these processes represent a continuum of severity of small airway and parenchymal reaction to cigarette smoke.[21] Pneumoconiosis, rheumatologic disease, and some drug reactions have also been associated with DIP.[22] Pathologically, intra-alveolar accumulation of pigmented macrophages is seen, and not desquamation of epithelial cells as previously thought.[23] Cystic lesions correspond with dilated alveolar ducts, bronchioles, and/or pulmonary cysts, as well as numerous macrophage-filled air spaces.[24]

On CT, ground-glass opacities are the predominant feature, with a slight peripheral and lower lung predilection.[25,26] Few small cystic areas may develop in areas of ground-glass opacity, which can resolve over time (**Fig. 4**).[24]

Pneumocystis jirovecii Pneumonia

P jirovecii pneumonia (PJP) characteristically affects patients with human immunodeficiency virus (HIV) infection with low CD4 counts (<200 cells/mm^3), as well as other immunosuppressed states.[27] It is typically an alveolar pathogen attaching to type I alveolar epithelium. Diffuse alveolar damage is thought to be caused by the host's own inflammatory response.[28]

Typical CT manifestations include diffuse, central, bilateral, and symmetric ground-glass opacities with a slight upper-lobe predilection. Septal lines, crazy paving, and consolidation may develop in advanced stages. Thin-walled cysts between 1 and 5 cm in diameter develop within

7 days within areas of ground-glass abnormality in up to 34% of patients; these cysts likely represent pneumatoceles (**Fig. 5**). Cysts mostly resolve after acute episodes of pneumonia.[27,29,30] The presence of cysts is reportedly lower in patients without HIV infection.[31]

Hypersensitivity Pneumonitis

HP represents a diffuse granulomatous response to inhaled organic antigens. A thorough clinical history is essential to making this diagnosis; however, the cause is often not identified. Most cases occur after months or years of inhaling the offending agent.[32] The pathophysiology for cyst formation in HP is unclear but may be due to the ball-valve effect from peribronchiolar infiltration.[33]

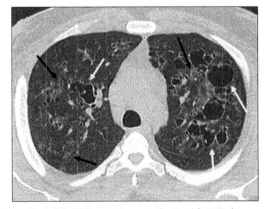

Fig. 5. Axial CT image in a patient with PJP demonstrates upper-lobe predominant ground-glass nodular opacities (*black arrows*) and cysts (*white arrows*).

Traditionally, HP is categorized as acute, subacute, and chronic, although these categories are not easily distinguished, and more recently, HP is separated instead into nonfibrotic and fibrotic forms.[34] Acute HP can present as subtle centrilobular nodules or bilateral central ground-glass opacities resembling acute pulmonary edema.[35] Subacute HP manifests as diffuse, patchy, ground-glass opacities, poorly defined small centrilobular nodules, and mosaic attenuation with patchy areas of air-trapping, ground-glass abnormality, and normal parenchyma, colloquially termed the "headcheese sign." Chronic HP demonstrates signs of pulmonary fibrosis, reticulations, architectural distortion, and traction bronchiectasis, superimposed on findings of subacute HP; the lung bases are characteristically spared.[32] Pulmonary cysts have been observed in a small percentage (13%) of patients with subacute HP (Fig. 6). The cysts are typically in a random distribution and measure between 3 and 25 mm in diameter.[33]

CYSTIC LUNG DISEASE ASSOCIATED WITH NODULES
Pulmonary Langerhans Cell Histiocytosis

Pulmonary Langerhans cell histiocytosis (PLCH) is a rare disease characterized by infiltration of myeloid cells that have similar characteristics with epidermal Langerhans cells. Pulmonary involvement typically occurs in young adult current or former smokers but can also be seen in systemic forms. Clinically, patients can present with cough, dyspnea, fever, weight loss, sweats, or spontaneous pneumothoraces.[36] Bronchiolar infiltration by Langerhans cells results in small airways obstruction and cyst formation.[37]

CT demonstrates bizarre-shaped, thin-walled cysts of various sizes, which are predominantly distributed within the upper and middle lung zones with relative sparing of the lung bases.[38] Centrilobular nodules and small cavitary nodules (1–10 mm) predominate in early disease, whereas cysts persist in end-stage PLCH. These imaging findings suggest a pattern of disease evolution from solid nodules to cavitary nodules to thick-walled cysts to thin-walled cysts (Fig. 7).[39] End-stage PLCH can present as isolated cystic lung disease. Mediastinal lymphadenopathy, consolidative opacities, and pleural effusions are unusual.[40] The nodules and cavities may be hypermetabolic on fluorodeoxyglucose (FDG)-PET, which may raise concern for malignancy. Extrapulmonary involvement in PLCH may occur in bone, skin, and lymph nodes.[41] Pulmonary hypertension is also a common complication of PLCH.[36]

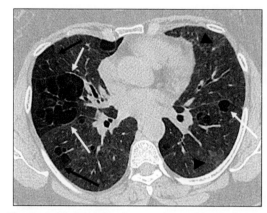

Fig. 6. Axial CT image in a patient with HP demonstrates mosaic attenuation with patchy areas of ground-glass abnormality (*arrowhead*) and air-trapping (*black arrows*). Clustered cysts (*white arrows*) are also present in both lungs.

Definitive diagnosis of PLCH requires lung biopsy; however, this may not be necessary in patients with characteristic clinical and CT features.[42]

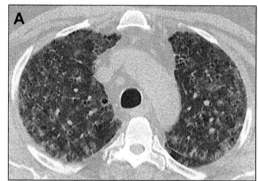

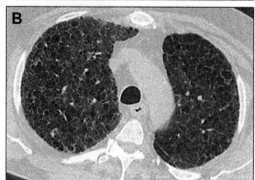

Fig. 7. Axial CT images 1 year apart in a patient with a significant smoking history and PLCH. Upper-lobe predominant ill-defined centrilobular nodules predominate early in the disease course (*A*), which progressively cavitate into bizarre-shaped cysts (*B*).

Amyloidosis

Amyloidosis is a rare disease with varied clinical and radiologic manifestations that is caused by extracellular accumulation of fibrillary proteins throughout the body. Pulmonary amyloidosis is most commonly a localized process and is typically classified as nodular parenchymal amyloidosis or diffuse alveolar septal amyloidosis.[43] Cysts are more commonly associated with the nodular parenchymal pattern[44–46] than the diffuse alveolar septal form.[47] The underlying mechanism for cyst formation is unclear but may be due to peribronchiolar infiltration and bronchiolar obstruction via the ball-valve effect.[48]

CT findings of nodular parenchymal amyloidosis include one or more pulmonary nodules with smooth, lobulated, or spiculated margins and occasional calcification. Cavitation is rare. Biopsy is often required for definitive diagnosis owing to its nonspecific appearance.[43] Alveolar septal amyloidosis is less common but more clinically significant, as these patients may progress to respiratory failure and pulmonary hypertension.[49] CT typically reveals well-defined 2- to 4-mm micronodules with reticular opacities, interlobar septal thickening, and confluent consolidations with basal and peripheral predominance.[43] Pulmonary cysts, when they occur, are often multiple and subpleural or perivascular in distribution[48] (Fig. 8).

Cancers Associated with Cystic Spaces

Although cancers associated with cystic spaces do not represent DCLD, it is important to be aware of this entity, as delayed diagnosis may lead to increased mortality. Cystic and pericystic primary lung cancers are predominantly adenocarcinomas. Cystic pulmonary metastases have been described with many cancers, including colorectal cancer[50] and soft tissue sarcoma,[51] and tend to progress faster than lung cancers. Pericystic lung cancers can be associated with various types of cystic structures within the lungs, including bullae, pleural blebs, or bronchiectatic airways. In most cases, lung cancers tend to arise along the walls of preexisting cysts, although evidence also suggests that microscopic disease can infiltrate bronchioles, causing cyst formation via the ball-valve effect. Solid primary or metastatic tumors may undergo cavitation or cystic transformation following treatment with chemotherapy or immunotherapy.[52]

Change in the morphology of a cyst or pericystic nodule should raise suspicion for malignancy, especially in a patient with a known history of malignancy or high risk for developing lung cancer. Suspicious changes can include an increase in

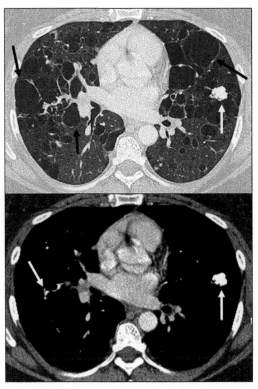

Fig. 8. Axial CT images in a patient with Sjögren syndrome and LIP demonstrate numerous perivascular cysts (*black arrows*) and scattered calcified nodules (*white arrows*). The calcified nodules represent nodular parenchymal amyloidosis. The cystic lesions demonstrate the same characteristics as those seen in LIP without accompanying amyloidosis.

cyst size, solid component, or wall thickness (Fig. 9). FDG-PET may be helpful if the nodular or solid component is greater than 1 cm in diameter. Because of the nonspecific imaging findings, percutaneous biopsy of the solid component is often required.[53]

Ultrarare CYSTIC LUNG DISEASES
Chronic Inflammatory Bronchiolitis

Chronic inflammatory bronchiolitis causing cyst formation is a recently described and poorly understood entity (Table 4). In several case series, cystic lung disease resembling LAM was found to have coexisting small airways disease on pathologic examination. Typical clinical, pathologic, and immunohistochemical features of LAM and PLCH were not identified.[54–56]

The cysts in chronic inflammatory bronchiolitis are diffusely distributed, and some cysts may demonstrate prominent vessels along the walls.[54,56]

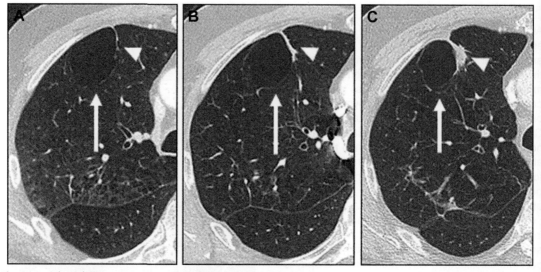

Fig. 9. Serial axial CT images approximately 1 year apart demonstrating the evolution of lung cancer (*arrowhead*) associated with a cystic space (*arrow*). The initial CT (*A*) shows a right upper-lobe bulla with minimal thickening along the medial wall. The subsequent CT (*B*) depicts increased thickening of the medial wall, and the final CT (*C*) demonstrates the development of a nodular component with mild spiculations. Biopsy revealed adenocarcinoma. Changes in the morphology of a cyst, such as increased wall thickness or the development of a solid or nodular component, should raise suspicion for malignancy.

Table 4
Ultrarare cystic lung diseases

	CT Appearance	Mimics	Clinical Associations
Chronic inflammatory bronchiolitis	Diffusely distributed cysts with prominent vessels along walls	LAM	Young nonsmoking women
LCDD	Scattered perivascular cysts, no calcification or lymphadenopathy	Amyloidosis	Lymphoproliferative and autoimmune disorders
NF1	Apical cysts/bullae, occasionally with lower lung ground-glass opacities	LAM	Pigmented hamartomas of the iris (Lisch nodules), café-au-lait spots, and neurofibromas
COPA syndrome	Variably distributed cysts, ground-glass opacities, and nodules also seen	LIP	Young child with arthritis and cough
Cowden syndrome	Randomly distributed cysts and nodules	BHD syndrome	Lhermitte-Duclos disease and mucocutaneous lesions, breast, thyroid, and endometrial cancer.

Light Chain Deposition Disease

In light chain deposition disease (LCDD), light chain fragments from monoclonal immunoglobulin produced by B-lymphocytes can cause damage via tissue deposition within the kidney, liver, and heart.[57] Although its pathogenesis is similar to that of amyloidosis, it lacks the ability to form amyloid fibrils.[58]

On CT, cysts and nodules may be present without zonal predominance (**Fig. 10**). Vessels are often seen along cyst walls. Unlike amyloidosis, lymphadenopathy and calcification are uncommon. In patients with lymphoproliferative disease or connective tissue disorders and the aforementioned CT findings, LCDD should be strongly considered.[59,60]

Neurofibromatosis

Neurofibromatosis type 1 (NF1) is an autosomal dominant disease caused by mutations in the NF1 gene. Clinically, NF1 is characterized by the triad of pigmented hamartomas of the iris (Lisch nodules), café-au-lait spots, and neurofibromas.[61] Thoracic manifestations include intrathoracic neurogenic tumors, meningoceles, kyphoscoliosis, pulmonary hypertension, and interstitial lung disease.[62,63]

Cystic lung disease in NF1 is characterized by apical predominant, thin-walled bullae/cysts (**Fig. 11**). Lower lung ground-glass opacities may occasionally be present.[61,63]

Coatamer Subunit Alpha (COPA) Syndrome

Coatamer subunit Alpha (COPA) syndrome is an autosomal dominant primary immunodeficiency affecting the coatomer complex-I alpha subunit, which is responsible for intracellular transport. Most patients present in childhood with arthritis or cough and tachypnea.[64] Kidneys are less commonly involved. Follicular bronchiolitis can be seen on lung biopsy.[65]

CT in patients with COPA syndrome demonstrate thin-walled cysts with a variable distribution. Ground-glass opacities and nodules have been observed in approximately half of patients. The ground-glass abnormality has been described to resemble nonspecific interstitial pneumonia,[66] although it may also represent diffuse alveolar hemorrhage.[65]

Cowden Syndrome

Cowden syndrome is a multisystem autosomal dominant disorder characterized by benign hamartomas of all 3 germ layers often related to mutations in the PTEN tumor suppressor gene. Major diagnostic criteria include PTEN mutation, Lhermitte-Duclos disease, mucocutaneous

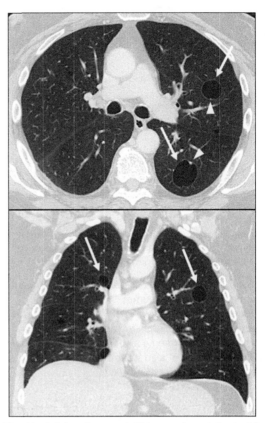

Fig. 10. Axial and coronal CT images in a patient with LCDD demonstrate scattered perivascular cysts (*arrows*). Note the vessels (*arrowheads*) along the cyst walls. CT features of LCDD can mimic those of amyloidosis or LIP. (*Courtesy of* S Hobbs, MD, Lexington, KY.)

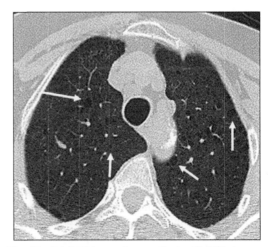

Fig. 11. Axial CT image in a patient with NF1 demonstrating numerous upper-lobe predominant tiny thin-walled cysts (*arrows*).

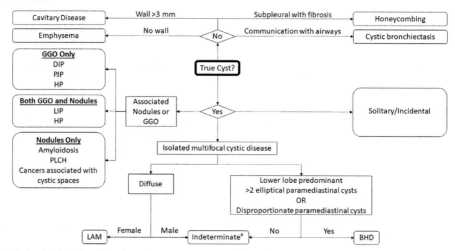

Fig. 12. Radiologic decision flowchart for common cystic lung disease. Ultrarare cystic lung diseases can mimic common cystic diseases and are discussed in **Table 4.** [a]Commonly, LIP or end-stage PLCH. Other cystic lung diseases should be considered based on clinical features.

lesions, macrocephaly, or cancers of the breast, thyroid, and endometrium.[67,68]

Pulmonary cysts occur in 80% of patients. They are typically few (<10), are randomly distributed, and measure between 4 and 63 mm. Solid pulmonary nodules are also common and randomly distributed.[69]

SUMMARY

Cystic lung disease can present a diagnostic dilemma for both the radiologist and the clinician. Accurate identification of true pulmonary cysts is the first step in the diagnostic approach. Following the recognition of true cystic lung disease, combining the appearance and distribution of cysts with ancillary imaging findings and clinical features can significantly narrow the differential and, occasionally, allow the radiologist to render a definitive diagnosis (**Fig. 12**).

CLINICS CARE POINTS

- Delayed diagnosis of cystic lesions can lead to complications such as recurrent pneumothorax or cancer.

- Other lucent lesions such as cavitary disease and bronchiectasis can mimic cystic lung disease and suggest alternative etiologies.

- Attention to associated imaging features such as ground glass opacities and nodules as well as clinical features such as gender and auto-immune disease is critical to narrowing the diagnosis.

- Consider open lung biopsy in cases with indeterminate clinical and imaging features.

DISCLOSURE

The authors have nothing to disclose.

REFERENCES

1. Boddu P, Parimi V, Taddonio M, et al. Pathologic and Radiologic Correlation of Adult Cystic Lung Disease: A Comprehensive Review. Pathol Res Int 2017;2017: e3502438. https://doi.org/10.1155/2017/3502438.

2. American College of Radiology. ACR–STR practice parameter for the performance of high resolution computed tomography (HRCT) of the lungs in adults. 2020. 9. Available at: https://www.acr.org/-/media/ACR/Files/Practice-Parameters/HRCT-Lungs.pdf. Accessed November 2, 2021.

3. Hansell DM, Bankier AA, MacMahon H, et al. Fleischner Society: Glossary of Terms for Thoracic Imaging. Radiology 2008;246(3):697–722.

4. Araki T, Nishino M, Gao W, et al. Pulmonary cysts identified on chest CT: Are they part of aging change or of clinical significance? Thorax 2015;70(12):1156–62.

5. Steagall WK, Pacheco-Rodriguez G, Darling TN, et al. The Lymphangioleiomyomatosis Lung Cell and Its Human Cell Models. Am J Respir Cell Mol Biol 2018;58(6):678–83.

6. Harari S, Torre O, Moss J. Lymphangioleiomyomatosis: what do we know and what are we looking for? Eur Respir Rev 2011;20(119):034–44.

7. Taveira-DaSilva AM, Moss J. Clinical features, epidemiology, and therapy of lymphangioleiomyomatosis. Clin Epidemiol 2015;7:249–57.

8. Efficacy and Safety of Sirolimus in Lymphangioleiomyomatosis | NEJM. Available at: https://www.nejm.org/doi/full/10.1056/nejmoa1100391. Accessed December 5, 2021.

9. Gupta N, Finlay GA, Kotloff RM, et al. Lymphangioleiomyomatosis Diagnosis and Management: High-Resolution Chest Computed Tomography,

Transbronchial Lung Biopsy, and Pleural Disease Management. An Official American Thoracic Society/Japanese Respiratory Society Clinical Practice Guideline. Am J Respir Crit Care Med 2017; 196(10):1337–48.

10. Pallisa E, Sanz P, Roman A, et al. Lymphangioleiomyomatosis: Pulmonary and Abdominal Findings with Pathologic Correlation. RadioGraphics 2002; 22(suppl_1):S185–98.

11. Agarwal PP, Gross BH, Holloway BJ, et al. Thoracic CT Findings in Birt-Hogg-Dubé Syndrome. Am J Roentgenol 2011;196(2):349–52.

12. Kennedy JC, Khabibullin D, Henske EP. Mechanisms of pulmonary cyst pathogenesis in Birt-Hogg-Dube syndrome: The stretch hypothesis. Semin Cell Dev Biol 2016;52:47–52.

13. Escalon JG, Richards JC, Koelsch T, et al. Isolated Cystic Lung Disease: An Algorithmic Approach to Distinguishing Birt-Hogg-Dubé Syndrome, Lymphangioleiomyomatosis, and Lymphocytic Interstitial Pneumonia. Am J Roentgenol 2019;212(6):1260–4.

14. Schmidt LS, Linehan WM. Molecular Genetics and Clinical Features of Birt-Hogg-Dubé-Syndrome. Nat Rev Urol 2015;12(10):558–69.

15. Ichikawa Y, Kinoshita M, Kotaro Oizumi TK, et al. Lung Cyst Formation in Lymphocytic Interstitial Pneumonia: CT Features. J Comput Assist Tomogr 1994;18(5):745–8.

16. Swigris JJ, Berry GJ, Raffin TA, et al. Lymphoid Interstitial Pneumonia: A Narrative Review. Chest 2002; 122(6):2150–64.

17. Johkoh T, Müller NL, Pickford HA, et al. Lymphocytic Interstitial Pneumonia: Thin-Section CT Findings in 22 Patients. Radiology 1999;212(2):567–72.

18. Louza GF, Nobre LF, Mançano AD, et al. Lymphocytic interstitial pneumonia: computed tomography findings in 36 patients. Radiol Bras 2020;53:287–92.

19. Johkoh T, Ichikado K, Akira M, et al. Lymphocytic Interstitial Pneumonia: Follow-up CT Findings in 14 Patients. J Thorac Imaging 2000;15(3):162–7.

20. Honda O, Johkoh T, Ichikado K, et al. Differential diagnosis of lymphocytic interstitial pneumonia and malignant lymphoma on high-resolution CT. AJR Am J Roentgenol 1999;173(1):71–4.

21. Heyneman LE, Ward S, Lynch DA, et al. Respiratory bronchiolitis, respiratory bronchiolitis-associated interstitial lung disease, and desquamative interstitial pneumonia: different entities or part of the spectrum of the same disease process? AJR Am J Roentgenol 1999;173(6):1617–22.

22. Godbert B, Wissler MP, Vignaud JM. Desquamative interstitial pneumonia: an analytic review with an emphasis on aetiology. Eur Respir Rev 2013; 22(128):117–23.

23. Attili AK, Kazerooni EA, Gross BH, et al. Smoking-related Interstitial Lung Disease: Radiologic-Clinical-Pathologic Correlation. RadioGraphics 2008;28(5):1383–96.

24. Akira M, Yamamoto S, Hara H, et al. Serial computed tomographic evaluation in desquamative interstitial pneumonia. Thorax 1997;52(4):333–7.

25. Wells AU, Hirani N. Interstitial lung disease guideline. Thorax 2008;63(Suppl 5):v1–58.

26. Hartman TE, Primack SL, Swensen SJ, et al. Desquamative interstitial pneumonia: thin-section CT findings in 22 patients. Radiology 1993;187(3): 787–90.

27. Kanne JP, Yandow DR, Meyer CA. Pneumocystis jiroveci Pneumonia: High-Resolution CT Findings in Patients With and Without HIV Infection. Am J Roentgenol 2012;198(6):W555–61.

28. Truong J, Ashurst JV. Pneumocystis Jirovecii Pneumonia. In: StatPearls. StatPearls Publishing; 2021. Available at: http://www.ncbi.nlm.nih.gov/books/NBK482370/. Accessed December 30, 2021.

29. Kuhlman JE, Kavuru M, Fishman EK, et al. Pneumocystis carinii pneumonia: spectrum of parenchymal CT findings. Radiology 1990;175(3):711–4.

30. Chow C, Templeton PA, White CS. Lung cysts associated with Pneumocystis carinii pneumonia: radiographic characteristics, natural history, and complications. Am J Roentgenol 1993;161(3): 527–31.

31. Hardak E, Brook O, Yigla M. Radiological Features of Pneumocystis jirovecii Pneumonia in Immunocompromised Patients with and Without AIDS. Lung 2010;188(2):159–63.

32. Silva CIS, Churg A, Müller NL. Hypersensitivity Pneumonitis: Spectrum of High-Resolution CT and Pathologic Findings. Am J Roentgenol 2007; 188(2):334–44.

33. Franquet T, Hansell DM, Senbanjo T, et al. Lung cysts in subacute hypersensitivity pneumonitis. J Comput Assist Tomogr 2003;27(4):475–8.

34. Raghu G, Remy-Jardin M, Ryerson CJ, et al. Diagnosis of hypersensitivity pneumonitis in adults. An official ats/jrs/alat clinical practice guideline. Am J Respir Crit Care Med 2020;202(3):e36–69.

35. Matar LD, McAdams HP, Sporn TA. Hypersensitivity Pneumonitis. Am J Roentgenol 2000;174(4):1061–6.

36. Vassallo R, Harari S, Tazi A. Current understanding and management of pulmonary Langerhans cell histiocytosis. Thorax 2017;72(10):937–45.

37. Juvet SC, Hwang D, Downey GP. Rare lung diseases III: Pulmonary Langerhans' cell histiocytosis. Can Respir J J Can Thorac Soc 2010;17(3):e55–62.

38. Brauner MW, Grenier P, Mouelhi MM, et al. Pulmonary histiocytosis X: evaluation with high-resolution CT. Radiology 1989;172(1):255–8.

39. Brauner MW, Grenier P, Tijani K, et al. Pulmonary Langerhans cell histiocytosis: evolution of lesions on CT scans. Radiology 1997;204(2):497–502.

40. Sundar KM, Gosselin MV, Chung HL, et al. Pulmonary Langerhans Cell Histiocytosis. Chest 2003; 123(5):1673–83.

41. Vassallo R, Ryu JH, Schroeder DR, et al. Clinical outcomes of pulmonary Langerhans'-cell histiocytosis in adults. N Engl J Med 2002;346(7):484–90.

42. Vassallo R, Ryu JH, Colby TV, et al. Pulmonary Langerhans'-cell histiocytosis. N Engl J Med 2000; 342(26):1969–78.

43. Czeyda-Pommersheim F, Hwang M, Chen SS, et al. Amyloidosis: Modern Cross-sectional Imaging. RadioGraphics 2015;35(5):1381–92.

44. Lantuejoul S, Moulai N, Quetant S, et al. Unusual cystic presentation of pulmonary nodular amyloidosis associated with MALT-type lymphoma. Eur Respir J 2007;30(3):589–92.

45. Baqir M, Kluka EM, Aubry MC, et al. Amyloid-associated cystic lung disease in primary Sjögren's syndrome. Respir Med 2013;107(4):616–21.

46. Chew KM, Clarke MJ, Dubey N, et al. Nodular pulmonary amyloidosis with unusual, widespread lung cysts. Singapore Med J 2013;54(5):e97–9.

47. Ohdama S, Akagawa S, Matsubara O, et al. Primary diffuse alveolar septal amyloidosis with multiple cysts and calcification. Eur Respir J 1996;9(7): 1569–71.

48. Zamora AC, White DB, Sykes AMG, et al. Amyloid-associated Cystic Lung Disease. Chest 2016; 149(5):1223–33.

49. Milani P, Basset M, Russo F, et al. The lung in amyloidosis. Eur Respir Rev 2017;26(145).

50. Simion NI, Pezzetta E. Cystic appearance: an uncommon feature of pulmonary metastasis of colorectal origin. BMJ Case Rep 2011;2011: bcr1020115063.

51. Itoh T, Mochizuki M, Kumazaki S, et al. Cystic pulmonary metastases of endometrial stromal sarcoma of the uterus, mimicking lymphangiomyomatosis: A case report with immunohistochemistry of HMB45. Pathol Int 1997;47(10):725–9.

52. Farooqi AO, Cham M, Zhang L, et al. Lung Cancer Associated With Cystic Airspaces. Am J Roentgenol 2012;199(4):781–6.

53. Sheard S, Moser J, Sayer C, et al. Lung Cancers Associated with Cystic Airspaces: Underrecognized Features of Early Disease. RadioGraphics 2018; 38(3):704–17.

54. Rowan C, Hansell DM, Renzoni E, et al. Diffuse Cystic Lung Disease of Unexplained Cause With Coexistent Small Airway Disease: A Possible Causal Relationship? Am J Surg Pathol 2012;36(2):228–34.

55. de Oliveira MR, Dias OM, Amaral AF. Diffuse cystic lung disease as the primary tomographic manifestation of bronchiolitis: A case series. Pulmonology 2020;26(6):403–6.

56. Gupta N, Colby TV, Meyer CA, et al. Smoking-Related Diffuse Cystic Lung Disease. Chest 2018; 154(2):e31–5.

57. Colombat M, Caudroy S, Lagonotte E, et al. Pathomechanisms of cyst formation in pulmonary light chain deposition disease. Eur Respir J 2008;32(5): 1399–403.

58. Ganeval D, Noël LH, Preud'homme JL, et al. Light-chain deposition disease: Its relation with AL-type amyloidosis. Kidney Int 1984;26(1):1–9.

59. Sheard S, Nicholson AG, Edmunds L, et al. Pulmonary light-chain deposition disease: CT and pathology findings in nine patients. Clin Radiol 2015; 70(5):515–22.

60. Baqir M, Moua T, White D, et al. Pulmonary nodular and cystic light chain deposition disease: A retrospective review of 10 cases. Respir Med 2020;164: 105896.

61. Zamora AC, Collard HR, Wolters PJ, et al. Neurofibromatosis-associated lung disease: a case series and literature review. Eur Respir J 2007;29(1):210–4.

62. Ryu JH, Parambil JG, McGrann PS, et al. Lack of Evidence for an Association Between Neurofibromatosis and Pulmonary Fibrosis. Chest 2005;128(4): 2381–6.

63. Dehal N, Arce Gastelum A, Millner PG. Neurofibromatosis-Associated Diffuse Lung Disease: A Case Report and Review of the Literature. Cureus 2020; 12(6):e8916.

64. Vece TJ, Watkin LB, Nicholas S, et al. Copa Syndrome: A Novel Autosomal Dominant Immune Dysregulatory Disease. J Clin Immunol 2016;36(4): 377–87.

65. Tsui JL, Estrada OA, Deng Z, et al. Analysis of pulmonary features and treatment approaches in the COPA syndrome. ERJ Open Res 2018;4(2): 00017–2018.

66. Noorelahi R, Perez G, Otero HJ. Imaging findings of COPA syndrome in a 12-year-old boy. Pediatr Radiol 2018;48(2):279–82.

67. Pilarski R. PTEN Hamartoma Tumor Syndrome: A Clinical Overview. Cancers 2019;11(6):844.

68. Pilarski R. Cowden Syndrome: A Critical Review of the Clinical Literature. J Genet Couns 2009;18(1): 13–27.

69. Parvinian A, Cox CW, Hartman TE. Cowden Syndrome: A Cause of Pulmonary Cysts. J Thorac Imaging 2018;33(6):W48.

Mosaic Attenuation Pattern
A Guide to Analysis with HRCT

Gregory M. Lee, MD[a], Melissa B. Carroll, MD[b], Jeffrey R. Galvin, MD[a],
Christopher M. Walker, MD[b],*

KEYWORDS

- Mosaic attenuation • Small airways disease • Constrictive bronchiolitis • Air trapping
- High-resolution computed tomography • Expiratory phase

KEY POINTS

- Mosaic attenuation is a frequently encountered finding in high-resolution computed tomography (HRCT). Differential possibilities can be broadly grouped into three categories: parenchymal disease, small airways disease, and vascular disease.
- Sharply demarcated mosaic attenuation suggests small airways or vascular disease. Decreased peripheral vascularity can be seen in both of these disease states.
- When mosaic attenuation is particularly severe and demarcated, constrictive bronchiolitis is often the cause. Imaging alone makes it difficult to differentiate among causes of constrictive bronchiolitis, emphasizing the importance of clinical history in establishing etiology.

INTRODUCTION

Mosaic attenuation, formerly mosaic perfusion or mosaic oligemia, is a commonly encountered imaging pattern on computed tomography (CT) of the chest. The Fleischner Society defines a mosaic attenuation pattern as a "patchwork of regions of differing attenuation that may represent patchy interstitial disease, obliterative small airways disease, or occlusive vascular disease."[1] Mosaic attenuation is not a specific disease process, but rather an imaging finding with a differential diagnosis.[2]

The difficulty in encountering this pattern is differentiating the areas of the lung parenchyma that are normal and abnormal. In some pathologic processes such as small airways disease or occlusive vascular disease, the abnormal lung is more lucent, whereas in parenchymal lung disease, the abnormal lung is more dense.[3] To complicate matters, certain diseases such as hypersensitivity

pneumonitis may have both parenchymal lung disease and small airways disease.[4]

Small airways disease may be a primary disorder or related to parenchymal, large airways or mixed disease. Any disease resulting in constriction or injury to the small airways may result in mosaic attenuation. Similarly, any process that results in variable perfusion to the lung may also cause a mosaic pattern. This review seeks to highlight the causes of mosaic attenuation and provide ancillary imaging and clinical features that allow for definitive diagnosis.

Normal Anatomy

The airways include the trachea, main bronchi, lobar bronchi, segmental and intrapulmonary bronchi, and the bronchioles. Airways are classified as conducting or gas-exchanging regions, separated by a transitional zone. The conducting membranous bronchiole is the terminal

[a] Department of Diagnostic Radiology and Nuclear Medicine, University of Maryland, 22 South Greene Street, Baltimore, MD 21201, USA; [b] Department of Radiology, University of Kansas Medical Center, 3901 Rainbow Blvd Kansas City, KS 66160, USA
* Corresponding author.
E-mail address: walk0060@gmail.com

Radiol Clin N Am 60 (2022) 963–978
https://doi.org/10.1016/j.rcl.2022.06.009
0033-8389/22/© 2022 Elsevier Inc. All rights reserved.

bronchiole. Respiratory bronchioles are transitional branches that lead to gas-exchanging alveolar ducts, alveolar sacs, and the alveoli. The acinus is lung parenchyma distal to the terminal bronchiole, composed of respiratory bronchioles, alveolar ducts, alveolar sacs and alveoli. The acinus is the largest unit of lung in that all airways participate in gas exchange. The small airways are composed of membranous and respiratory bronchioles, measure <2 mm in internal diameter, and lack cartilage.[5]

Membranous bronchioles are lined by ciliated columnar cells and non-ciliated club cells that are exocrine cells unique to bronchioles.[6] Elastic fibers attached to the adventitia of bronchioles from adjacent alveoli provide mechanical support and prevent small airways collapse in the final phase of expiration.[7] Respiratory bronchioles arise distal to the terminal membranous bronchioles and are partially alveolated, transitional airways.

The secondary pulmonary lobule (SPL) is the smallest functional unit of the lung that is bound by connective tissue septa, supplied centrally by a lobular bronchiole and arteriole, and drained peripherally by veins and lymphatics in the interlobular septa. Each SPL measures 1 to 2.5 cm in size and contains 3 to 12 acini. While not normally visible by CT, the SPL is a key anatomic structure in the lung.[8,9]

Imaging Technique and Normal Findings at CT

Thin-section high-resolution computed tomography (HRCT) with high spatial frequency reconstruction has improved the characterization of the lung parenchyma and is used to evaluate interstitial lung disease and differentiate among the causes of mosaic attenuation. Expiratory and prone images are often part of the full HRCT protocol. Scans obtained in the prone position allow for differentiation between dependent atelectasis and early interstitial lung disease, and expiratory images assess for air trapping.

Various reconstructions of the CT imaging data can be manipulated to assist the radiologist in determining the cause of mosaic attenuation. For example, maximum-intensity projection (MIP) images project voxels with the highest attenuation values that aid in the characterization of small nodules and opacities, such as ill-defined centrilobular nodules that may be present in diseases such as hypersensitivity pneumonitis. Minimum-intensity projection (MinIP) images (Fig. 1) project voxels with the lowest attenuation values that improve visualization of subtle areas of mosaic attenuation or expiratory air trapping that may be difficult to identify with standard CT techniques. Additionally, coronal and sagittal reformatted images help visualize apicobasal or anterior-posterior gradients of parenchymal disease.

Mild mosaic attenuation can occur in normal patients and is often accentuated when imaged mid-inspiration or during expiration.[10] There is also mildly increased attenuation of the lung parenchyma in the most dependent portions of the lobes, relative to the non-dependent portions of the lung.[11] Furthermore, lung in the upper lobes adjacent to the major fissure is often of slightly higher attenuation than the superior segments of the adjacent lower lobes.[12]

Expiratory images are used to evaluate for small airways disease that manifests with air trapping.[3] There are several pitfalls regarding expiratory CT acquisition. Poor coaching of the patient by the technologist and lack of patient effort may lead to inadequate images that do not appropriately depict end-expiration. To confirm an adequate expiration phase, look at the posterior wall of the trachea and main bronchi that should collapse inward because of their non-cartilaginous posterior walls. Some degree of air trapping may be physiologic and occurs irrespective of the patient's current smoking status. Physiologic air trapping generally affects one or a few secondary pulmonary lobules, usually occurs in the lung bases and superior segments of the lower lobes, and increases with aging (Fig. 2).[10,13] Air trapping should be considered pathologic when affecting an entire pulmonary segment or multiple segments, however, even this degree of air trapping is occasionally seen in a small percentage of normal individuals.[10,14]

Similar to inspiration, there is often variation in density at end-expiration with the dependent lung having a higher attenuation than the nondependent lung (see Fig. 2).[12,15]

The use of intravenous contrast and CT angiographic techniques is helpful in evaluating vascular causes of mosaic attenuation. Standard CT angiography allows for good visualization of the pulmonary vessels to the subsegmental level. Normally, the pulmonary trunk is smaller than the adjacent ascending aorta and measures less than 30 mm, as measured at the level of the bifurcation in the axial plane.[16] Normal pulmonary vessels taper gradually toward the periphery as the pulmonary vasculature divides into the segmental and subsegmental arteries, with vessel size similar to that of the adjacent bronchus, assuming no bronchiectasis. Intravascular contrast is also critical for the identification of filling defects or vascular occlusion that may be present in chronic thromboembolic pulmonary hypertension (CTEPH).[17]

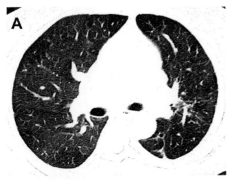
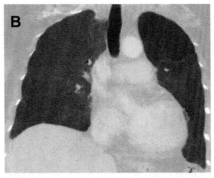

Fig. 1. A 58-year-old woman with pulmonary arterial hypertension (PAH) and sickle cell disease. (A) Axial CT shows mosaic attenuation of the lung parenchyma. Note smaller vessel size in areas of low attenuation lung and sharp demarcation between the two portions of lung. (B) MinIP coronal CT shows mosaic attenuation to better advantage. The patient underwent right heart catheterization that demonstrated severe pre-capillary pulmonary hypertension and was found to have high-output heart failure related to sickle cell disease.

Pulmonary Function Testing

Pulmonary function testing is one of the main diagnostic tools for pulmonologists and evaluates function as a sum collection of the airways. Unfortunately, pulmonary function testing has a wide range of normal (ie, 80%–120% of predicted values is considered normal range).[18] In other words, a patient could have 20% to 30% of airways destroyed and be several dyspneic, whereas pulmonary function values would remain in normal range. Another confounding factor is that some diseases may have opposing physiologic processes. For example, small airways disease and alveolar fibrosis tend to normalize each other in terms of lung size. In this case, FEV1 could be 100% of the predicted value, but the patient may be severely dyspneic. Pathologists may also have difficulty diagnosing small airways disease as histopathological evaluation may be insensitive and depends on the area of tissue biopsied. Some disease processes may destroy the airway and thus render the disease invisible to the microscope. Conversely, CT imaging can visualize and localize individual abnormal airways that may manifest indirectly as mosaic attenuation.

Toxic injury in airways disease often affects other compartments within the lungs, including alveolar walls, blood vessels, and the pleura. This contributes to pulmonary function tests (PFTs) more confounding to the clinical picture than clinicians would ideally want. One such confusing situation is the contingent of soldiers returning from Iraq and Afghanistan with severe dyspnea. These soldiers experience chronic difficulty breathing with relatively normal PFTs, likely caused by constrictive bronchiolitis, termed "Iraq lung," after exposures to various toxic inhalants such as sulfur, dust storms and burn pits (Fig. 3).[19–21] The role of the radiologist is paramount in such circumstances as mosaic attenuation on CT may be the only diagnostic finding in otherwise unexplained dyspnea.

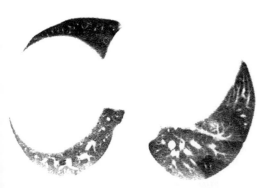

Fig. 2. A 16-year-old woman presenting with abdominal pain. Expiratory axial CT image through the lung bases shows incidental lobular air trapping within the left lower lobe. The remainder of the lower lobes demonstrate an expected increase in density during expiration. Note the more dependent areas of the lower lobes are of increased density relative to the non-dependent portions. Findings are without clinical significance in this patient and considered nonpathologic.

CLINICAL APPLICATIONS/DIAGNOSTIC CRITERIA
Helpful Clues in Mosaic Attenuation Pattern: What is Normal and What is Abnormal?

When you encounter a mosaic attenuation pattern, you must first determine which portion of the lung is abnormal—the areas of increased attenuation,

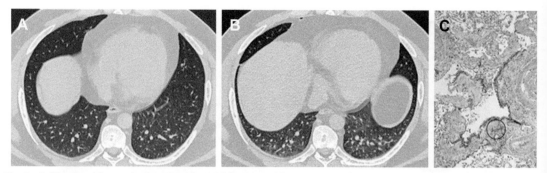

Fig. 3. A 40-year-old man deployed to the Middle East with exposure to burn pits and progressive dyspnea. Inspiratory axial chest CT image through the lung bases is normal (*A*). Expiratory phase imaging through the same region (*B*) reveals scattered air trapping. Surgical lung biopsy (*C*) demonstrates a markedly distorted respiratory bronchiole with subepithelial fibrosis and associated dust particles (black circle). (*Courtesy of* T Franks, MD, Silver Spring, MD.)

decreased attenuation, or both (**Fig. 4**). There are three broad categories under the mosaic attenuation pattern that can be seen: small airways disease, vascular disease, and parenchymal disease.

In parenchymal disease, the areas of high attenuation lung are abnormal and visible on CT as regions of ground-glass opacity. In contrast, in the setting of small airways disease or vascular

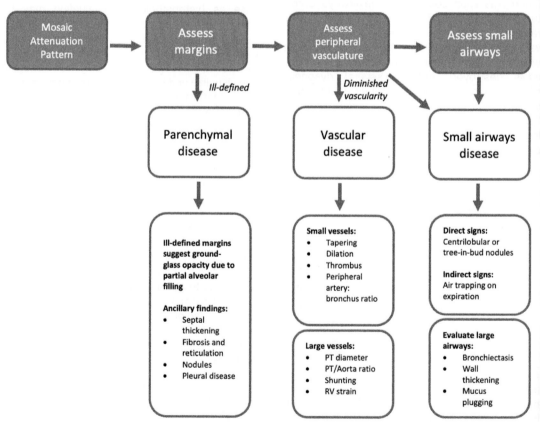

Fig. 4. Simplified flowchart to evaluate mosaic attenuation pattern encountered on HRCT. There is considerable overlap of imaging findings in many encountered disease processes. Mixed diseases exist as well, further complicating the diagnosis. Decreased peripheral vascularity is seen in both small airways and vascular disease states. Additionally, both dilated as well as corkscrew-like peripheral vessels have been described in pulmonary hypertension, a vascular disease. This flowchart is meant to provide general guidelines for approaching this pattern rather than a steadfast rule. PT, pulmonary trunk; RV, right ventricle.

disease, the darker lung is abnormal. In pulmonary vascular disease, areas of regional hypoperfusion and oligemia manifest as low attenuation regions of the lung. Air-trapping because of obstructed small airways also results in abnormal low attenuation regions. Secondary vasoconstriction in regions of air-trapping results in reduced perfusion and further blurs the distinction between these two causes of mosaic attenuation.[22]

One of the most helpful imaging findings to differentiate among the causes of mosaic attenuation is the presence of sharp demarcation between areas of high and low attenuations of the lung. If the cause is because of small airways or vascular disease, the margins between the abnormal lucent lung and normal lung tend to be sharply defined. Although the mosaicism is related to ground-glass opacity, the margins are often fuzzy or ill-defined, as the underlying histopathology is caused by the partial filling of the alveoli (**Fig. 5**).

Another helpful clue is the size of the peripheral vessels in the hypoattenuated portions of the lung. If the vessels in the darker lung regions are smaller relative to other peripheral pulmonary vessels, the mosaic pattern is likely from small airways or vascular disease. If the vessels are of a normal size throughout or if the vessels in the dark portions of the lung are equal to other areas, the cause is likely because of ground-glass opacity with parenchymal infiltration (see **Fig. 5**).[23]

Expiration phase images are useful in differentiating small airways disease from other causes of mosaic attenuation.[24] There should be a diffuse increase in lung attenuation during expiration in patients with normal lungs and non-small-airways-related causes of mosaic attenuation. In other words, in cases of vascular or interstitial causes of mosaic attenuation, there should be increased attenuation throughout the lungs, even in locations whereby there is abnormally low or high attenuation of the lung, respectively. Conversely, in a patient with small-airways disease, expiration phase CT images accentuate the differences between the abnormal lucent lung and normal lung (ie, the whiter lung becomes whiter and the darker lung stays dark), indicating the presence of air-trapping.[25] (**Fig. 6**) In small airways disease, air cannot readily escape the obstructed small airways but can still enter the lung via various collateral channels such as the pores of Kohn, canals of Lambert, and channels of Martin.[26]

Various ancillary imaging findings also suggest the underlying pathology of mosaic attenuation. The presence of dilated central pulmonary arteries, that can be seen with pulmonary hypertension, suggests a vascular cause. Other findings such as an increased segmental pulmonary artery to bronchial ratio, eccentric filling defects in the pulmonary arteries, and enlarged bronchial arteries would further support a vascular cause. Right heart enlargement or right ventricular (RV) wall thickening has also been observed with occlusive vascular disease (**Fig. 7**). Direct evidence of small airways involvement, such as tree-in-bud opacities, centrilobular nodules, or abnormally dilated or thickened small airways, mostly indicates underlying small airways disease. Close inspection of the large airways and bronchi is also helpful; if there is an abnormality of the large airways, there is often disease involving the small airways.

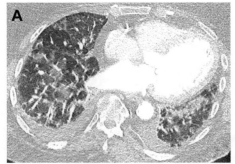 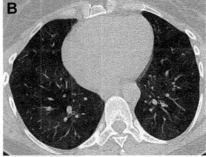

Fig. 5. A 79-year-old woman with cardiogenic pulmonary edema and severe aortic stenosis. (*A*) Axial CT image shows patchy ground-glass opacity, interlobular septal thickening and small pleural effusions representing pulmonary edema. Note ill-defined borders around the ground-glass opacity and the similar sized peripheral pulmonary arteries suggesting a parenchymal cause of the mosaic attenuation pattern. (*B*) 45-year-old woman with diffuse idiopathic pulmonary neuroendocrine cell hyperplasia (DIPNECH). Axial CT image shows sharply demarcated areas of hyperlucent lung with decreased size of the vessels compatible with either a vascular or small airways cause of mosaic attenuation. The presence of multiple pulmonary nodules makes DIPNECH with associated constrictive bronchiolitis the most likely diagnosis that was confirmed with biopsy.

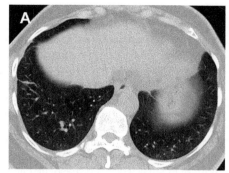
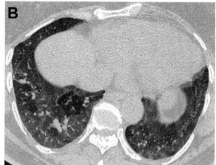

Fig. 6. A 64-year-old woman with follicular bronchiolitis and rheumatoid arthritis. (*A*) Axial CT image during inspiration demonstrates faint areas of mosaic attenuation at the lung bases. (*B*) Expiratory CT shows bilateral well-demarcated areas of air trapping. The patient demonstrated restriction on pulmonary function testing with biopsy showing follicular bronchiolitis. While this is not the typical appearance of follicular bronchiolitis, that usually manifests with centrilobular nodules and tree-in-bud opacities, these images demonstrate the considerable overlap of these imaging findings and importance of correlation with clinical and histopathologic findings.

DISEASE ENTITIES MANIFESTING AS MOSAIC ATTENUATION

Several diseases that may manifest as mosaic attenuation are discussed in more detail elsewhere in this issue. These include acute lung injury and organizing pneumonia (see Kligerman and colleagues), hypersensitivity pneumonitis (see Chung and colleagues) (**Figs. 8** and **9**), and connective tissue diseases (see Kallianos and colleagues).

GROUND-GLASS OPACITY

In contrast to consolidation, ground-glass opacity is defined as "an area of hazy increased opacity within the lung with preservation of bronchial and vascular structures." Ground-glass opacity is caused by partial filling of the airspaces, interstitial thickening, partial collapse of the alveoli,

increased capillary blood volume, or a combination of factors. The common denominator is the partial displacement of air.[27]

Ground-glass opacity is caused by acute and chronic disease processes (**Box 1**). Acute causes include pulmonary edema (see **Fig. 5**), pulmonary hemorrhage, certain infections, diffuse alveolar damage, and eosinophilic pneumonia. Subacute to chronic causes include organizing pneumonia (OP), hypersensitivity pneumonitis, certain infections, diffuse alveolar damage (DAD), and fibrotic lung diseases such as nonspecific interstitial pneumonia.[27,28]

Differentiating interstitial and alveolar causes of ground-glass opacity is difficult because of the overlap of imaging appearances and many diseases having both interstitial and alveolar components. For example, infection, DAD, and OP can result in interstitial and alveolar abnormalities.

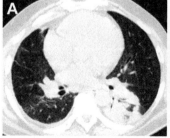
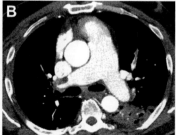
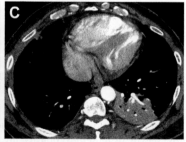

Fig. 7. A 59-year-old man with CTEPH and vascular abnormalities. (*A*) Axial CT image on lung windows (*A*) shows mosaic attenuation of the lung parenchymal bilaterally. Consolidation in the left lower lobe represented pneumonia. (*B*) The pulmonary trunk is enlarged measuring 47 mm. Thrombus is present in the pulmonary arteries bilaterally, some eccentric in location within the vessel. (*C*) Note dilated right ventricle with leftward bowing of the interventricular septum suggesting right heart dysfunction. The constellation of findings suggests a vascular cause of mosaic attenuation.

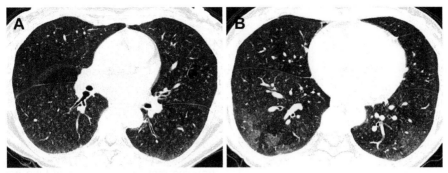

Fig. 8. A 53-year-old woman presenting with dyspnea and cough related to nonfibrotic hypersensitivity pneumonitis. Axial CT images (*A* and *B*) demonstrate diffuse ill-defined centrilobular ground-glass nodules. Note lower lung zone mosaic attenuation with patchwork of three different densities, representing the three-density or headcheese sign. The three-density sign indicates a mixed infiltrative and obstructive process, with the lucent areas representing air trapping and the denser areas representing infiltration by inflammatory cells. The three-density sign can be seen in multiple conditions but was classically described in the setting of hypersensitivity pneumonitis.

The clinical history and laboratory information can aid in the final diagnosis of the underlying cause of acute ground-glass opacity. For example, cultures from the bronchoalveolar lavage (BAL) or elevated lung eosinophils may suggest a specific diagnosis such as pneumonia or eosinophilic pneumonia, respectively. Procalcitonin is a serum biomarker that is elevated with bacterial pneumonia but not elevated from non-bacterial causes of infection or inflammation. Serum procalcitonin levels increase several hours following a bacterial infection, typically peaking at 24 to 48 h, with the peak correlated with the severity of infection.[29] Ground-glass opacities with or without pulmonary cysts in a patient with human immunodeficiency virus (HIV) infection and reduced CD4 count suggest the presence of *Pneumocystis jirovecii* pneumonia (**Fig. 10**).[30] Coronavirus disease 2019 (COVID-19) often manifests as peripheral ground-glass opacities with

patients having a positive reverse transcriptase polymerase chain reaction (RT-PCR) assay.[31] Elevated brain natriuretic peptide (BNP) levels are often seen with cardiogenic pulmonary edema and may be used to differentiate between this disease and DAD/acute respiratory distress syndrome (ARDS).[32]

In the subacute to chronic setting, bronchoscopy along with BAL, biopsy or both remain powerful tools in evaluating ground-glass opacity.

SMALL AIRWAYS DISEASE

Hogg and colleagues coined the term "small airways disease" over 40 years ago regarding inflammation in the peripheral airways of patients, primarily smokers with chronic obstructive pulmonary disease, who had moderate to severe airflow limitation.[5] Usage of this term has varied over the decades since, but generally is concerning a

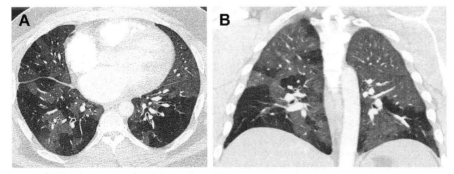

Fig. 9. A 35-year-old man with nonfibrotic hypersensitivity pneumonitis. Axial and coronal CT images (*A* and *B*) show sharply marginated areas of hyperlucency at the bases representing mosaic attenuation likely secondary to small airways disease. Note diffuse ground-glass opacity with more dense nodules, best appreciated in the upper zones on the coronal reconstruction.

Box 1
Causes of mosaic attenuation related to ground-glass opacity

Acute causes

Acute eosinophilic pneumonia

Diffuse alveolar damage

Edema

Infection (eg, viruses, mycoplasma, pneumocystis)

Hemorrhage

Subacute/chronic causes

Diffuse alveolar damage

Hypersensitivity pneumonitis

Infections

Nonspecific interstitial pneumonia

Organizing pneumonia

disease that primarily involves the bronchiole, or as components of interstitial or alveolar lung disease.

The peripheral airways only contribute 10% to 20% of total airway resistance because the total cross-sectional area of the small airways is much greater than the total cross-sectional area of the central airways.[5,33] However, when pathology is present, these small airways disproportionately contribute to increased airway resistance. As a result, measurement of airway resistance may be normal in the setting of significant obstruction of the peripheral small airways, and therefore may not be evident on PFTs until late in their course.[34]

Normally, the small airways are invisible on CT because of their diminutive size. However, both direct and indirect signs suggest the presence of small airways disease. Direct signs include visualization of the diseased airways themselves, whether it is the obliteration of the airway, filling in of the airway, or thickening of the wall.

Indirect signs refer to abnormalities of the lung parenchyma distal to the diseased small airways and primarily manifest as mosaic attenuation on inspiration and air trapping on expiratory CT. Air-trapping manifests as areas of lung parenchyma with a less than normal increase in attenuation and with a lack of volume reduction with sharply defined contours that follow the outlines of underlying SPLs (see **Fig. 6**). When identified, the presence of air-trapping confirms a small-airways cause of the mosaic attenuation.

There have been various classification systems proposed to group small airways disease. One system separates small airways disease into histologic groupings of proliferative (cellular) or fibrotic (constrictive) bronchiolitis. It is important to differentiate constrictive bronchiolitis, a fibrotic extrinsic bronchiolar lesion, from proliferative bronchiolitis, predominantly an inflammatory intrinsic bronchiolar lesion, because their outcome and treatment options are markedly different. The constrictive fibrotic lesion develops external to the airway, causing a concentric constriction. The clinically significant disease is usually associated with complete obliteration of the airway lumen. In contrast, the proliferative lesion develops internally from the wall, filling the lumen with inflammatory cells.

Cellular Bronchiolitis

Cellular bronchiolitis is characterized by inflammatory cells as the predominant histopathologic feature. Multiple types of cellular bronchiolitis are recognized: aspiration bronchiolitis, infectious bronchiolitis, follicular bronchiolitis, respiratory bronchiolitis, hypersensitivity pneumonitis, and diffuse panbronchiolitis. Common to these types of bronchiolitis is the presence of centrilobular micronodules and tree-in-bud opacities. The presence of ill-defined ground-glass centrilobular nodules can narrow the differential and is most often seen with respiratory bronchiolitis and hypersensitivity pneumonitis.

Infectious and Aspiration-Related Bronchiolitis

Infectious bronchiolitis is the most common type of bronchiolitis encountered in imaging. In its acute form, it is typically caused by viruses and less commonly by bacteria. Chronic infectious

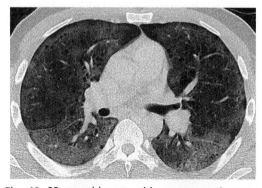

Fig. 10. 32-year-old man with pneumocystis pneumonia and human immunodeficiency virus (HIV) infection. Axial CT image shows patchy areas of ground-glass opacity with multiple cysts. In a patient with HIV, no pleural effusion and low CD4 count, the constellation of findings is typical of pneumocystis pneumonia that was confirmed by BAL.

bronchiolitis is often related to nontuberculous mycobacterial or *Pseudomonas aeruginosa* infections, especially when seen in conjunction with middle lobe and lingular-predominant bronchiectasis. Imaging findings of infectious bronchiolitis include tree-in-bud opacities, endobronchial mucous plugging and bronchial wall thickening. Mosaic attenuation and bronchiectasis are more common with chronic infectious bronchiolitis but may also be seen acutely.[25]

Aspiration bronchiolitis is the second most common type of bronchiolitis. Diagnosis can be challenging because findings are non-specific and similar to infectious bronchiolitis. Identification of this disease process is important because, if left untreated, it may result in permanent lung injury with fibrosis and bronchiectasis. Conditions associated with increased risk for aspiration include neurologic conditions, head and neck cancer, prior irradiation, gastric surgery, and esophageal abnormalities such as dysmotility or a hiatal hernia.[35]

Respiratory Bronchiolitis

Respiratory bronchiolitis (RB) is a histologic finding in most cigarette smokers. It is characterized by inflammation and accumulation of pigmented macrophages within respiratory bronchioles and alveoli. RB manifests on CT as ill-defined, centrilobular ground-glass nodules with upper zone predominance with or without mosaic attenuation or more confluent ground-glass opacities (**Fig. 11**). MIP reformatted imaging techniques may make the micronodules more pronounced and conspicuous. RB is part of a spectrum of smoking-related lung disease that includes respiratory bronchiolitis-interstitial lung disease (RB-ILD) and desquamative interstitial pneumonia (DIP).[36]

Follicular Bronchiolitis

Follicular bronchiolitis (FB), also known as pulmonary lymphoid hyperplasia, hyperplasia of the bronchus-associated lymphoid tissue, or hyperplasia of the mucosa-associated lymphoid tissue, is a type of cellular bronchiolitis characterized by peribronchial lymphoid follicles. FB has associations with congenital or acquired immunodeficiency syndromes, collagen vascular diseases such as rheumatoid arthritis, systemic hypersensitivity reactions, infection, lymphoproliferative disease, and diffuse panbronchiolitis.

Imaging findings include diffuse, small, ill-defined centrilobular nodules. Perilymphatic nodules, patchy ground-glass opacity, bronchial wall thickening, and mosaic attenuation may also be seen (see **Fig. 6**).[37]

Diffuse Panbronchiolitis

Diffuse panbronchiolitis (DPB) is a progressive form of cellular bronchiolitis that occurs nearly exclusively in Japanese adults and is associated with chronic inflammation of the paranasal sinuses and colonization of the respiratory tract by *P aeruginosa*. Imaging features have significant overlap with other inflammatory airway diseases, such as cystic fibrosis (CF), inflammatory bowel disease (IBD), constrictive bronchiolitis, and follicular bronchiolitis. Histopathologically, there is infiltration of the interstitium and peribronchiolar tissue by foamy macrophages, lymphocytes, and plasma cells.

CT demonstrates small, usually diffuse, centrilobular and tree-in-bud opacities, bronchiolectasis and bronchiectasis, as well as mosaic attenuation. Cystic spaces, air-trapping, and mosaicism predominate in the later stages.[38]

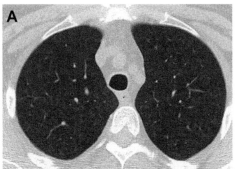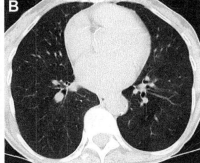

Fig. 11. A 67-year-old woman with extensive history of smoking. Axial CT images (*A* and *B*) demonstrate mosaic attenuation, best visualized in the left lower lobe. Faint upper zone predominant ground-glass nodules are compatible with respiratory bronchiolitis.

Constrictive Bronchiolitis

Constrictive bronchiolitis, synonyms bronchiolitis obliterans and obliterative bronchiolitis, was first used to describe lesions characterized by submucosal and peribronchiolar fibrosis. Inflammatory cell infiltrates may also be present but are variable in composition. Patients with constrictive bronchiolitis present with chronic dyspnea and cough, typically following a progressive course. In contrast to inflammatory causes of small airways disease that are often reversible, the fibrotic change in constrictive bronchiolitis leads to irreversible obstruction of the small airways.[39]

There are numerous conditions associated with constrictive bronchiolitis (Box 2). Common causes include infection, inhalational lung injury, collagen vascular disorders, and chronic lung allograft dysfunction following lung transplantation. Classic imaging findings include mosaic attenuation and expiratory air-trapping. Bronchial abnormalities are common, often later in the disease course, and include bronchiectasis and bronchial wall thickening.

When disease is severe and widespread, it is often difficult to appreciate any abnormality because the lung is nearly diffusely abnormal. In such cases, the imaging findings often underestimate the extent and severity of the patient's symptoms. When mosaic attenuation is particularly severe and well-demarcated, the cause is often constrictive bronchiolitis.

SPECIFIC CAUSES OF CONSTRICTIVE BRONCHIOLITIS
Lung Transplantation

Constrictive bronchiolitis is a common complication of lung and heart-lung transplantation

---

Box 2
Causes of constrictive (obliterative) bronchiolitis and associated disorders

Graft versus host disease following bone marrow/stem cell transplantation

Chronic rejection following lung transplantation

Connective tissue disorders

Drug reaction

Idiopathic

Inflammatory bowel disease

Inhalation injury/Toxic exposure

Paraneoplastic pemphigus

Post-infection

Neuroendocrine cell hyperplasia

Stevens-Johnson syndrome

---

affecting up to 60% of patients who survive 5 years after transplantation and is considered a form of chronic lung allograft dysfunction (CLAD) or chronic rejection. A clinical classification system based on FEV1, referred to as bronchiolitis obliterans syndrome (BOS), was created because the disease was so common and transbronchial biopsies of these lesions were often limited value. Pathogenesis of this lesion relates to injury and inflammation of the bronchiolar airway epithelial cells, resulting in excessive fibroproliferation. BOS classically manifests 6 to 18 months after transplantation with an irreversible decline of FEV1. On inspiration, the chest CT findings are often normal. Expiratory CT images classically depict air-trapping. If the disease is severe, BOS will manifest with mosaic attenuation on inspiration, accentuated on expiration (air-trapping).[40–42] A helpful imaging clue indicating lung transplantation is the presence of a clamshell sternotomy (Fig. 12).

Connective Tissue Disease

Constrictive bronchiolitis is an uncommon complication of several autoimmune diseases, including rheumatoid arthritis (Fig. 13), systemic lupus erythematosus, and systemic sclerosis. Several imaging clues may suggest an underlying autoimmune disease because of the patient's constrictive bronchiolitis, such as humeral head erosions (rheumatoid arthritis), esophageal dysmotility or dilation (scleroderma), or pleural/pericardial effusions (lupus).

Inhalation Lung Injury/Toxic Exposure

Diagnosis of constrictive bronchiolitis related to occupational and other toxic exposures is difficult clinically as these often manifest with an indolent course rather than acutely. A high index of suspicion should be maintained for this disease in young dyspneic patients with complaints out of proportion to PFT values. Both physiologic and radiologic studies are insensitive to biopsy-proven cases of constrictive bronchiolitis. For these reasons, the burden of disease of exposure-related CB is likely larger than what is actually diagnosed.[43]

A non-exhaustive list of exposure-related causes of constrictive bronchiolitis includes butter flavoring-related (diacetyl), sulfur dioxide, mustard gas, iron oxide, nitrogen oxide, ammonia, and chlorine.[44,45] An association between dust exposure after the collapse of the World Trade Center on September 11, 2001, and interstitial lung disease has been described in the literature.[46] Many patients with constrictive bronchiolitis and

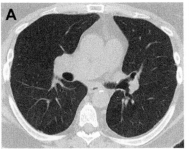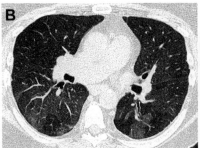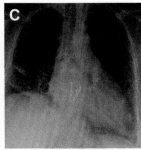

Fig. 12. A 60-year-old woman with bronchiolitis obliterans syndrome (BOS) following lung transplantation. (*A*) Axial CT image during inspiration shows subtle mosaic attenuation. (*B*) Expiratory CT shows accentuation of the pattern that confirms air trapping. Bronchiolitis obliterans (syn constrictive bronchiolitis) as a form of chronic rejection was confirmed by transbronchial biopsy. (*C*) Frontal chest radiograph shows transverse sternal wires in keeping with clamshell sternotomy, the standard incision for bilateral lung transplantation. Clamshell sternal wires may also have a "butterfly" morphology.

associated adverse health effects have been described in workers and volunteers exposed to the dense cloud of dust containing high levels of airborne pollutants after the collapse.

Diffuse Idiopathic Pulmonary Neuroendocrine Cell Hyperplasia

Diffuse idiopathic pulmonary neuroendocrine cell hyperplasia (DIPNECH) is part of a spectrum of conditions of pulmonary neuroendocrine cell hyperplasia predominantly affecting middle-aged women. While it remains rare, it is identified with increasing frequency and is likely underdiagnosed. Histologically, there is pathologic proliferation of the normal neuroendocrine cells within the airway mucosa, leading to airflow obstruction caused by constrictive bronchiolitis. DIPNECH manifests with mosaic attenuation on inspiratory CT and air trapping on expiratory CT. The main clue to the diagnosis is the presence of numerous small, non-calcified randomly distributed pulmonary nodules representing carcinoid tumorlets (<5 mm in size) and carcinoid tumors ($\geq$ 5 mm) (**Figs. 14**

and **15**). These nodules are generally stable on serial CT scans but when compared with remote scans (ie, >2 years), many nodules often show slow growth.[47]

Postinfectious Constrictive Bronchiolitis

Constrictive bronchiolitis following infection continues to occur, resulting in irreversible airflow obstruction. Some infections that may result in fibrotic bronchiolar lesions include *Mycoplasma pneumoniae* and viruses such as adenovirus, influenza, and parainfluenza. Mosaic attenuation, hyperattenuating lung regions, and air-trapping are the primary CT findings. Bronchiectasis, patchy ground-glass opacity, and centrilobular nodules are less common. Swyer–James–MacLeod syndrome follows a childhood respiratory viral infection and is characterized by a unilateral, asymmetrically small and hyperlucent lung with diminished vascularity.[48] Obstructive lung disease and air trapping are recognized findings in post-acute sequelae of COVID-19 pneumonia.[49]

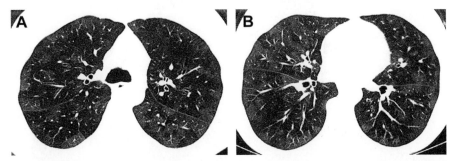

Fig. 13. A 57-year-old woman with constrictive bronchiolitis and rheumatoid arthritis. (*A* and *B*) Axial CT images show sharply demarcated areas of mosaic attenuation and bronchiectasis representing biopsy confirmed constrictive bronchiolitis. Often the most obvious examples of mosaic attenuation are secondary to constrictive bronchiolitis. Note small vessel size in areas of hyperlucent lung indicating a small airways or vascular cause of mosaic attenuation.

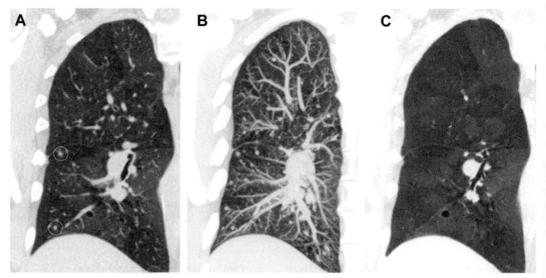

Fig. 14. A 58-year-old woman with wheezing and chronic dyspnea diagnosed with diffuse idiopathic pulmonary neuroendocrine cell hyperplasia (DIPNECH). Coronal CT image (*A*) acquired during full inspiration reveals diffuse mosaic attenuation and 2 soft tissue nodules (*yellow circles*). Coronal maximum intensity projection image (*B*) demonstrates numerous nodules that involve both upper and lower lung zones. Coronal minimum intensity projection image from the same inspiratory acquisition (*C*) more clearly demonstrates the mosaic attenuation.

PULMONARY VASCULAR DISEASE

Pulmonary vascular disease may result in mosaic attenuation because of regional differences in lung perfusion. The most common cause is CTEPH, whereas other etiologies of pulmonary arterial hypertension (PAH) are less common. Rare causes include pulmonary veno-occlusive

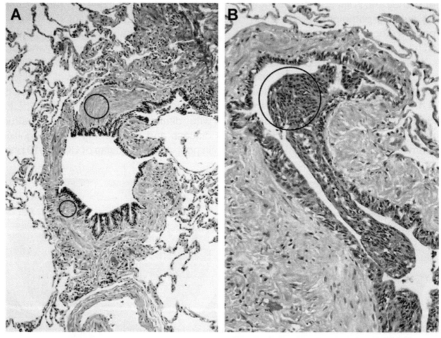

Fig. 15. Surgical lung biopsy acquired from the same patient in **Fig. 14** demonstrates a respiratory bronchiole with subepithial fibrosis (*black circles in A*) and second bronchiole (*B*) with numerous neuroendocrine cells (*black circle*) that partially obstruct the airway lumen. Both processes contribute to the mosaic pattern seen in **Fig. 14C**. (*Courtesy of* T Franks, MD, Silver Spring, MD.)

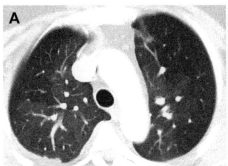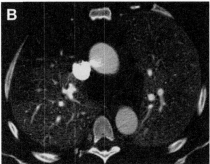

Fig. 16. A 51-year-old woman with chronic thromboembolic pulmonary hypertension (CTEPH). (*A*) Axial CT image of the lung apices demonstrate mosaic attenuation. In this patient with recurrent pulmonary embolism, this is likely vascular in etiology and related to regional differences in perfusion. There is variation in vessel size because the segmental and subsegmental vessels in the region of oligemic lung are abnormally narrowed and attenuated relative to the adjacent bronchi. (*B*) Iodine density perfusion map obtained with spectral CT shows decreased perfusion to portions of the anterior segment of the right upper lobe.

disease (PVOD) and pulmonary capillary hemangiomatosis (PCH), that may be suggested when seen in association with interlobular septal thickening or poorly defined centrilobular nodules. Both PVOD and PCH are post-capillary causes of pulmonary hypertension. Findings in PVOD include a small left atrium from reduced return, pleural effusion, enlarged mediastinal nodes and normal wedge pressure on right heart catheterization. Common to these disease processes is the reduction in vessel caliber within areas of decreased lung attenuation.[50]

Chronic Thromboembolic Pulmonary Hypertension

In patients with pulmonary hypertension, CTEPH is the most common cause of significant mosaic attenuation and is because of regional differences in lung perfusion.[50] Ancillary features that suggest this diagnosis include pulmonary arterial eccentric filling defects, linear webs and complete or partial vascular occlusion (**Fig. 16**). Less common findings include post-stenotic dilation or vascular beading. Subpleural peripheral opacities and reticulation often indicate remote pulmonary infarcts.[51] The presence of dilated bronchial arteries may be helpful in suggesting this diagnosis over other causes of pulmonary hypertension.[52] For reasons not entirely clear, bronchial artery dilation is uncommon in patients with primary pulmonary hypertension.[53]

Pulmonary Arterial Hypertension

Idiopathic PAH (a group 1 PH cause under ERS classification) is characterized by angioproliferative lesions of the endothelial cells and hypertrophy of the pre-capillary arteriole vessel walls.[54] In addition to enlargement of the central pulmonary arteries, most cases of PAH have pruning of the distal peripheral pulmonary arteries, generally without mediastinal or parenchymal abnormalities. Mosaic attenuation can also be seen but is less common than in CTEPH (see **Fig. 1**).[55–58]

The presence of centrilobular ground-glass nodules in pulmonary hypertension has been well-described. They are considered a manifestation of severe PH and may represent cholesterol granulomas or plexogenic arteriopathy.[55,59] When present, they tend to occur in patients undergoing long-term treatment with vasodilator therapy.[60]

A pulmonary trunk diameter measurement of greater than 29 mm had a sensitivity of 87% for the prediction of pulmonary hypertension, although the presence of a normal-sized pulmonary trunk did not exclude the diagnosis of pulmonary hypertension.[61] There is a very high probability of pulmonary arterial hypertension if the ratio of the diameters of the pulmonary trunk and the ascending aorta is >1.[62] Most cases of pulmonary arterial hypertension demonstrate pruning of the peripheral vasculature. However, occasionally, dilated peripheral pulmonary arteries may also be seen. A segmental artery-to-bronchus diameter ratio greater than 1:1 in three or more lobes is more specific for pulmonary hypertension.[60,61,63]

SUMMARY

Mosaic attenuation is not a disease process, rather a clue into the underlying pathology. When mosaicism is present, imaging plays a vital role in the work-up of dyspnea and can provide vital insight into the disease process whereby other diagnostic tools such as the PFT may be insufficient.

Although mosaicism is a commonly encountered imaging pattern, once the radiologist identifies its presence, close attention should be paid to other imaging findings to allow for definitive diagnosis. Correlation with symptoms, exposures, laboratory results and other comorbidities is helpful. Tissue sampling is uncommonly needed for definitive diagnosis.

CLINICS CARE POINTS

- Causes of mosaic attenuation pattern can be broadly separated into categories of small-airways disease, pulmonary vascular disease and parenchymal disease.

- Evaluation of the airways, vasculature, parenchyma and heart may provide vital clues to the underlying cause of mosaic attenuation.

- Expiratory phase imaging is helpful to identify air trapping and small airways disease related causes of mosaic attenuation.

- Mosaic attenuation and air trapping may be the only clues for airways disease in cases of severe dyspnea with normal pulmonary function tests.

- Constrictive bronchiolitis should be considered when mosaic attenuation is particularly pronounced and is the end result of a wide variety of disease processes.

DISCLOSURE

C.M Walker disclosures: Speakers' Bureau: Boehringer Ingelheim, Royalties: Elsevier. The remaining investigators have nothing to disclose.

REFERENCES

1. Hansell DM, Bankier AA, MacMahon H, et al. Fleischner Society: Glossary of Terms for Thoracic Imaging. Radiology 2008;246(3):697–722.
2. Kligerman SJ, Henry T, Lin CT, et al. Mosaic Attenuation: Etiology, Methods of Differentiation, and Pitfalls. RadioGraphics 2015;35(5):1360–80.
3. Stern EJ, Frank MS. Small-airway diseases of the lungs: findings at expiratory CT. Am J Roentgenol 1994;163(1):37–41.
4. Franks TJ, Galvin JR. Hypersensitivity Pneumonitis: Essential Radiologic and Pathologic Findings. Surg Pathol Clin 2010;3(1):187–98.
5. Hogg JC, Macklem PT, Thurlbeck WM. Site and Nature of Airway Obstruction in Chronic Obstructive Lung Disease. N Engl J Med 1968;278(25):1355–60.
6. Boers JE, Ambergen AW, Thunnissen FBJM. Number and Proliferation of Clara Cells in Normal Human Airway Epithelium. Am J Respir Crit Care Med 1999;159(5):1585–91.
7. Colby TV. Bronchiolitis: Pathologic Considerations. Am J Clin Pathol 1998;109(1):101–9.
8. Hogg JC, McDonough JE, Suzuki M. Small Airway Obstruction in COPD. Chest 2013;143(5):1436–43.
9. Müller NL, Miller RR. Diseases of the bronchioles: CT and histopathologic findings. Radiology 1995;196(1):3–12.
10. Park CS, Müller NL, Worthy SA, et al. Airway obstruction in asthmatic and healthy individuals: inspiratory and expiratory thin-section CT findings. Radiology 1997;203(2):361–7.
11. Verschakelen JA, Van fraeyenhoven L, Laureys G, et al. Differences in CT density between dependent and nondependent portions of the lung: influence of lung volume. Am J Roentgenol 1993;161(4):713–7.
12. Webb WR, Stern EJ, Kanth N, et al. Dynamic pulmonary CT: findings in healthy adult men. Radiology 1993;186(1):117–24.
13. Lee KW, Chung SY, Yang I, et al. Correlation of Aging and Smoking with Air Trapping at Thin-Section CT of the Lung in Asymptomatic Subjects. Radiology 2000;214(3):831–6.
14. Tanaka N, Matsumoto T, Miura G, et al. Air Trapping at CT: High Prevalence in Asymptomatic Subjects with Normal Pulmonary Function. Radiology 2003;227(3):776–85.
15. Arakawa H, Niimi H, Kurihara Y, et al. Expiratory High-Resolution CT. AJR Am J Roentgenol 2000;7.
16. Munden RF, Carter BW, Chiles C, et al. Managing Incidental Findings on Thoracic CT: Mediastinal and Cardiovascular Findings. A White Paper of the ACR Incidental Findings Committee. J Am Coll Radiol 2018;15(8):1087–96.
17. Frazier AA, Galvin JR, Franks TJ, et al. From the Archives of the AFIP: Pulmonary Vasculature: Hypertension and Infarction. RadioGraphics 2000;20(2):491–524.
18. Stocks J, Quanjer PhH. Reference values for residual volume, functional residual capacity and total lung capacity. Eur Respir J 1995;8(3):492–506.
19. Stack M. The Soldiers Came Home Sick. The Government Denied It Was Responsible. The New York times Magazine. Available at: https://www.nytimes.com/2022/01/11/magazine/military-burn-pits.html, 2022. Accessed Febuary 1, 2022.
20. King MS, Eisenberg R, Newman JH, et al. Constrictive Bronchiolitis in Soldiers Returning from Iraq and Afghanistan. N Engl J Med 2011;365(3):222–30.
21. Gutor SS, Richmond BW, Du RH, et al. Postdeployment Respiratory Syndrome in Soldiers With Chronic Exertional Dyspnea. Am J Surg Pathol 2021;45(12):1587–96.

22. Worthy SA, Müller NL, Hartman TE, et al. Mosaic attenuation pattern on thin-section CT scans of the lung: differentiation among infiltrative lung, airway, and vascular diseases as a cause. Radiology 1997;205(2):465–70.

23. Stern EJ, Swensen SJ, Hartman TE, et al. CT mosaic pattern of lung attenuation: distinguishing different causes. Am J Roentgenol 1995;165(4): 813–6.

24. Arakawa H, Webb WR, McCowin M, et al. Inhomogeneous lung attenuation at thin-section CT: diagnostic value of expiratory scans. Radiology 1998; 206(1):89–94.

25. Pipavath SJ, Lynch DA, Cool C, et al. Radiologic and Pathologic Features of Bronchiolitis. Am J Roentgenol 2005;15.

26. Terry PB, Traystman RJ. The Clinical Significance of Collateral Ventilation. Ann Am Thorac Soc 2016; 13(12):2251–7.

27. Engeler CE, Tashjian JH, Trenkner SW, et al. Ground-glass opacity of the lung parenchyma: a guide to analysis with high-resolution CT. Am J Roentgenol 1993;160(2):249–51.

28. Gluecker T, Capasso P, Schnyder P, et al. Clinical and Radiologic Features of Pulmonary Edema. RadioGraphics 1999;19(6):1507–31.

29. Assicot M, Bohuon C, Gendrel D, et al. High serum procalcitonin concentrations in patients with sepsis and infection. Lancet 1993;341(8844):515–8.

30. Kanne JP, Yandow DR, Meyer CA. Pneumocystis jiroveci Pneumonia: High-Resolution CT Findings in Patients With and Without HIV Infection. Am J Roentgenol 2012;198(6):W555–61.

31. Parekh M, Donuru A, Balasubramanya R, et al. Review of the Chest CT Differential Diagnosis of Ground-Glass Opacities in the COVID Era. Radiology 2020;297(3):E289–302.

32. Burnett JC, Kao PC, Hu DC, et al. Atrial Natriuretic Peptide Elevation in Congestive Heart Failure in the Human. Science 1986;231(4742):1145–7.

33. Macklem PT, Mead J. Resistance of central and peripheral airways measured by a retrograde catheter. J Appl Physiol 1967;22(3):395–401.

34. Cosio M, Ghezzo H, Hogg JC, et al. The Relations between Structural Changes in Small Airways and Pulmonary-Function Tests. N Engl J Med 1978; 298(23):1277–81.

35. Winningham PJ, Martínez-Jiménez S, Rosado-de-Christenson ML, et al. Bronchiolitis: A Practical Approach for the General Radiologist. RadioGraphics 2017;37(3):777–94.

36. Heyneman LE, Ward S, Lynch DA, et al. Respiratory bronchiolitis, respiratory bronchiolitis-associated interstitial lung disease, and desquamative interstitial pneumonia: different entities or part of the spectrum of the same disease process? Am J Roentgenol 1999;173(6):1617–22.

37. Howling SJ, Hansell DM, Wells AU, et al. Follicular Bronchiolitis: Thin-Section CT and Histologic Findings. Radiology 1999;212(3):637–42.

38. Poletti V. Diffuse panbronchiolitis. Eur Respir J 2006; 28(4):862–71.

39. Cordier JF. Challenges in pulmonary fibrosis 2 : Bronchiolocentric fibrosis. Thorax 2007;62(7): 638–49.

40. Leung AN, Fisher K, Valentine V, et al. Bronchiolitis Obliterans After Lung Transplantation. Chest 1998; 113(2):365–70.

41. Worthy SA, Park CS, Kim JS, et al. Bronchiolitis obliterans after lung transplantation: high-resolution CT findings in 15 patients. Am J Roentgenol 1997; 169(3):673–7.

42. de Jong PA, Dodd JD, Coxson HO, et al. Bronchiolitis obliterans following lung transplantation: early detection using computed tomographic scanning. Thorax 2006;61(9):799–804.

43. Falvo MJ, Sotolongo AM, Osinubi OY, et al. Diagnostic Workup of Constrictive Bronchiolitis in the Military Veteran. Mil Med 2020;185(11–12):472–5.

44. Kreiss K. Occupational causes of constrictive bronchiolitis. Curr Opin Allergy Clin Immunol 2013;13(2): 167–72.

45. Lockey JE, Hilbert TJ, Levin LP, et al. Airway obstruction related to diacetyl exposure at microwave popcorn production facilities. Eur Respir J 2009;34(1):63–71.

46. Mann JM, Sha KK, Kline G, et al. World Trade Center dyspnea: Bronchiolitis obliterans with functional improvement: A Case Report. Am J Ind Med 2005; 48(3):225–9.

47. Davies SJ, Gosney JR, Hansell DM, et al. Diffuse idiopathic pulmonary neuroendocrine cell hyperplasia: an under-recognised spectrum of disease. Thorax 2007;62(3):248–52.

48. Moore AD, Godwin JD, Dietrich PA, et al. Swyer-James syndrome: CT findings in eight patients. Am J Roentgenol 1992;158(6):1211–5.

49. Solomon JJ, Heyman B, Ko JP, et al. CT of Post-Acute Lung Complications of COVID-19. Radiology 2021;301(2):E383–95.

50. Hansell DM. Small-Vessel Diseases of the Lung: CT-Pathologic Correlates. Radiology 2002;225(3): 639–53.

51. King MA, Ysrael M, Bergin CJ. Chronic thromboembolic pulmonary hypertension: CT findings. Am J Roentgenol 1998;170(4):955–60.

52. Schwickert HC, Schweden F, Schild HH, et al. Pulmonary arteries and lung parenchyma in chronic pulmonary embolism: preoperative and postoperative CT findings. Radiology 1994;191(2):351–7.

53. Walker CM, Rosado-de-Christenson ML, Martínez-Jiménez S, et al. Bronchial Arteries: Anatomy, Function, Hypertrophy, and Anomalies. RadioGraphics 2015;35(1):32–49.

54. Simonneau G, Montani D, Celermajer DS, et al. Hae-modynamic definitions and updated clinical classification of pulmonary hypertension. Eur Respir J 2019;53(1):1801913.

55. Grosse C, Grosse A. CT Findings in Diseases Associated with Pulmonary Hypertension: A Current Review. RadioGraphics 2010;30(7):1753–77.

56. Barbosa EJM, Gupta NK, Torigian DA, et al. Current Role of Imaging in the Diagnosis and Management of Pulmonary Hypertension. Am J Roentgenol 2012;198(6):1320–31.

57. Devaraj A, Wells AU, Meister MG, et al. Detection of Pulmonary Hypertension with Multidetector CT and Echocardiography Alone and in Combination. Radiology 2010;254(2):609–16.

58. Sherrick AD, Swensen SJ, Hartman TE. Mosaic pattern of lung attenuation on CT scans: frequency among patients with pulmonary artery hypertension of different causes. Am J Roentgenol 1997;169(1):79–82.

59. Edwards WD, Edwards JE. Clinical primary pulmonary hypertension: three pathologic types. Circulation 1977;56(5):884–8.

60. Aluja Jaramillo F, Gutierrez FR, Díaz Telli FG, et al. Approach to Pulmonary Hypertension: From CT to Clinical Diagnosis. RadioGraphics 2018;38(2): 357–73.

61. Tan RT, Kuzo R, Goodman LR, et al. Utility of CT Scan Evaluation for Predicting Pulmonary Hypertension in Patients With Parenchymal Lung Disease. Chest 1998;113(5):1250–6.

62. Ng CS, Wells AU, Padley SPG. A CT Sign of Chronic Pulmonary Arterial Hypertension: The Ratio of Main Pulmonary Artery to Aortic Diameter. J Thorac Imaging 1999;14(4):270–8.

63. Peña E, Dennie C, Veinot J, et al. Pulmonary Hypertension: How the Radiologist Can Help. RadioGraphics 2012;32(1):9–32.

Imaging Patterns in Occupational Lung Disease—When Should I Consider?

Yasmeen K. Tandon, MD, Lara Walkoff, MD*

KEYWORDS

• Pneumoconiosis • Occupational lung disease • Inhalational lung disease

KEY POINTS

- Despite workplace safety regulations, occupational lung diseases (OLDs) remain a leading cause of work-related illnesses.
- Substantial overlap exists between the imaging appearance of many OLDs and other entities; therefore, an OLD should be considered when formulating a differential.
- Diagnosing OLDs often requires a multidisciplinary approach, which includes a detailed clinical history, imaging findings, and sometimes histopathology.

INTRODUCTION

Occupational lung diseases (OLDs) encompass a broad group of entities related to workplace exposures that result from the inhalation of organic or inorganic antigens.[1] Pneumoconioses are a subgroup of OLDs caused by the inhalation of inorganic mineral dusts. Despite safety regulations, OLDs remain a leading cause of work-related illness and mortality.[2] Manifestations of OLDs depend on the properties of the inhaled substance, intensity and duration of exposure, and the susceptibility of an individual.[3,4]

Diagnosing OLDs can be challenging due to the absence of an exposure history, potentially long latency between exposure and manifestation, entities unrelated to occupational exposures producing similar imaging findings, single agents resulting in variety of manifestations, and some OLDs that can result from multiple different inhaled antigens.[4] Additionally, symptoms are often nonspecific and may not occur until late in the course of the disease.[5] Establishing the correct diagnosis often requires a multidisciplinary approach and depends on the integration of a thorough exposure history, laboratory results, diagnostic imaging, pulmonary function testing, and sometimes biopsy.[5] Because imaging plays such a key role in diagnosis, it is imperative that radiologists consider OLDs in the differential and remain apprised of evolving industrial practices.

IMAGING TECHNIQUE

Imaging is central in the diagnosis and monitoring of OLDs. Because chest radiographs are widely available, inexpensive, and relatively low radiation dose, they remain the primary imaging modality for both the initial evaluation of suspected OLDs and occupational exposure surveillance programs.[6] However, numerous studies have shown radiographs to be both less sensitive and less specific than CT for the detection and characterization of many OLDs.[7–10] The International Labor Organization (ILO) has a standardized classification system based on the posteroanterior (PA) chest radiograph evaluating multiple subcategories of pleural and parenchymal abnormalities to codify changes related to pneumoconioses for epidemiologic research, screening, surveillance, and clinical

Mayo Clinic Department of Radiology, 200 First Street Southwest, Rochester, MN 55905, USA
* Corresponding author.
E-mail address: Walkoff.Lara@mayo.edu

Radiol Clin N Am 60 (2022) 979–992
https://doi.org/10.1016/j.rcl.2022.06.011
0033-8389/22/© 2022 Elsevier Inc. All rights reserved.

Abbreviations	
CWP	coal worker's pneumoconiosis
NSIP	nonspecific interstitial pneumonia
UIP	usual interstitial pneumonial
PF	idiopathic pulmonary fibrosis

Table 1
Typical thoracic high-resolution computed tomography patterns in occupational lung diseases

Pulmonary parenchyma	
Fibrosis	Aluminosis[56]
	Asbestosis[24]
	CBD[46]
	Chronic HP[61]
	Chronic silicosis[31]
	CWP[31]
	HMP[52]
	Inhalational talcosis[35]
Centrilobular nodules	Acute silicosis[33]
	Aluminosis[56]
	Chronic silicosis[35]
	CWP[35]
	Inhalational talcosis[49]
	Siderosis[51]
	Subacute HP[61]
Perilymphatic nodules	CBD[46]
	Chronic silicosis[35]
	CWP[35]
Consolidative opacities	Acute HP[3]
	Acute silicosis[33]
	HMP[52]
GGOs	Acute silicosis[33]
	CBD[46]
	HMP[52]
	Subacute or chronic HP[61,63]
Conglomerate masses	CBD[46]
	Complicated silicosis[31]
	Complicated CWP[31]
	Inhalational talcosis[50]
Rounded atelectasis	Asbestos exposure[27]
Cysts	Chronic HP[63]
Air trapping	Subacute or chronic HP[61,63]
	Work-related asthma[6]
Pleura	
Effusion	Asbestos exposure[13]
Thickening	Asbestos exposure[13]
Plaques	Asbestos exposure[13]
	CBD (pseudoplaques)[45]
	Chronic silicosis (pseudoplaques)[4]
	CWP (pseudoplaques)[4]
	Inhalational talcosis[49]
Other	
Calcified lymph nodes	CBD[39]
	Chronic silicosis[31]
	Chronic CWP[31]

purposes, although no diagnosis is assigned.[11] High-resolution computed tomography (HRCT) is primarily is used to characterize abnormalities identified on radiographs, evaluate equivocal radiographs, and assess symptomatic patients.[6] (18)F-fluorodeoxyglucose (FDG) PET and MR imaging are not routinely used for screening or surveillance of OLDs, however may have utility in specific situations, such as in the evaluation of associated bronchogenic malignancies or mesothelioma.

IMAGING PROTOCOLS

When radiographs are used for the evaluation for OLDs 2 views, both PA and lateral, should be obtained, if possible. A HRCT protocol for the evaluation of OLDs should include thin-section noncontrast supine inspiratory views, expiratory imaging to evaluate for air trapping, and prone imaging to differentiate dependent atelectasis from fibrosis.

IMAGING FINDINGS

The most common HRCT patterns associated with various OLDs are summarized in **Table 1**.

ASBESTOS

Inhalation of asbestos fibers occurs in occupations such as asbestos mining, asbestos abatement, or industries such as ship building, brake manufacturing, insulation, and construction.[4] Pathogenesis depends on asbestos fiber shape and size, fiber dose, duration of exposure, concurrent exposures, and host immune factors.[12] Both pulmonary parenchymal and pleural manifestations of asbestos exposure tend to have long latency periods on the order of decades.

Asbestos-Related Pleural Disease

Benign asbestos-related pleural effusions are typically the earliest asbestos-related pleural change with onset as early as 10 years exposure; however, they are less common than pleural plaques.[13,14] The effusions are usually small, exudative (may be hemorrhagic), can be unilateral or bilateral, and can persist, resolve, and/or recur over time.[14,15] In the absence of other imaging findings of prior asbestos exposure, the appearance mimics other causes of exudative effusions including infection and malignancy. Mesothelioma should be considered in cases of late developing or recurrent pleural effusions.[13]

Diffuse pleural thickening (DPT) is due to thickening of the visceral pleura[11] and most commonly involves the posterior and posteromedial pleura over the lower lobes.[16] DPT is a less specific indicator of prior asbestos exposure than pleural plaques and can also occur in the setting of prior infection, hemothorax, and connective tissue disease.[13] Unlike pleural plaques, DPT rarely calcifies, although it may coexist with calcified pleural plaques (CPP; **Fig. 1**).[17] Some variation in the definition of DPT exists; however, McLoud and colleagues defined DPT on chest radiography as "a smooth, non-interrupted pleural density extending over at least one-fourth of the chest wall, with or without costophrenic angle obliteration,"[18] although the ILO definition must include an obliterated costophrenic angle.[11] On CT, DPT has been defined by Lynch and colleagues as "a continuous sheet of pleural thickening more than 5 cm wide, more than 8 cm in craniocaudal extent,

and more them 3 mm thick."[16] In contrast to well-circumscribed pleural plaques, the margin between the DPT and adjacent lung is commonly irregular due to underlying fibrosis.[19]

Asbestos-related pleural plaques, focal protrusions of hyaline fibrosis arising from the parietal pleura that often calcify, are the most common manifestation of prior asbestos exposure.[13] Plaques are typically not detected radiographically until at least 20 years after exposure.[17] Pleural plaques commonly involve the hemidiaphragms (virtually pathognomonic), with other characteristic locations including the mid to lower posterior and posterolateral chest wall, paravertebral pleura, and sometimes the mediastinal pleura. Asbestos-related pleural plaques rarely involve the apices or costophrenic sulci, unlike DPT.[17] Plaques are usually present bilaterally but may have an asymmetric distribution. On frontal radiographs, pleural plaques can appear as a focal opacity projected over the lung when present along the anterior and posterior chest wall and viewed en face. A high attenuation, serpentine, peripheral margin of calcification may be visible, resembling a holly leaf.[20] When viewed in profile the plaques have a more linear configuration (**Fig. 2**). Subpleural fat,

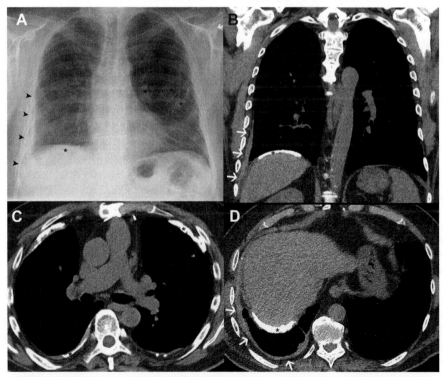

Fig. 1. DPT and pleural plaques. Frontal chest radiograph (*A*) demonstrates CPP bilaterally (*) and smooth linear opacity, DPT, along the inferior third of the right hemithorax extending into the lateral costophrenic sulcus (*arrowheads*). Coronal (*B*) and axial (*C, D*) CT images demonstrate DPT in this patient with prior asbestos exposure (*arrows, B* and *D*). CPP are also present bilaterally (*).

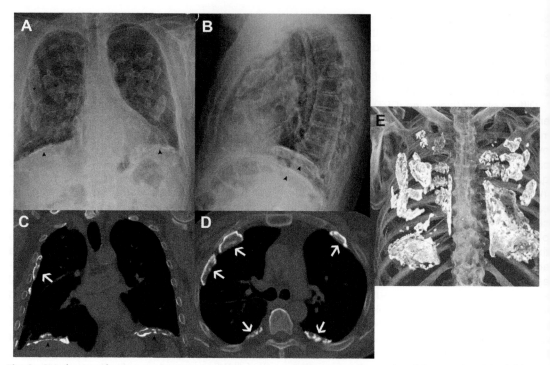

Fig. 2. CPP due to asbestos exposure. Frontal (*A*) and lateral (*B*) chest radiographs with extensive CPP visible en face along the chest wall (eg, * in *A*). CPP are also present along both hemidiaphragms, (*arrowheads*). Coronal (*C*) and axial (*D*) CT images show partially calcified plaques along the chest wall (*arrows*) and hemidiaphragms (*arrowheads*). Coronal 3D MIP rendering (*E*) shows the extent and distribution of the plaques.

rib fractures, and companion shadows from chest wall musculature can mimic pleural plaques on frontal radiograph.[17] On CT, pleural plaques are focal circumscribed areas of pleural thickening separated from the underlying ribs and other extrapleural structures by a thin layer of fat. Punctate, linear, or coalescent calcification may be present.[19] CT is more sensitive than radiograph for the detection of both pleural plaques and DPT.[9]

Malignant Pleural Mesothelioma

Asbestos is a known carcinogen, which increases the risk of malignant pleural mesothelioma (MPM; as well as bronchogenic malignancies), with the most MPM cases related to prior asbestos exposure.[21] MPM is typically not diagnosed until 20 to 40 years after exposure.[3] Pleural thickening and pleural effusions are common (**Fig. 3**). CT features that are more often present in MPM compared with benign pleural disease such as DPT include mediastinal pleural thickening, pleural rind, pleural nodularity, and parietal pleural thickening measuring more than 1 cm in thickness.[22]

Parenchymal

Asbestosis is diffuse pulmonary fibrosis, which typically occurs in individuals with prolonged and high concentration exposure to asbestos fibers. A dose-dependent relationship between exposure and fibrosis exists. Asbestosis usually occurs 20 years or greater after exposure.[3] Radiographs show small bilateral reticular opacities with a lower lung and peripheral predominance, which become more diffuse and as fibrosis progresses. The earliest HRCT manifestation of asbestosis is small, round, branching subpleural centrilobular opacities reflecting fibrosis in the walls of the respiratory bronchiole.[23] Typical HRCT findings include intralobular lines, interlobular septal thickening, ground glass opacities (GGOs), subpleural curvilinear opacities, and parenchymal bands (**Fig. 4**). Subpleural curvilinear opacities are linear densities paralleling the inner chest wall located within 1 cm of the pleura. Parenchymal bands are linear densities measuring 2 to 5 cm in length coursing through the lung to contact the pleural surface, often associated with parenchymal distortion, which do not resolve on prone imaging.[24] Subpleural curvilinear opacities and parenchymal bands are not specific for asbestosis, although have been observed more commonly in asbestosis than in some other causes of fibrosing pneumonia.[25] Honeycombing may occur in advanced disease. IPF and other causes of a UIP pattern can have similar manifestations. However,

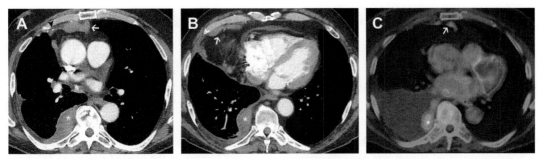

Fig. 3. MPM (epithelioid). Axial CT images (*A, B*) and axial FDG PET/CT fusion image (*C*) showing lobulated soft tissue masses along the right posteromedial pleural space with increased FDG activity (***). Enlarged and mildly FDG avid right cardiophrenic angle lymph nodes are also present (*arrows*). Note a small CPP (*arrowhead, A*) compatible with history of prior asbestos exposure. Note the accumulation of right pleural fluid between the CT and PET/CT performed 3 months apart.

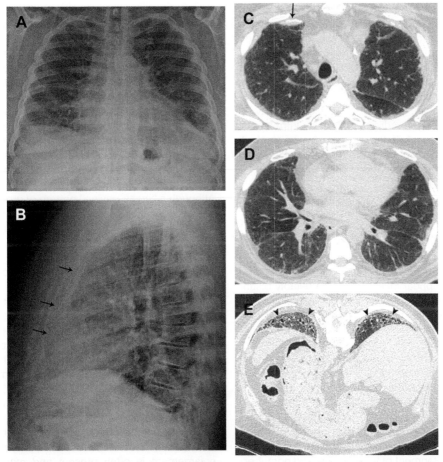

Fig. 4. Asbestosis. PA (*A*) and lateral (*B*) chest radiograph images demonstrate lower lung zone predominant fine reticular opacities and partially CPP (*arrow, B*). Axial CT images from the upper (*C*), mid (*D*), and lower (*E*) lungs also show lower lung predominant reticulations with associated ground glass and traction bronchiectasis (*arrowheads, E*). Note persistence of findings on the prone image through the lung bases (*E*), consistent with fibrosis. CPP are also visible on CT (*arrow, C*).

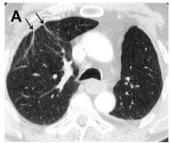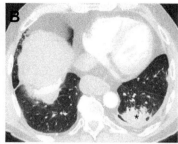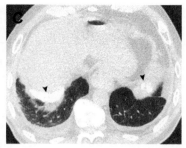

Fig. 5. Asbestos-related pleural and parenchymal changes. Axial CT image at the level of the carina (*A*) shows linear parenchymal bands coursing through right lung (*arrows*). Axial CT images through the lung bases (*B, C*) demonstrate a rounded atelectasis in the posterior left lower lobe (*, B*). CPP are present along both hemidiaphragms (*arrowheads, C*). Note small bilateral pleural effusions and mild fibrosis in the right lung base (*C*).

asbestos-related pleural abnormalities are present in most individuals with asbestosis,[24] which can indicate an alternative diagnosis to IPF and suggest asbestosis.[26]

Rounded atelectasis is a round or oval opacity with volume loss adjacent to a pleural abnormality, often a pleural effusion, plaque, or thickening (**Fig. 5**). Rounded atelectasis is most common in the posterior lower lungs and can be diagnosed on CT if all of the following features are present: rounded or ovoid shape, volume loss, contact with the pleural surface, and vessels converging on the opacity with a curvilinear appearance (comet tail sign).[27] Uniform enhancement may be present after the administration of intravenous contrast material. If the appearance is atypical, FDG-PET/CT can be performed, which should not demonstrate increased FDG activity.[28]

SILICOSIS AND COAL WORKERS' PNEUMOCONIOSIS

Silicosis and CWP are 2 pathologically distinct entities occurring secondary to the inhalation of different inorganic dusts; however, the radiograph and HRCT appearances cannot be reliably distinguished.[3] Silicosis results from inhalation of crystalline silicone dioxide (silica). Occupations associated with silica exposure include tunneling, foundry work, sandblasting, mining, quarrying, drilling, stone cutting, polishing, brick lining, and ceramics manufacturing.[29] More recently, outbreaks of silicosis have been documented in association with engineered stone, a quartz based composite material.[30] CWP occurs in coal miners and is caused by the inhalation of coal dust free of silica. Both silicosis and CWP are risk factors for the development of tuberculosis and nontuberculous mycobacterial infections.[31,32]

There are 4 subtypes of silicosis: acute silicosis (silicoproteinosis), chronic simple silicosis, chronic complicated silicosis (progressive massive fibrosis

[PMF]), and accelerated silicosis, depending on both the duration and intensity of the exposure, although more than one of these subtypes can coexist concurrently.[31]

Acute silicosis develops following acute exposure to very high concentrations of silica dust over months to several years, which results in filling of air spaces with proteinaceous material similar to idiopathic pulmonary alveolar proteinosis.[33] Radiograph findings include diffuse reticulonodular opacites and airspace consolidations, with or without air bronchograms, which may have a predilection for the upper lungs.[34] HRCT may show consolidations, greatest in the posterior lungs, and poorly defined soft tissue or ground glass centrilobular nodules. Foci of calcification are common, although are usually not seen in other entities presenting with acute consolidation, such as bacterial pneumonia or lymphoma.[33] Although a "crazy-paving" pattern of ground glass and superimposed septal thickening is associated with idiopathic pulmonary alveolar proteinosis, it is not typical for acute silicosis.[33]

Chronic simple silicosis and CWP typically develop 10 to 20 years after lower concentration exposure.[31] Radiographs demonstrate multiple solid, well-defined, small (<5 mm) pulmonary nodules that are most profuse in the upper posterior lung zones and may calcify.[6,35] HRCT appearance is most commonly small (<5 mm) bilateral pulmonary nodules with a predilection for the upper and posterior lung zones and either a centrilobular or perilymphatic distribution (**Fig. 6**).[35,36] Coalescence of subpleural nodules may result in pseudo-plaques in both silicosis and CWP.[4] Pleural thickening has also been reported in both silicosis and CWP.[37,38] Mediastinal and hilar lymph node enlargement is often present and may demonstrate calcifications. Despite the commonly reported association with eggshell peripheral lymph node calcification, diffuse, punctate, and central patterns of calcification are actually more

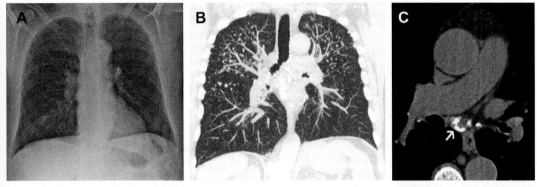

Fig. 6. Chronic simple silicosis. PA chest radiograph (*A*) and MIP coronal CT image (*B*) demonstrate numerous small, solid, perilymphatic distribution nodules with an upper lung predominance. Axial CT image (*C*) shows a mildly enlarged subcarinal lymph node with peripheral calcifications (*arrow*).

prevalent in silicosis. Eggshell calcifications are even less common in CWP.[36,39] Eggshell lymph node calcification can also be seen in chronic beryllium disease (CBD), sarcoidosis, amyloidosis, and some infections.[39]

Chronic complicated disease, or PMF, occurs more commonly with silicosis than CWP because silica is more fibrogenic than coal dust. PMF arises when small nodules coalesce into conglomerate nodules and masses that measure greater than 1 cm in diameter.[39] PMF can mimic the appearance of the conglomerate masses that form in advanced sarcoidosis.[6] In contrast to simple disease, PMF typically results in functional respiratory impairment.[6] The typical appearance of PMF on imaging is large bilateral opacities at the periphery of the upper lobes on a background of small nodules (**Figs. 7** and **8**). Paracicatricial emphysema may develop between the pleura and the

opacities. Calcification is often present. Cavitation may occur due to ischemic necrosis or superimposed TB.[6,35] PMF may mimic lung cancer on imaging. MR imaging may be useful to help distinguish malignancy from PMF[40] but PET/CT has limited use because PMF may be FDG avid, even in the absence of superimposed malignancy or infection.[41] Biopsy or continued imaging surveillance may also be used in patients with PMF and concern for an underlying malignant mass.

Accelerated silicosis occurs with high-intensity exposure to silica dust, has shorter latency period of 4 to 10 years, and manifests similar to the complicated form of silicosis.[31,39]

CHRONIC BERYLLIUM DISEASE

Beryllium is a lightweight metal used in many industries including aerospace, ceramics, dentistry,

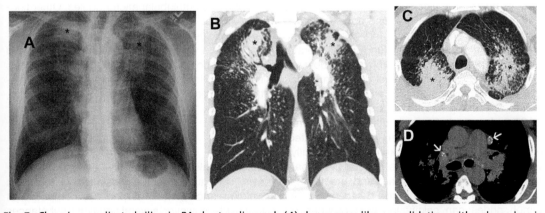

Fig. 7. Chronic complicated silicosis. PA chest radiograph (*A*) shows mass-like consolidation with volume loss in both upper lobes (*) on background of smaller upper lung predominant nodules. Coronal (*B*) and axial (*C*) chest CT images reveal innumerable small solid pulmonary nodules with an upper lung predominance and upper lung PMF (*). Axial CT soft tissue window image (*D*) demonstrates mildly enlarged lymph nodes with calcifications (*white arrows*).

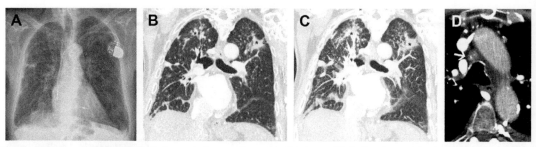

Fig. 8. Chronic complicated CWP. Frontal chest radiograph *(A)* shows ill-defined opacities in the bilateral upper lungs with associated volume loss and surrounding nodularity, as well as linear scarring and/or atelectasis in the mid and lower lungs. Thin section *(B)* and MIP *(C)* coronal CT images demonstrate PMF in both upper lobes (*) with surrounding small nodules. Axial CT image through the mediastinum *(D)* shows small calcifications in a paratracheal lymph node *(white arrow)*.

nuclear, and electronics.[6] Acute berylliosis has been nearly eliminated in the United States due workplace regulations.[42] CBD occurs after exposure to beryllium or its salts, which may be in the form of dusts, fumes, or mists.[42] CBD is due to an immune-mediated delayed hypersensitivity response with the proliferation of beryllium-specific T cells.[43] CBD primarily affects the lungs; however, other organs may also be involved.[4] No clear dose–response relationship exists;CBD may occur after short-term, low-level exposure or may not develop even after long-term high-level exposure.[44] The diagnosis of CBD is based on exposure history, imaging, and the beryllium lymphocyte proliferation test. The beryllium lymphocyte proliferation test performed on blood or bronchiolar lavage fluid is quite sensitive and specific for CBD and useful in distinguishing CBD from mimics such as sarcoidosis.[42] As with silica and asbestos, beryllium exposure is thought to be a risk factor for developing lung carcinoma.[5]

Radiographs may appear normal in mild or early disease; however, patients with abnormal findings may have small irregular or round opacities, usually symmetric, and in either a mid-to-upper lung or diffuse distribution. Upper lung conglomerate masses, septal thickening, emphysema, upward hilar retraction with architectural distortion, linear scarring, hilar lymph node enlargement, and pleural thickening may also be observed.[42,45] HRCT findings include small nodules in a perilymphatic distribution, which are often associated with interlobular septal thickening. Additionally, conglomerate masses, GGOs, pleural abnormalities, bronchial wall thickening, and mediastinal and hilar lymphadenopathy may be seen (**Fig. 9**). Lymph nodes can calcify in an amorphous or eggshell pattern. As the disease progresses, fibrosis and occasionally honeycombing may occur.[35,46] In one study of a group of patients initially diagnosed with sarcoidosis, 40% were

reclassified as having CBD after reevaluation.[47] Due to the overlap in imaging appearance, CBD should be considered when imaging findings are suggestive of sarcoidosis.

TALCOSIS

Talc is a hydrated magnesium silicate used in a variety of industries including rubber, plastics, textiles, and cosmetics.[4] The 3 forms of inhalational talc-related pulmonary diseases are pure talcosis, talcosilicosis, and talcoasbestosis. The fourth form of talcosis is due to the intravenous injection of crushed oral talc-containing medication tablets.[48] Talcosis produces a nonnecrotizing granulomatous reaction that may progress to fibrosis.[35] In the inhalational subtypes of talcosis, small diffuse rounded nodules are the most commonly described radiographic abnormality; however, larger nodular opacities greater than 1 cm and reticulations are also reported.[49] On HRCT, the most common finding is diffusely distributed centrilobular micronodules. Other findings include septal and subpleural lines, GGOs, large opacities with areas of high attenuation secondary to talc deposition, pleural plaques, and lymph node enlargement.[49,50] Talcoasbestosis and talcosilicosis often have imaging manifestations similar to asbestosis and silicosis, respectively.[48]

SIDEROSIS

Siderosis, also called "arc-welders' pneumoconiosis," is caused by the inhalation of inorganic welding smoke, which is primarily composed of iron oxide; however, several additional substances may also be present.[51] On chest radiograph, micronodules are sometimes visible.[51] The most common HRCT manifestation is defined pulmonary micronodules, often in a centrilobular

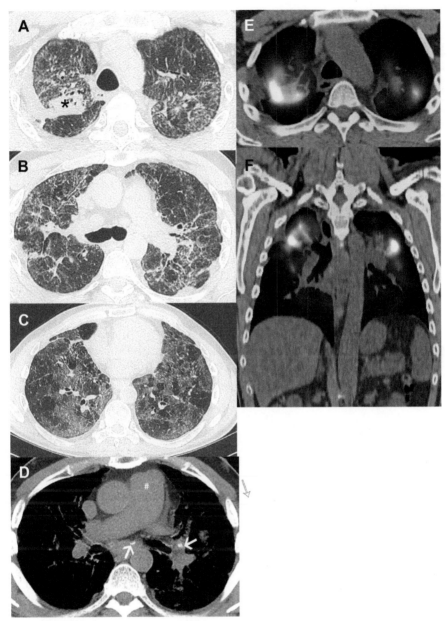

Fig. 9. CBD in a beryllium oxide machinist. Axial CT slices from the upper (*A*), mid (*B*), and lower (*C*) lungs demonstrate a conglomerate mass in the right upper lobe (*, A) with associated volume loss. Perihilar predominant perilymphatic nodularity, architectural distortion, interlobular septal thickening, and traction bronchiectasis are also present, greatest in the upper and mid lung zones. Diffuse GGOs and mosaic attenuation are present throughout the lungs but most conspicuous in the lung bases. Axial CT image on mediastinal window setting (*D*) reveals calcifications within hilar and subcarinal lymph nodes (*white arrows*). A dilated main pulmonary artery (#) is visible in the setting of known pulmonary hypertension. Axial (*E*) and coronal (*F*) FDG-PET/CT fusion images demonstrate increased FDG activity in the bilateral upper lungs associated with the conglomerate masses and more confluent regions of fibrosis.

distribution, reflecting accumulation of iron oxide particles in macrophages along peribronchiolar lymphatic vessels (**Fig. 10**).[51–53] Branching linear opacities have also been described and less commonly GGOs.[53] Ill-defined centrilobular micronodules and linear branching opacities are slightly more common in the upper lung zones, however relatively evenly distributed axially.[53] Findings can resemble hypersensitivity pneumonitis (HP), although mosaic attenuation may be a

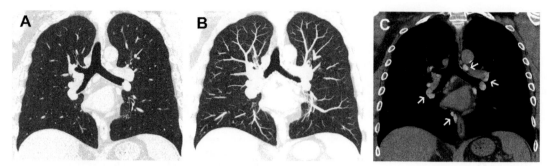

Fig. 10. Siderosis in a welder. Coronal CT thin section (*A*) and MIP (*B*) images demonstrate diffuse centrilobular micronodules throughout both lungs. Mediastinal window coronal CT image (*C*) shows numerous high attenuation mediastinal and bilateral hilar lymph nodes, some of which are enlarged.

more prominent feature in HP. Respiratory bronchiolitis and other infectious/inflammatory bronchiolitides are also on the differential.[43] Fibrosis is not a typical feature; however, it may result with additives to the welding process, such as silica.[53]

HARD METAL PNEUMOCONIOSIS

Hard metal pneumoconiosis (HMP) is caused by the inhalation of the dusts from alloys of tungsten, carbon, and cobalt, sometimes with the addition of small quantities of other metals; cobalt is the

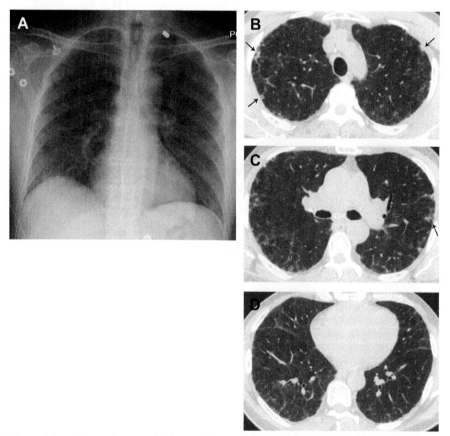

Fig. 11. Hard metal lung disease in a machinist working with tungsten carbide and cobalt-based alloys. Frontal chest radiograph (*A*) shows ill-defined bilateral linear and small nodular consolidative opacities in the periphery of both lungs. Axial chest CT images through the upper (*B*), mid (*C*), and lower (*D*) lungs show peripheral reticular opacities with mild architectural distortion and small areas of mildly nodular consolidation (*arrows, B, C*). Subtle ill-defined GGOs and interlobular septal thickening are also present (*C, D*).

primary component implicated in the pulmonary toxicity.[3,4] These durable and heat-resistant alloys are used in polishing, drilling, grinding, and cutting metals or other hard materials due to their durability and heat-resistant properties. Exposure can result in interstitial pneumonitis and fibrosis.[3] On histopathology, HMP can take several forms; however, giant cell interstitial pneumonia is nearly pathognomonic, when present.[54] Chest radiograph appearance is nonspecific and may be normal, show small nodules and reticular opacities, or fibrosis.[35] HRCT findings include consolidative opacities, which may contain air bronchograms and traction bronchiectasis, and multilobular or panlobular GGOs (Fig. 11).[52] Reticulation, subpleural cystic spaces, and nodular peribronchovascular thickening with traction bronchiectasis have also been reported.[55] Thus, HMP can appear similar to sarcoidosis, NSIP, and/or UIP on imaging.[55] The diagnosis of HMP requires a combination of exposure history, clinical symptoms, radiologic findings of interstitial lung disease, and histologic findings of interstitial lung disease or giant cell pneumonia, as well as histopathologic findings of metal in lung tissue.[35]

ALUMINOSIS

Aluminosis is caused by the inhalation of aluminum powder and aluminum oxide[56] with exposures including alumina abrasive manufacture and pyrotechnic manufacture.[57] In early disease, radiographs may be unrevealing or demonstrate upper or mid lung predominant small rounded and irregular opacities. In later disease, upper lung fibrotic changes may be visible.[31,56] HRCT findings of early aluminosis include small rounded ill-defined centrilobular opacities measuring 3 mm or less with an upper lung predominance. This pattern may resemble HP, silicosis, CWP, or respiratory bronchiolitis.[31,56] In advanced disease, HRCT may demonstrate upper lung predominant reticular and nodular interstitial fibrosis with subpleural emphysema, mimicking silicosis, CWP, sarcoidosis, or HP.[31,56] Increased attenuation within mediastinal and hilar lymph nodes due to aluminum deposition has been reported.[58]

HYPERSENSITIVITY PNEUMONITIS

HP is an immunologically mediated process caused by the inhalation of organic antigens, which can occur due to occupational or

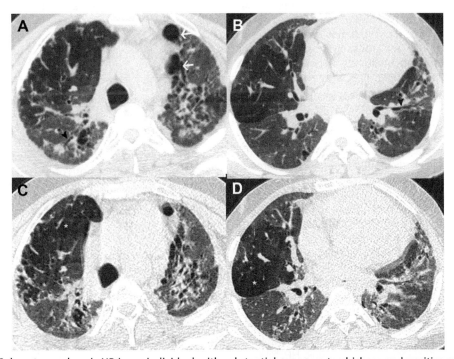

Fig. 12. Subacute on chronic HP in an individual with substantial exposure to chickens and positive avian antigens. Axial inspiratory CT images through the mid and lower lungs (A, B) with expiratory CT images at corresponding locations (C, D, respectively) demonstrate mosaic attenuation of the lung parenchyma with areas of air trapping (*, C, D). Peripheral and peribronchovascular distribution irregular opacities with architectural distortion, volume loss, and traction bronchiectasis (*arrowheads*, A, B) are also present, consistent with fibrosis. Subpleural cysts are also present (*arrow*, A).

nonoccupational exposures. HP develops in susceptible individuals following sensitization and subsequent repeated exposure to a variety of organic antigens, including those from animals, plants, bacteria, fungi, and some chemicals. HP subtypes are often named to reflect the causative agent, for example, "bird fancier's lung" and "farmer's lung." The most common inciting antigens in a study from the United States were avian antigens, followed by hot tub-related *Mycobacterium avium* complex; however, no specific antigen was identified in one-quarter of cases.[59] A diagnosis of HP considers clinical, imaging, laboratory, and sometimes histopathologic data.[60] HP has historically been characterized as either acute, subacute, or chronic; however, classification into fibrotic versus nonfibrotic subtypes is now preferred.[60]

Consistent imaging findings in acute HP are less well reported but airspace consolidations may be seen.[3]

HRCT findings of subacute HP include patchy or diffuse ground-glass opacities and small (<5 mm) poorly defined centrilobular nodules, which may be uniformly distributed or be more pronounced in the mid to lower lungs. Inspiratory images demonstrate mosaic attenuation corresponding with air trapping on expiratory images.[61] The head-cheese sign, named for its resemblance to the processed meat product, has been described in subacute HP and reflects a patchwork of different lung attenuations: hyperlucent lung caused by air trapping, GGOs due to interstitial pneumonitis, and regions of normal lung attenuation.[62]

Chronic HP is characterized by fibrosis visible as reticulations, ground glass, volume loss, and traction bronchiectasis in patchy, subpleural, or peribronchovascular distribution (**Fig. 12**). Fibrosis may have an upper or lower lung predominance or no zonal predilection; however, the costophrenic sulci and apices may be spared.[63] Subpleural honeycombing is a marker of advanced disease and more often upper lobe predominant; this is in contrast to IPF characterized by basilar predominant honeycombing.[63] Air trapping on expiratory images is common, which may be helpful in distinguishing HP from IPF or NSIP.[63,64] Cysts are also substantially more prevalent in HP than in IPF or NSIP.[63] Studies also have demonstrated high rates of emphysema in nonsmoking farmers and bird fanciers with chronic HP.[65,66]

WORK-RELATED ASTHMA

Work-related asthma is the most common form of OLD and includes both work-exacerbated asthma

(preexisting asthma worsened by workplace exposures) and occupational asthma (asthma caused by airborne dusts, vapors gases, or fumes in the workplace).[6] Imaging findings cannot be differentiated from nonoccupational causes of small airways disease. On radiographs, pulmonary hyperinflation and bronchial wall thickening may be visible. HRCT findings are those of small airways disease including mosaic attenuation, bronchial wall thickening, and air trapping on expiratory images.[6]

SUMMARY

Despite regulations, OLDs remain a leading cause of work-related illnesses. Establishing a diagnosis of an OLD often requires a multidisciplinary approach, incorporating a thorough exposure of history and other diagnostic data, including imaging. Although radiographs remain the standard for screening and surveillance, HRCT is often both more sensitive and specific for evaluation. Substantial overlap in imaging findings exists between many OLDs and other entities including fibrotic interstitial lung diseases, sarcoidosis, and infectious processes. As a result, the radiologist should be familiar with the myriad of imaging appearances and consider OLDs when formulating a differential.

CLINICS CARE POINTS

- Because substantial overlap exists between the imaging appearances of OLDs and other nonoccupational entities, OLDs should be considered when formulating a differential.

- Establishing the diagnosis of an OLD often requires a multidisciplinary approach and integration of a thorough exposure history, laboratory results, diagnostic imaging, pulmonary function testing, and sometimes biopsy.

- HRCT is often both more sensitive and specific for the evaluation of OLDs than radiographs.

DISCLOSURE

The authors have nothing to disclose.

REFERENCES

1. Vlahovich KP, Sood AA. 2019 Update on Occupational Lung Diseases: A Narrative Review. Pulm Ther 2021;7(1):75–87.

2. Weston A. Work-related lung diseases. IARC Sci Publ 2011;163:387–405.

3. Kim KI, Kim CW, Lee MK, et al. Imaging of occupational lung disease. Radiographics 2001;21(6):1371–91.

4. Ahuja J, Kanne JP, Meyer CA. Occupational lung disease. Semin Roentgenol 2015;50(1):40–51.

5. Cox CW, Rose CS, Lynch DA. State of the art: Imaging of occupational lung disease. Radiology 2014; 270(3):681–96.

6. Champlin J, Edwards R, Pipavath S. Imaging of Occupational Lung Disease. Radiol Clin North Am 2016;54(6):1077–96.

7. Remy-Jardin M, Degreef JM, Beuscart R, et al. Coal worker's pneumoconiosis: CT assessment in exposed workers and correlation with radiographic findings. Radiology 1990;177(2):363–71.

8. Gevenois PA, Pichot E, Dargent F, et al. Low grade coal worker's pneumoconiosis. Comparison of CT and chest radiography. Acta Radiol 1994;35(4): 351–6.

9. al Jarad N, Poulakis N, Pearson MC, et al. Assessment of asbestos-induced pleural disease by computed tomography–correlation with chest radiograph and lung function. Respir Med 1991;85(3):203–8.

10. Aberle DR, Gamsu G, Ray CS. High-resolution CT of benign asbestos-related diseases: clinical and radiographic correlation. AJR Am J Roentgenol 1988;151(5):883–91.

11. Guidelines for the use of the ILO International classification of radiographs of pneumoconioses. Geneva: International Labour Office; 2011. p. 2011. Available at: https://www.ilo.org/wcmsp5/groups/public/—ed_protect/—protrav/—safework/documents/publication/wcms_168260.pdf.

12. Mossman BT, Churg A. Mechanisms in the pathogenesis of asbestosis and silicosis. Am J Respir Crit Care Med 1998;157(5 Pt 1):1666–80.

13. Peacock C, Copley SJ, Hansell DM. Asbestos-related benign pleural disease. Clin Radiol 2000; 55(6):422–32.

14. Epler GR, McLoud TC, Gaensler EA. Prevalence and incidence of benign asbestos pleural effusion in a working population. JAMA 1982;247(5):617–22.

15. Hillerdal G, Ozesmi M. Benign asbestos pleural effusion: 73 exudates in 60 patients. Eur J Respir Dis 1987;71(2):113–21.

16. Lynch DA, Gamsu G, Aberle DR. Conventional and high resolution computed tomography in the diagnosis of asbestos-related diseases. Radiographics 1989;9(3):523–51.

17. Fletcher DE, Edge JR. The early radiological changes in pulmonary and pleural asbestosis. Clin Radiol 1970;21(4):355–65.

18. McLoud TC, Woods BO, Carrington CB, et al. Diffuse pleural thickening in an asbestos-exposed population: prevalence and causes. AJR Am J Roentgenol 1985;144(1):9–18.

19. Hobbs SB. Asbestos-Related Disease. In: Walker CM, Chung JH, Hobbs SB, et al, editors. Müller's imaging of the chest. 2nd edition. Philadelphia, PA: Elsevier Health Sciences; 2019. p. 775–92.

20. Cugell DW, Kamp DW. Asbestos and the pleura: a review. Chest 2004;125(3):1103–17.

21. Yates DH, Corrin B, Stidolph PN, et al. Malignant mesothelioma in south east England: clinicopathological experience of 272 cases. Thorax 1997;52(6):507–12.

22. Leung AN, Muller NL, Miller RR. CT in differential diagnosis of diffuse pleural disease. AJR Am J Roentgenol 1990;154(3):487–92.

23. Akira M, Yokoyama K, Yamamoto S, et al. Early asbestosis: evaluation with high-resolution CT. Radiology 1991;178(2):409–16.

24. Aberle DR, Gamsu G, Ray CS, et al. Asbestos-related pleural and parenchymal fibrosis: detection with high-resolution CT. Radiology 1988;166(3): 729–34.

25. al-Jarad N, Strickland B, Pearson MC, et al. High resolution computed tomographic assessment of asbestosis and cryptogenic fibrosing alveolitis: a comparative study. Thorax 1992;47(8):645–50.

26. Raghu G, Remy-Jardin M, Myers JL, et al. Diagnosis of Idiopathic Pulmonary Fibrosis. An Official ATS/ERS/JRS/ALAT Clinical Practice Guideline. Am J Respir Crit Care Med 2018;198(5):e44–68.

27. Batra P, Brown K, Hayashi K, et al. Rounded atelectasis. J Thorac Imaging 1996;11(3):187–97.

28. McAdams HP, Erasums JJ, Patz EF, et al. Evaluation of patients with round atelectasis using 2-[18F]-fluoro-2-deoxy-D-glucose PET. J Comput Assist Tomogr 1998;22(4):601–4.

29. Bang KM, Attfield MD, Wood JM, et al. National trends in silicosis mortality in the United States, 1981-2004. Am J Ind Med 2008;51(9):633–9.

30. Rose C, Heinzerling A, Patel K, et al. Severe Silicosis in Engineered Stone Fabrication Workers - California, Colorado, Texas, and Washington, 2017-2019. MMWR Morb Mortal Wkly Rep 2019;68(38):813–8.

31. Hobbs SB. Silicosis and Coal Workers' Pneumoconiosis. In: Walker C, Chung J, Hobbs S, et al, editors. Müller's imaging of the chest. 2nd edition. Philadelphia, PA: Elsevier Health Sciences; 2019. p. 793–808.

32. Cowie RL. The epidemiology of tuberculosis in gold miners with silicosis. Am J Respir Crit Care Med 1994;150(5 Pt 1):1460–2.

33. Marchiori E, Souza CA, Barbassa TG, et al. Silicoproteinosis: high-resolution CT findings in 13 patients. AJR Am J Roentgenol 2007;189(6):1402–6.

34. Dee P, Suratt P, Winn W. The radiographic findings in acute silicosis. Radiology 1978;126(2):359–63.

35. Chong S, Lee KS, Chung MJ, et al. Pneumoconiosis: comparison of imaging and pathologic findings. Radiographics 2006;26(1):59–77.

36. Antao VC, Pinheiro GA, Terra-Filho M, et al. High-resolution CT in silicosis: correlation with radiographic findings and functional impairment. J Comput Assist Tomogr 2005;29(3):350–6.

37. Young RC Jr, Rachal RE, Carr PG, et al. Patterns of coal workers' pneumoconiosis in Appalachian former coal miners. J Natl Med Assoc 1992;84(1):41–8.

38. Arakawa H, Honma K, Saito Y, et al. Pleural disease in silicosis: pleural thickening, effusion, and invagination. Radiology 2005;236(2):685–93.

39. Batra K, Aziz MU, Adams TN, et al. Imaging Of Occupational Lung Diseases. Semin Roentgenol 2019;54(1):44–58.

40. Ogihara Y, Ashizawa K, Hayashi H, et al. Progressive massive fibrosis in patients with pneumoconiosis: utility of MRI in differentiating from lung cancer. Acta Radiol 2018;59(1):72–80.

41. Chung SY, Lee JH, Kim TH, et al. 18F-FDG PET imaging of progressive massive fibrosis. Ann Nucl Med 2010;24(1):21–7.

42. Aronchick JM, Rossman MD, Miller WT. Chronic beryllium disease: diagnosis, radiographic findings, and correlation with pulmonary function tests. Radiology 1987;163(3):677–82.

43. Hobbs SB, Uncommon Pneumoconioses. In: Walker CM, Chung JH, Hobbs SB, et al., Eds Müller's Imaging of the Chest. 2nd ed. Elsevier Philadelphia, PA; 2019:809-821.

44. Kreiss K, Mroz MM, Zhen B, et al. Epidemiology of beryllium sensitization and disease in nuclear workers. Am Rev Respir Dis 1993;148(4 Pt 1): 985–91.

45. Sharma N, Patel J, Mohammed TL. Chronic beryllium disease: computed tomographic findings. J Comput Assist Tomogr 2010;34(6):945–8.

46. Newman LS, Buschman DL, Newell JD Jr, et al. Beryllium disease: assessment with CT. Radiology 1994;190(3):835–40.

47. Muller-Quernheim J, Gaede KI, Fireman E, et al. Diagnoses of chronic beryllium disease within cohorts of sarcoidosis patients. Eur Respir J 2006;27(6): 1190–5.

48. Feigin DS. Talc: understanding its manifestations in the chest. AJR Am J Roentgenol 1986;146(2): 295–301.

49. Akira M, Kozuka T, Yamamoto S, et al. Inhalational talc pneumoconiosis: radiographic and CT findings in 14 patients. AJR Am J Roentgenol 2007;188(2): 326–33.

50. Marchiori E, Souza Junior AS, Muller NL. Inhalational pulmonary talcosis: high-resolution CT findings in 3 patients. J Thorac Imaging 2004;19(1):41–4.

51. Takahashi M, Nitta N, Kishimoto T, et al. Computed tomography findings of arc-welders' pneumoconiosis: Comparison with silicosis. Eur J Radiol 2018; 107:98–104.

52. Akira M. Uncommon pneumoconioses: CT and pathologic findings. Radiology 1995;197(2):403–9.

53. Han D, Goo JM, Im JG, et al. Thin-section CT findings of arc-welders' pneumoconiosis. Korean J Radiol 2000;1(2):79–83.

54. Ohori NP, Sciurba FC, Owens GR, et al. Giant-cell interstitial pneumonia and hard-metal pneumoconiosis. A clinicopathologic study of four cases and review of the literature. Am J Surg Pathol 1989;13(7): 581–7.

55. Gotway MB, Golden JA, Warnock M, et al. Hard metal interstitial lung disease: high-resolution computed tomography appearance. J Thorac Imaging 2002;17(4):314–8.

56. Kraus T, Schaller KH, Angerer J, et al. Aluminosis–detection of an almost forgotten disease with HRCT. J Occup Med Toxicol 2006;1:4.

57. Guidotti T. Pulmonary aluminosis-a review. Toxicol Pathol 1975;3:16–8.

58. Vahlensieck M, Overlack A, Muller KM. Computed tomographic high-attenuation mediastinal lymph nodes after aluminum exposition. Eur Radiol 2000; 10(12):1945–6.

59. Hanak V, Golbin JM, Ryu JH. Causes and presenting features in 85 consecutive patients with hypersensitivity pneumonitis. Mayo Clin Proc 2007;82(7):812–6.

60. Raghu G, Remy-Jardin M, Ryerson CJ, et al. Diagnosis of Hypersensitivity Pneumonitis in Adults. An Official ATS/JRS/ALAT Clinical Practice Guideline. Am J Respir Crit Care Med 2020;202(3):e36–69.

61. Glazer CS, Rose CS, Lynch DA. Clinical and radiologic manifestations of hypersensitivity pneumonitis. J Thorac Imaging 2002;17(4):261–72.

62. Torres PP, Moreira MA, Silva DG, et al. High-resolution computed tomography and histopathological findings in hypersensitivity pneumonitis: a pictorial essay. Radiol Bras 2016;49(2):112–6.

63. Silva CI, Muller NL, Lynch DA, et al. Chronic hypersensitivity pneumonitis: differentiation from idiopathic pulmonary fibrosis and nonspecific interstitial pneumonia by using thin-section CT. Radiology 2008;246(1):288–97.

64. Silva CI, Churg A, Muller NL. Hypersensitivity pneumonitis: spectrum of high-resolution CT and pathologic findings. AJR Am J Roentgenol 2007;188(2): 334–44.

65. Remy-Jardin M, Remy J, Wallaert B, et al. Subacute and chronic bird breeder hypersensitivity pneumonitis: sequential evaluation with CT and correlation with lung function tests and bronchoalveolar lavage. Radiology 1993;189(1):111–8.

66. Erkinjuntti-Pekkanen R, Rytkonen H, Kokkarinen JI, et al. Long-term risk of emphysema in patients with farmer's lung and matched control farmers. Am J Respir Crit Care Med 1998;158(2):662–5.

Diagnosis and Treatment of Lung Cancer in the Setting of Interstitial Lung Disease

Dane A. Fisher, MD[a], Mark C. Murphy, MB, BCh, BAO[a],
Sydney B. Montesi, MD[b], Lida P. Hariri, MD, PhD[c], Robert W. Hallowell, MD[b],
Florence K. Keane, MD[d], Michael Lanuti, MD[e], Meghan J. Mooradian, MD[f],
Florian J. Fintelmann, MD[a],*

KEYWORDS

- Interstitial lung disease • Idiopathic pulmonary fibrosis • Lung cancer • Radiation therapy
- Percutaneous thermal ablation

KEY POINTS

- Interstitial lung disease (ILD) including idiopathic pulmonary fibrosis increases the risk of developing lung cancer.
- Diagnosis and staging of lung cancer in patients with ILD require complementary imaging modalities and minimally invasive tissue sampling.
- Treatment of lung cancer in patients with ILD requires multidisciplinary evaluation; well-defined management guidelines are lacking.
- Treatment options include surgery, radiation therapy, percutaneous thermal ablation, and systemic therapy; however, ILD increases the risks and complications associated with each treatment option.

INTRODUCTION

Lung cancer is the second most common malignancy in both men and women and the leading cause of cancer death in the United States.[1] The American Cancer Society expects 236,740 new lung cancer diagnoses in 2022.[1] A retrospective analysis of the SEER-Medicare database found that among 54,453 patients with non-small cell lung cancer (NSCLC), 1.6% had both lung cancer and idiopathic pulmonary fibrosis (IPF).[2]

The gold standard definitive treatment of early-stage NSCLC is anatomic resection and lymph node dissection.[3] In addition to surgery, localized treatment options include radiation therapy and percutaneous thermal ablation with palliative systemic therapies—including chemotherapy and immunotherapy—often used in recurrent and/or metastatic disease. Management of NSCLC at any stage is challenging in patients with underlying interstitial lung disease (ILD), especially IPF. Regardless of the treatment, patients with IPF

[a] Department of Radiology, Division of Thoracic Imaging and Intervention, Massachusetts General Hospital, 55 Fruit Street, Boston, MA 02114, USA; [b] Division of Pulmonology and Critical Care Medicine, Massachusetts General Hospital, 55 Fruit Street, Boston, MA 02114, USA; [c] Department of Pathology, Massachusetts General Hospital, 55 Fruit Street, Boston, MA 02114, USA; [d] Department of Radiation Oncology, Massachusetts General Hospital, 55 Fruit Street, Boston, MA 02114, USA; [e] Department of Surgery, Division of Thoracic Surgery, Massachusetts General Hospital, 55 Fruit Street, Boston, MA 02114, USA; [f] Massachusetts General Hospital Cancer Center, 55 Fruit Street, Boston, MA 02114, USA
* Corresponding author.
E-mail address: fintelmann@mgh.harvard.edu

Radiol Clin N Am 60 (2022) 993–1002
https://doi.org/10.1016/j.rcl.2022.06.010

and NSCLC experience higher treatment-related morbidity and mortality, primarily due to acute exacerbation (AE) of IPF and the risk of respiratory failure.[4] This review discusses the epidemiology of NSCLC in the setting of ILD, strategies for diagnosis and treatment, and the benefits and risks of available treatment options.

Nature of the Problem

Patients with ILD are at increased risk for developing NSCLC.[4] The primary proposed mechanism for cancer development is a proinflammatory state induced by the underlying ILD. Inflammatory cells produce an array of cytokines that stimulate epithelial cell proliferation.[5] This increased proliferation can lead to genetic alterations that can activate oncogenes, transform apoptotic genes, and inhibit tumor suppressor genes.[6,7] In ILD associated lung cancer, *p53* is the most common mutation, whereas epidermal growth factor receptor (*EGFR*) mutations are rare.[6] Although lung cancer is associated with several ILD subtypes, the remainder of this review will focus primarily on IPF and NSCLC.

Although adenocarcinoma is the most common NSCLC histology in the general population, squamous cell carcinoma is the most common subtype in patients with IPF, followed by adenocarcinoma.[8] In a retrospective study of 2,309 cases of lung adenocarcinoma including 44 patients with IPF, the authors reported a high prevalence of invasive mucinous adenocarcinoma in IPF versus non-IPF patients (29.5% vs 3.9%).[9] Unfortunately, the prognosis for patients with NSCLC in the setting of IPF is worse than that of patients with IPF or NSCLC in isolation. Differences in survival following NSCLC diagnosis by the presence or absence of IPF persist even when controlling for baseline lung function.[10,11]

Epidemiology

Accounting for age, sex, and smoking history, the lung cancer risk in patients with IPF is higher compared with the non-IPF population.[4,7] An analysis of 670,258 patients in the national Korean Health Insurance Review and Assessment Service database estimated that the prevalence of NSCLC in patients with IPF was 17.5 times greater than in the general population.[7] Patients with connective tissue disease (CTD)-related ILD are 1.7 to 2 times more likely to develop lung cancer than ILD patients without CTD.[12] The relative risk increase in patients with any ILD ranges from 3.5 to 7.3.[6] In terms of incidence, NSCLC occurs in 10% to 20% of patients with ILD and more than 15% of patients with ILD are likely to die from NSCLC.[6]

A retrospective longitudinal cohort study showed that the cumulative incidence of NSCLC in patients with IPF was 3.3%, 15.4%, and 54.7% at 1, 5, and 10 years of clinical follow-up from time of IPF diagnosis, respectively.[13] A retrospective analysis of 160 patients showed that NSCLC developed on average 888 days following the diagnosis of ILD, including both IPF and non-IPF subtypes.[14] Finally, the prognosis of NSCLC is also worse in patients with IPF compared with patients with NSCLC in the general population (Table 1).[15]

Evaluation

Diagnosing NSCLC in patients with ILD is challenging because the clinical signs of NSCLC overlap with those of ILD and include shortness of breath, cough, fatigue, decreased functional capacity, and weight loss.[16] Radiographic assessment is complex due to the inherent ILD-associated parenchymal abnormalities.

Imaging

There are no consensus guidelines on imaging surveillance for patients with ILD.[17] In a 2017 expert opinion piece in the Lancet, an international multidisciplinary group of authors suggested annual high resolution chest CT (thin axial slices in the supine and prone position, plus inspiratory and expiratory images) and more frequent follow-up for pulmonary nodules measuring up to 8 mm in patients with IPF, as well as fluorodeoxyglucose (FDG) positron emission tomography (PET) computed tomography (CT) for nodules greater than 8 mm.[18]

Table 1
Survival of non-small cell lung cancer by stage and the presence of idiopathic pulmonary fibrosis

Stage	IPF (%)	Non-IPF (%)
IA	59	87
IB	42	74
IIA	43	62
IIB	29	50
IIIA	25	41
IIIB	17	28
IV	17	28

Data from Sato T, Watanabe A, Kondo H, Kanzaki M, Okubo K, Yokoi K, Matsumoto K, Marutsuka T, Shinohara H, Teramukai S, Kishi K, Ebina M, Sugiyama Y, Meinoshin O, Date H; Japanese Association for Chest Surgery. Long-term results and predictors of survival after surgical resection of patients with lung cancer and interstitial lung diseases. J Thorac Cardiovasc Surg. 2015 Jan;149(1):64 to 9, 70.e1-2.

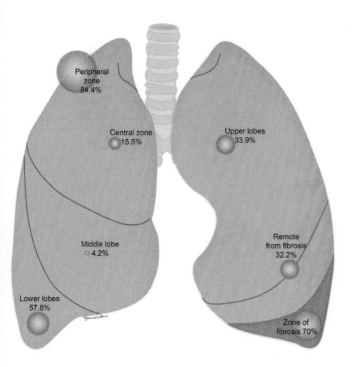

Fig. 1. Distribution of lung cancers in patients with interstitial lung disease.

Peripheral zone 84.4%

Central zone 15.5%

Upper lobes 33.9%

Middle lobe 4.2%

Remote from fibrosis 32.2%

Lower lobes 57.8%

Zone of fibrosis 70%

Retrospective analyses on the radiographic appearance of NSCLC in ILD report that NSCLC is most likely to develop in the peripheral and lower lung zones near or within regions of fibrosis (Fig. 1) as opposed to the upper lobes as seen in the general population.[6,19] Lung cancer will often present as discrete nodules or masses that compress adjacent honeycombing.[20] Comparison to earlier examinations is essential since nodule growth is key for differentiating cancer from reactive intrapulmonary lymph nodes and focal fibrosis.[20] In patients with ILD, median doubling times of 77 days have been reported for NSCLC.[21]

Fibrosis creates architectural distortion of the lung parenchyma, which affects the evaluation of lung nodules and the average tumor size can be underestimated by 10.3% versus 3.2% in controls.[6] The specificity of CT for diagnosing mediastinal nodal metastases is limited because reactive lymph node enlargement is present in 55% to 93% of patients with ILD (Fig. 2).[6] In the setting of IPF, the specificity of CT was only 47% compared with 84% in the general population.[6] Under these circumstances, the addition of FDG PET/CT to contrast-enhanced CT increases the accuracy for identifying mediastinal nodal metastases by 33%.[22] However, specificity for mediastinal nodal metastases is also reduced on PET by the virtue of reactive lymph node enlargement (see Fig. 2).

Additional Testing

Tissue sampling is typically necessary to confirm a suspected diagnosis of NSCLC. CT-guided percutaneous thoracic needle biopsy (PTNB) as well as electromagnetic navigational bronchoscopy (ENB) and endobronchial ultrasound (EBUS)-guided transbronchial needle aspiration (TBNA) allow for minimally invasive lung cancer diagnosis and staging (Table 2).

Sampling of peripheral lung nodules can often be performed via a percutaneous approach. PTNB allows for sampling of lung nodules via fine needle aspiration and core needle biopsy with a high sensitivity for malignancy.[23,24] A retrospective study of 91 PTNB in patients with IPF found the success rates to approach those of patients without ILD and reported diagnostic accuracy, sensitivity, and specificity of 89%, 90%, and 84%; nondiagnostic rate was 34%.[25] However, patients with IPF are generally poor candidates for PTNB due to limited respiratory status and the risk of pneumothorax increases if the biopsy path traverses regions of honeycombing.[25] Additionally, in patients with IPF, biopsy targets are more likely to be in the lower lobes, which are considered more challenging for PTNB due to increased respiratory motion.[23] Overall complication and major complication rates for PTNB in patients

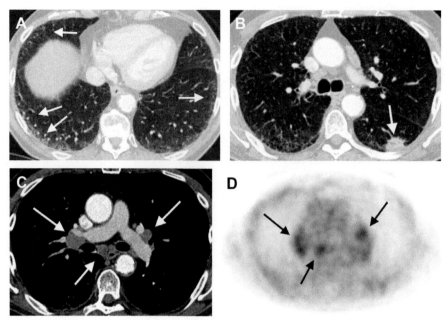

Fig. 2. A 64-year-old male patient with interstitial lung disease and lung cancer. Contrast-enhanced axial CT images demonstrate (*A*) subpleural reticular opacities and mild architectural distortion at the lung bases (*arrows*); (*B*) a solid left lower lobe nodule corresponding to an adenocarcinoma (*arrow*); (*C*) enlarged subcarinal and bilateral hilar lymph nodes (*arrows*). (*D*) Concurrent FDG PET image demonstrates increased uptake in enlarged lymph nodes (*arrows*) but no malignant cells were found at subsequent resection.

Table 2 Noninvasive and invasive strategies for diagnosing and staging lung cancer in the setting of interstitial lung disease	
Noninvasive	**CT** • Diagnosis is challenging due to background architectural distortion • Lung cancer in patients with IPF more often peripheral and in the lower lung zone • Nodules often occur at fibrotic zone of transition and demonstrate rapid growth • Reactive lymph node enlargement common in interstitial lung disease and may or may not represent metastases FDG PET/CT **FDG PET/CT** • Increased sensitivity for diagnosing local and distant metastases • Reactive lymph nodes often FDG avid
Invasive	**CT-guided PTNB** • Outpatient procedure performed with moderate sedation • Ideal for peripheral lesions • Higher risk in IPF (particularly for pneumothorax) • Similar success rate for non-IPF and IPF patients **ENB and EBUS TBNA** • Outpatient procedure performed under general anesthesia • EBUS ideal for central lesions and mediastinal lymph nodes; ENB able to target more peripheral lesions • Lower risk in IPF relative to PTNB • Limited data comparing success in patients without and with ILD

CT, computed tomography; EBUS, endobronchial ultrasound; ENB, electromagnetic navigational bronchoscopy; FDG, fluorodeoxyglucose; ILD, interstitial lung disease; IPF, idiopathic pulmonary fibrosis; PTNB, percutaneous thoracic needle biopsy; TBNA, transbronchial needle aspiration.

with IPF have been reported as high (51% and 12%, respectively).[25]

EBUS TBNA can sample mediastinal lymph nodes adjacent to the bronchial tree.[26] In an analysis of 1,299 patients with known or suspected NSCLC, EBUS TBNA had a sensitivity of 90% for diagnosing nodal metastases in the general population.[27] In a review of 15 trials including 1,033 biopsied nodules, ENB demonstrated overall diagnostic accuracy of 73.9% and a 71.1% sensitivity in the general population.[28] Data in the setting of ILD are lacking.

Approach

Treating NSCLC in patients with ILD is challenging and requires multidisciplinary evaluation. Potential local and/or systemic options include surgical resection, radiation therapy, percutaneous thermal ablation, and systemic therapy. ILD increases the risks associated with each treatment option, especially AE of the underlying ILD.

Surgery

Lobectomy with mediastinal lymph node dissection remains the oncologic gold standard for the treatment of early-stage NSCLC (Table 3).[3] A retrospective study of 711 patients with NSCLC documented increased postoperative morbidity and mortality for patients with versus without IPF (26% vs 9.1% and 8% vs 0.8%, respectively).[29] ILD may preclude lobectomy because patients often have insufficient respiratory reserve to tolerate the permanent reduction in lung function.

A retrospective study of 1,763 patients with ILD and NSCLC treated with lobectomy or sublobar resection documented AE in 9.3% of cases and mortality up to 43.9%.[30] The risk of postoperative AE increases with age greater than 75 years, IPF versus other types of ILD, and honeycombing on CT.[6] Other CT findings predictive of AE include ground glass opacities occupying more than 5% of the lungs, any consolidation, and main pulmonary artery diameter greater than 28 mm.[31]

Surgical technique and medical management can influence the risk of AE. For example, intraoperative time greater than 4 hours and extent of lung resection increase the risk of AE.[6] In a retrospective analysis of 101 patients with IPF and lung cancer (NSCLC and SCLC), the authors reported AE in 10% of patients following lobectomy or sublobar resection.[11] Another retrospective study of 101 patients observed a 20% rate of AE following pneumonectomy and lobectomy but none following sublobar resection.[32] Perioperative strategies investigated to reduce the risk of AE include delivery of lower oxygen concentrations, avoidance of intraoperative lung hyperinflation with careful attention to barotrauma and mean airway pressures, corticosteroids, and prophylactic antibiotics to reduce the risk of pneumonia.[33] Antifibrotic drugs also seem to affect the incidence of postoperative AE in patients with IPF and NSCLC: AE incidence was 3.2% in patients receiving pirfenidone after both wedge and anatomic resections compared with 21.1% in patients not receiving pirfenidone.[34]

Table 3
Comparison of available lung cancer treatments in the setting of interstitial lung disease

Treatment	Definitive Therapy?	Benefits	Risk of acute exacerbation	Unique Risks
Surgery	Yes	Gold standard	0%–20%, increases with extent of resection and perioperative factors	Most invasive; permanent reduction in lung function
Stereotactic body radiotherapy	Yes	Noninvasive	18%–20.5%	Pneumonitis; can reduce lung function
Percutaneous thermal ablation	Yes	Minimally invasive, no permanent decrease in lung function (in absence of acute exacerbation)	18%	Less invasive and risky than surgery
Systemic therapy	No	Noninvasive	13%–50%	Immunosuppression from certain agents/regimens

Beyond the acute postoperative period, the prognosis of patients with IPF and NSCLC remains poor. The median overall survival following lobar and sublobar resection of NSCLC in patients with IPF is 42 vs 90 months for patients without IPF.[11] A systemic review of NSCLC outcomes in the setting of ILD reported that 3-year overall survival following surgical resection was 31% to 75% for patients with ILD vs 79% to 95% for patients without ILD.[35] A retrospective analysis of 1,763 patients with stage IA NSCLC and IPF documented 5-year overall survival of 33.2% after wedge resection, 61.0% after segmentectomy, and 68.4% after lobectomy.[15]

Radiation therapy

Radiation therapy with stereotactic body radiation therapy (SBRT) is the standard of care for treatment of early-stage NSCLC in patients who are not surgical candidates (see **Table 3**).[36] However, for patients with ILD, SBRT is associated with an increased risk of toxicity, which presents as radiation pneumonitis (RP).[35] Retrospective data on the use of radiotherapy in patients with ILD are limited because studies primarily included patients with subclinical ILD, defined as radiographic characteristics consistent with ILD on pretreatment imaging, or, less commonly, patients with a history of ILD but not on active treatment. In a retrospective study of 101 patients with IPF and lung cancer (NSCLC and SCLC), RP occurred in 18% of patients following SBRT.[11] A single-center retrospective study of 537 patients including 39 patients with ILD found that the risk of RP was significantly higher in patients with ILD (including both IPF and non-IPF subtypes) vs patients without ILD (grade ≥2, 20.5% vs 5.8%; grade ≥3, 10.3% vs 1.0%).[37] In a retrospective study of 242 patients with stage I NSCLC and ILD treated with SBRT, the authors reported grade 3 to 5 and grade 5 RP in 12.4% and 6.9% of patients, respectively.[38] In a retrospective analysis of 71 metastatic or primary tumors treated with SBRT, subclinical ILD was the only factor significantly associated with grade 2 to 5 RP.[39] RP was not associated with the location of ILD (within vs outside radiated lung), age, sex, lobe, and number of SBRT fractions. In this study, 2 of 4 patients with honeycombing on CT died of grade 5 RP.[39]

Charged particle therapy, such as proton beam therapy (PBT), is less widely used than SBRT.[40] PBT is characterized by rapid dose fall-off, which may minimize exposure of normal tissues to radiotherapy, an appealing potential option in patients with IPF. In a retrospective study including 30 patients with early-stage NSCLC and IPF treated with either PBT or SBRT, the authors found that severe treatment-related pulmonary complications were less common with PBT (12.5% vs 40.9%).[41] There were 4 SBRT-related deaths and no PBT-related deaths and better 1-year overall survival for PBT (50% vs 26%).[41] In a retrospective single-center study of 16 patients with NSCLC treated with PBT, RP occurred in 19.8% of patients with IPF.[42] There was one case of grade 5 RP (6.3%).

Treatment of patients with locally advanced NSCLC is especially complex, given the large treatment fields required to encompass both the primary tumor and involved lymph nodes. In a series of 87 patients with subclinical ILD including 61 patients with Stage III NSCLC, the rate of grade 2 or greater RP was 51.7%.[43]

Selection of patients with ILD and NSCLC for the treatment with radiotherapy is complex and requires multidisciplinary evaluation. In a retrospective study including 100 patient with NSCLC stages I–III, the authors determined that patients were 6.9 times more likely to experience at least grade 2 RP if pretreatment FDG PET/CT demonstrated SUV_{95} greater than 1.5 for all lung parenchyma.[44] In a series of patients with Stage III NSCLC, the rate of grade 3 or greater RP was higher in patients with subclinical ILD involving 25% or greater of lung volume.[43]

Percutaneous image-guided thermal ablation

Percutaneous image-guided thermal ablation (IGTA) is a minimally invasive option for definitive treatment of early-stage NSCLC using either heat-based modalities (radiofrequency ablation [RFA], microwave ablation [MWA]) or cryoablation (**Fig. 3**).[36,45] In the setting of ILD, IGTA is attractive because long-term pulmonary function is preserved as long as no AE occurs (see **Table 2**). Moreover, local control of IGTA is comparable with sublobar resection and radiation therapy in the general population.[46,47]

As with other lung cancer treatments in patients with ILD, AE is of paramount concern. Data on IGTA following treatment of NSCLC in patients with ILD are limited. A retrospective analysis of 420 patients including 42 patients with ILD who underwent RFA for either NSCLC or pulmonary metastases reported that 3 of 4 deaths were due to AE of ILD resulting in 7.1% morality for patients with preexisting ILD.[48] In a systematic review including 3 retrospective studies and a total of 46 inoperable patients treated with RFA for early-stage NSCLC or oligo metastases, mortality was 8.7% and ILD-specific toxicity of 25%.[35] The same review found that although ILD-specific toxicity was the same for RFA and SBRT, mortality associated with RFA was 45% lower compared with SBRT.

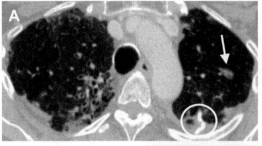
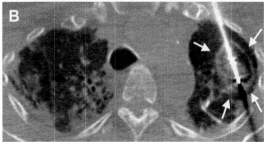
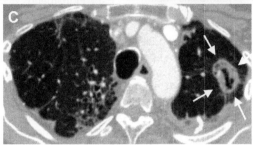

Fig. 3. An 83-year-old woman with interstitial lung disease and recurrent lung cancer status after left upper lobe wedge resection. (*A*) Contrast-enhanced axial CT image demonstrates an enlarging part solid left upper lobe nodule (*arrow*) anterior to and distinct from a chain suture (*circle*), consistent with a metachronous primary lung cancer. (*B*) Intraprocedural CT image shows percutaneous cryoablation probe in the nodule and ice ball formation (*arrows*). (*C*) Contrast-enhanced axial CT image 1 month after cryoablation demonstrates expected appearance of the treatment zone (*arrows*) that extends beyond the margins of the target. Cavitation after thermal ablation does not indicate disease progression, and the patient did not develop AE.

In the general population, percutaneous cryoablation of lung tumors is associated with significantly lower morbidity compared with RFA and MWA, suggesting it may be an appealing potential treatment option for NSCLC in patients with IPF.[49] A 2017 conference abstract reported AE and death in 2 of 11 patients (18%) with IPF following percutaneous cryoablation of T1N0M0 NSCLC with oral corticosteroids and chest tube as predictors of AE and death.[50] However, no detailed report is available, and the future role of cryoablation in the management of patients in with lung cancer and ILD remains to be determined.

Systemic therapy
Treatment of metastatic or unresectable NSCLC centers on the use of systemic therapy. The treatment paradigm continues to evolve since the advent of immune checkpoint inhibitors (ICIs), particularly programmed cell death 1 inhibitors (PD-1/PD-1L1 inhibitors).

Before the advent of ICIs, patients received first-line chemotherapy with a platinum-based doublet with carboplatin or cisplatin paired with a histology-based partner such as pemetrexed, paclitaxel, docetaxel, or etoposide.[6] In the setting of ILD, the optimal chemotherapy regimen is uncertain and toxicity is an important consideration.

Pulmonary toxicity has been reported for gemcitabine, taxanes, and topoisomerase-1 inhibitors.[16] In a retrospective study of 69 patients with IPF and lung cancer treated with cytotoxic chemotherapy, 30% of patients developed AE while only 8% of patients with non-IPF subtype of ILD experienced AE.[51] In another retrospective study of 101 patients with IPF and either NSCLC or SCLC, AE occurred in 13% of patients treated with cytotoxic chemotherapy.[11] Interestingly, the risk of AE not only varies with subtype of ILD but also varies with cancer histology: A retrospective analysis of 122 patients reported AE after first-line therapy for NSCLC in 31% compared with 63% patients with SCLC.[51] Increased FDG avidity in the contralateral lung on FDG PET/CT correlates with the risk of chemotherapy-related AE and may help identify high-risk patients.[52] Overall, these data highlight the value of pretreatment imaging and histologic diagnosis to optimize treatment strategy while also reducing morbidity.

Standard treatment of patients with locally advanced, inoperable NSCLC consists of both chemoradiotherapy and radiotherapy, which increase the risk of pneumonitis. A retrospective study of 37 patients found that 46% of patients with underlying ILD treated with either sequential or concurrent radiotherapy developed at least grade 3 pneumonitis within 1 year following completion of radiation therapy and the incidence was higher in patients with IPF.[53] A review from the International Association for the Study of Lung Cancer Advanced Radiation Technology Committee concluded that the risks of severe side effects from concurrent or sequential chemoradiotherapy are highest for patients with IPF and therefore these patients should be carefully selected.[54]

ICIs have been approved as a first-line therapy option for patients with metastatic NSCLC with or without chemotherapy, regardless of PD-1/L1 tumor proportion score.[55] Compared with chemotherapy, PD-1/PD-1L1 inhibitors have been associated with an increased pneumonitis risk.[56] However, data regarding the safety of ICIs in patients with ILD is limited as patients with preexisting ILD were excluded from initial clinical trials using ICIs. In a retrospective case series of 41 patients (73% with lung cancer) with ILD who received PD-1 therapy, 7.3% developed ICI-related pneumonitis.[57] At 1 year, more patients (87%) died from cancer or other non-ILD-related causes than from respiratory failure secondary to ILD or pneumonitis (13%).[57]

It is important to consider if ILD-directed therapies could mitigate the risk of AE in a patient with ILD and NSCLC. The antifibrotic agent nintedanib has been shown to decrease the risk of AE of IPF in patients without lung cancer.[58] The LUME-Lung 1 and LUME-Lung 2 trials assessed the efficacy of nintedanib in combination with cytotoxic chemotherapy for the treatment of advanced NSCLC. Whether or not nintedanib may have a future role in the management of patients in with lung cancer and ILD remains to be determined.

SUMMARY

In the setting of ILD, patients are at increased risk for lung cancer. The diagnosis and treatment of lung cancer at any stage is challenging in the setting of ILD, especially in patients with IPF. Given the poor prognosis of certain ILDs, especially IPF, and the increased morbidity and mortality associated with all lung cancer treatments in the setting of ILD, each patient requires multidisciplinary evaluation and a personalized treatment plan tailored to their goals of care.

CLINICS CARE POINTS

- Lung cancer in the setting of ILD requires multidisciplinary evaluation because treatment guidelines are not well defined.
- Lung cancer in the setting of ILD occurs more commonly in the lower lobes, within or along regions of fibrosis.
- In the setting of ILD, reactive lymphadenopathy decreases the accuracy of imaging for the detection of nodal metastases.

- Patients with ILD, especially IPF, are at risk for AE following lung cancer treatment with surgery, radiation, thermal ablation, and systemic therapy.

CONFLICTS OF INTEREST

F.J. Fintelmann and M.J. Mooradian receive research funding from the William M. Wood Foundation. M.J. Mooradian has served as a consultant/received honorarium from AstraZeneca, Bristol Myers Squibb, Istari Oncology, Nektar Therapeutics, and Immunai. S.B. Montesi is funded by NIH/NHLBI [K23HL15033] and receives research funding from Merck, United Therapeutics and Pliant Therapeutics, consulting fees from Dev-Pro Biopharma, Gilead Sciences, and Roche, and royalties form Wolters Kluwer. L.P. Hariri receives research funding from Boehringer Ingelheim and has received personal consulting fees from Boehringer Ingelheim, Pliant Therapeutics, Bioclinica and Biogen Idec. R.W. Hallowell has received personal consulting fees from Boehringer Ingelheim, Genentech, Dynamed, and Wolters Kluwer and has received indirect clinical research funding from Boehringer Ingelheim, Regeneron, and Galapagos. He has served on an advisory board for Boehringer Ingelheim. The other authors declare no relevant conflicts of interest.

REFERENCES

1. Key statistics for lung cancer. In: American cancer society. Available at: Cancer.org. Accessed January 15, 2022.
2. Whittaker Brown SA, Padilla M, Mhango G, et al. Outcomes of older patients with pulmonary fibrosis and non-small cell lung cancer. Ann Am Thorac Soc 2019;16(8):1034–40.
3. Hartwig MG, D'Amico TA. Thoracoscopic lobectomy: the gold standard for early-stage lung cancer? Ann Thorac Surg 2010;89(6):S2098–101.
4. Brown SAW, Dobelle M, Padilla M, et al. Idiopathic pulmonary fibrosis and lung cancer. a systematic review and meta-analysis. Ann Am Thorac Soc 2019; 16(8):1041–51.
5. Joo S, Kim DK, Sim HJ, et al. Clinical results of sublobar resection versus lobectomy or more extensive resection for lung cancer patients with idiopathic pulmonary fibrosis. J Thorac Dis 2016;8(5):977–84.
6. Naccache JM, Gibiot Q, Monnet I, et al. Lung cancer and interstitial lung disease: a literature review. J Thorac Dis 2018;10(6):3829–44.
7. Jung HI, Park JS, Lee MY, et al. Prevalence of lung cancer in patients with interstitial lung disease is higher than in those with chronic obstructive

pulmonary disease. Medicine (Baltimore) 2018; 97(11):e0071.

8. Song MJ, Kim DJ, Paik HC, et al. Impact of idiopathic pulmonary fibrosis on recurrence after surgical treatment for stage I–III non-small cell lung cancer. PLoS One 2020;15(6):e0235126.

9. Masai K, Tsuta K, Motoi N, et al. Clinicopathological, immunohistochemical, and genetic features of primary lung adenocarcinoma occurring in the setting of usual interstitial pneumonia pattern. J Thorac Oncol 2016;11(12):2141–9.

10. Yoon JH, Nouraie M, Chen X, et al. Characteristics of lung cancer among patients with idiopathic pulmonary fibrosis and interstitial lung disease – analysis of institutional and population data. Respir Res 2018;19(1):195.

11. Kim HC, Lee S, Song JW. Impact of idiopathic pulmonary fibrosis on clinical outcomes of lung cancer patients. Sci Rep 2021;11(1):8312.

12. Choi WI, Lee DY, Choi HG, et al. Lung Cancer development and mortality in interstitial lung disease with and without connective tissue diseases: a five-year Nationwide population-based study. Respir Res 2019;20(1):117.

13. Ozawa Y, Suda T, Naito T, et al. Cumulative incidence of and predictive factors for lung cancer in IPF. Respirology 2009;14(5):723–8.

14. Barczi E, Nagy T, Starobinski L, et al. Impact of interstitial lung disease and simultaneous lung cancer on therapeutic possibilities and survival. Thorac Cancer 2020;11(7):1911–7.

15. Sato T, Watanabe A, Kondo H, et al. Long-term results and predictors of survival after surgical resection of patients with lung cancer and interstitial lung diseases. J Thorac Cardiovasc Surg 2015; 149(1):64–9, 70.e1-2.

16. Ryerson Christopher. Evaluation and management of lung cancer in patients with interstitial lung disease. In: King T, editor. UpToDate. 2021. Available at: https://www.uptodate.com/contents/evaluation-and-management-of-lung-cancer-in-patients-with-interstitial-lung-disease/print 2021. Accessed September 12, 2021.

17. Nambiar AM, Walker CM, Sparks JA. Monitoring and management of fibrosing interstitial lung diseases: a narrative review for practicing clinicians. Ther Adv Respir Dis 2021;15. 17534666211039772.

18. Tzouvelekis A, Spagnolo P, Bonella F, et al. Patients with IPF and lung cancer: diagnosis and management. Lancet Respir Med 2018;6(2):86–8.

19. Lee KJ, Chung MP, Kim YW, et al. Prevalence, risk factors and survival of lung cancer in the idiopathic pulmonary fibrosis: Idiopathic pulmonary fibrosis with lung cancer. Thorac Cancer 2012;3(2):150–5.

20. Lloyd CR, Walsh SLF, Hansell DM. High-resolution CT of complications of idiopathic fibrotic lung disease. Br J Radiol 2011;84(1003):581–92. https://doi.org/10.1259/bjr/65090500.

21. Oh SY, Kim MY, Kim JE, et al. Evolving early lung cancers detected during follow-up of idiopathic interstitial pneumonia: serial CT features. AJR Am J Roentgenol 2015;204(6):1190–6. https://doi.org/10.2214/AJR.14.13587.

22. Jeon TY, Lee KS, Yi CA, et al. Incremental value of PET/CT over ct for mediastinal nodal staging of non–small cell lung cancer: comparison between patients with and without idiopathic pulmonary fibrosis. Am J Roentgenol 2010;195(2):370–6.

23. Bourgouin PP, Rodriguez KJ, Fintelmann FJ. Image-guided percutaneous lung needle biopsy: how we do it. Tech Vasc Interv Radiol 2021;24(3):100770.

24. Fintelmann FJ, Troschel FM, Kuklinski MW, et al. Safety and success of repeat lung needle biopsies in patients with epidermal growth factor receptor-mutant lung cancer. Oncologist 2019;24(12): 1570–6.

25. Shin YJ, Yun G, Yoon SH, et al. Accuracy and complications of percutaneous transthoracic needle lung biopsy for the diagnosis of malignancy in patients with idiopathic pulmonary fibrosis. Eur Radiol 2021;31(12):9000–11.

26. Green DB, Groner LK, Lee JJ, et al. Overview of interventional pulmonology for radiologists. RadioGraphics 2021;41(7):1916–35.

27. Navani N, Nankivell M, Lawrence DR, et al. Lung cancer diagnosis and staging with endobronchial ultrasound-guided transbronchial needle aspiration compared with conventional approaches: an open-label, pragmatic, randomised controlled trial. Lancet Respir Med 2015;3(4):282–9.

28. Gex G, Pralong JA, Combescure C, et al. Diagnostic yield and safety of electromagnetic navigation bronchoscopy for lung nodules: a systematic review and meta-analysis. Respir Int Rev Thorac Dis 2014;87(2): 165–76.

29. Kawasaki H, Nagai K, Yoshida J, et al. Postoperative morbidity, mortality, and survival in lung cancer associated with idiopathic pulmonary fibrosis. J Surg Oncol 2002;81(1):33–7.

30. Sato T, Teramukai S, Kondo H, et al. Impact and predictors of acute exacerbation of interstitial lung diseases after pulmonary resection for lung cancer. J Thorac Cardiovasc Surg 2014;147(5):1604–11.e3.

31. Ozawa Y, Shibamoto Y, Hiroshima M, et al. Preoperative CT findings for predicting acute exacerbation of interstitial pneumonia after lung cancer surgery: a multicenter case-control study. Am J Roentgenol 2021;217(4):859–69.

32. Okamoto T, Gotoh M, Masuya D, et al. Clinical analysis of interstitial pneumonia after surgery for lung cancer. Jpn J Thorac Cardiovasc Surg 2004;52(7): 323–9.

33. Watanabe A, Higami T, Ohori S, et al. Is lung cancer resection indicated in patients with idiopathic pulmonary fibrosis? J Thorac Cardiovasc Surg 2008; 136(5):1357–63.e1-2.

34. Iwata T, Yoshida S, Fujiwara T, et al. Effect of Perioperative Pirfenidone Treatment in Lung Cancer Patients With Idiopathic Pulmonary Fibrosis. Ann Thorac Surg 2016;102(6):1905–10.

35. Chen H, Senan S, Nossent EJ, et al. Treatment-related toxicity in patients with early-stage non-small cell lung cancer and coexisting interstitial lung disease: a systematic review. Int J Radiat Oncol 2017; 98(3):622–31.

36. National Comprehensive Cancer Network. Non-small cell lung cancer (Version 1.2022). Available at: https://www.nccn.org/guidelines/guidelines-detail?category=1&id=1450. Accessed February 18, 2022.

37. Glick D, Lyen S, Kandel S, et al. Impact of pretreatment interstitial lung disease on radiation pneumonitis and survival in patients treated with lung stereotactic body radiation therapy (SBRT). Clin Lung Cancer 2018;19(2):e219–26.

38. Onishi H, Yamashita H, Shioyama Y, et al. stereotactic body radiation therapy for patients with pulmonary interstitial change: high incidence of fatal radiation pneumonitis in a retrospective multi-institutional study. Cancers 2018;10(8):257.

39. Okubo M, Itonaga T, Saito T, et al. Predicting risk factors for radiation pneumonitis after stereotactic body radiation therapy for primary or metastatic lung tumours. Br J Radiol 2017;90(1073):20160508.

40. Simone CB, Rengan R. The Use of Proton Therapy in the Treatment of Lung Cancers. Cancer J 2014; 20(6):427–32.

41. Kim H, Pyo H, Noh JM, et al. Preliminary result of definitive radiotherapy in patients with non-small cell lung cancer who have underlying idiopathic pulmonary fibrosis: comparison between X-ray and proton therapy. Radiat Oncol 2019;14(1):19.

42. Ono T, Hareyama M, Nakamura T, et al. The clinical results of proton beam therapy in patients with idiopathic pulmonary fibrosis: a single center experience. Radiat Oncol 2016;11(1):56.

43. Li F, Liu H, Wu H, et al. Risk factors for radiation pneumonitis in lung cancer patients with subclinical interstitial lung disease after thoracic radiation therapy. Radiat Oncol 2021;16(1):70.

44. Castillo R, Pham N, Ansari S, et al. Pre-radiotherapy FDG PET predicts radiation pneumonitis in lung cancer. Radiat Oncol Lond Engl 2014;9:74. https://doi.org/10.1186/1748-717X-9-74.

45. Murphy MC, Wrobel MM, Fisher DA, et al. Update on Image-Guided Thermal Lung Ablation: Society Guidelines, Therapeutic Alternatives, and Postablation Imaging Findings. AJR Am J Radiol 2022;(June):1–15. https://doi.org/10.2214/AJR.21.27099.

46. Kwan SW, Mortell KE, Talenfeld AD, et al. thermal ablation matches sublobar resection outcomes in older patients with early-stage non–small cell lung cancer. J Vasc Interv Radiol 2014;25(1):1–9.e1.

47. Zemlyak A, Moore WH, Bilfinger TV. Comparison of survival after sublobar resections and ablative therapies for stage I non–small cell lung cancer. J Am Coll Surg 2010;211(1):68–72.

48. Kashima M, Yamakado K, Takaki H, et al. Complications after 1000 lung radiofrequency ablation sessions in 420 patients: a single center's experiences. Am J Roentgenol 2011;197(4):W576–80.

49. Jiang B, Mcclure MA, Chen T, et al. Efficacy and safety of thermal ablation of lung malignancies: A Network meta-analysis. Ann Thorac Med 2018; 13(4):243–50.

50. Ohtsuka T, Asakura K, Masai K, et al. OA12.03 Percutaneous cryoablation for lung cancer patients for whom surgery or radiotherapy is contraindicated due to idiopathic pulmonary fibrosis. J Thorac Oncol 2017;12(1):S290.

51. Kenmotsu H, Naito T, Kimura M, et al. the risk of cytotoxic chemotherapy-related exacerbation of interstitial lung disease with lung cancer. J Thorac Oncol 2011;6(7):1242–6. https://doi.org/10.1097/JTO.0b013e318216ee6b.

52. Akaike K, Saruwatari K, Oda S, et al. Predictive value of 18F-FDG PET/CT for acute exacerbation of interstitial lung disease in patients with lung cancer and interstitial lung disease treated with chemotherapy. Int J Clin Oncol 2020;25(4):681–90.

53. Kobayashi H, Naito T, Omae K, et al. Impact of interstitial lung disease classification on the development of acute exacerbation of interstitial lung disease and prognosis in patients with stage iii non-small-cell lung cancer and interstitial lung disease treated with chemoradiotherapy. J Cancer 2018;9(11):2054–60.

54. Goodman CD, Nijman SFM, Senan S, et al. A primer on interstitial lung disease and thoracic radiation. J Thorac Oncol 2020;15(6):902–13.

55. Wang GX, Kurra V, Gainor JF, et al. immune checkpoint inhibitor cancer therapy: spectrum of imaging findings. Radiogr Rev Publ Radiol Soc N Am Inc 2017;37(7):2132–44.

56. Su Q, Zhu EC, Wu J Bo, et al. Risk of pneumonitis and pneumonia associated with immune checkpoint inhibitors for solid tumors: a systematic review and meta-analysis. Front Immunol 2019;10:108.

57. Dobre IA, Frank AJ, D'Silva KM, et al. Outcomes of patients with interstitial lung disease receiving programmed cell death 1 inhibitors: a retrospective case series. Clin Lung Cancer 2021;22(5):e738–44.

58. Richeldi L, du Bois RM, Raghu G, et al. Efficacy and safety of nintedanib in idiopathic pulmonary fibrosis. N Engl J Med 2014;370(22):2071–82.

Advances in Imaging of the ChILD – Childhood Interstitial Lung Disease

Olivia DiPrete, MD[a], Abbey J. Winant, MD[b], Sara O. Vargas, MD[c],
Vanessa Rameh, MD[b], Apeksha Chaturvedi, MD[d],
Edward Y. Lee, MD, MPH[b],*

KEYWORDS

- Interstitial lung disease • Diffuse lung disease • New classification system • Imaging techniques
- Children • Pediatric patients

KEY POINTS

- There has been substantial improvement in the understanding of childhood interstitial lung disease (chILD) over the past several years, largely due to improved clinical, imaging, and pathologic correlation for diagnosis.
- These advances have led to a new structured classification system for chILD, which categorizes infant ILD by etiology and childhood ILD by disorders of the immunocompetent and immunocompromised host.
- The crucial role of imaging in the diagnosis of chILD is to confirm its presence, characterize its extent and distribution, narrow the differential diagnosis, and suggest an optimal biopsy site.
- Due to substantial morbidity and mortality associated with chILD, it is essential for radiologists to be familiar with this spectrum of disorders and associated imaging characteristics to aid in prompt diagnosis and initiation of appropriate treatment.

INTRODUCTION

Interstitial (diffuse) lung disease of infants and children (also known as chILD) encompasses a heterogeneous group of individually rare parenchymal lung disorders with a wide range of etiologies including developmental, genetic, infectious, inflammatory, and reactive. The most common clinical signs and symptoms in affected infants include dyspnea, tachypnea, crackles, and hypoxemia.[1,2] Older children may present similarly or may have a more insidious presentation with exercise intolerance and failure to thrive.[3] Many of these diseases result in substantial morbidity and mortality, making prompt and accurate diagnosis essential for optimal patient care.

Although chILD was previously associated with diagnostic challenges due to limited evidence-based information, there has been considerable improvement in the understanding of pediatric interstitial lung disease over the past several years, mostly due to improved thoracoscopic lung biopsy techniques, established pathologic criteria for diagnosis, and a new structured classification system.[1,2,4] A multidisciplinary approach to diagnosis, including clinical, imaging, and pathologic correlation, is essential for accurate and reproducible diagnosis, and the critical role of imaging involves characterizing or confirming the disorder, generating a differential diagnosis, and guiding location for lung biopsy. Reiterative review of imaging findings to correlate with any subsequent relevant

---

[a] Department of Radiology, Beth Israel Deaconess Medical Center, 330 Brookline Avenue, Boston, MA 02115, USA; [b] Department of Radiology, Boston Children's Hospital, 300 Longwood Avenue, Boston, MA 02115, USA; [c] Department of Pathology, Boston Children's Hospital, 300 Longwood Avenue, Boston, MA 02115, USA; [d] Department of Imaging Sciences, University of Rochester Medical Center, 601 Elmwood Avenue, Rochester, NY 14642, USA
* Corresponding author.
E-mail address: Edward.Lee@childrens.harvard.edu

Radiol Clin N Am 60 (2022) 1003–1020
https://doi.org/10.1016/j.rcl.2022.06.008
0033-8389/22/© 2022 Elsevier Inc. All rights reserved.

clinical, pathologic, or genetic data can also be helpful.

In this review, the epidemiology, diagnostic challenges, imaging techniques, and new classification system of chILD, with a focus on the characteristic imaging findings of various clinically important pediatric interstitial (diffuse) lung disorders, are presented.

EPIDEMIOLOGY OF PEDIATRIC INTERSTITIAL LUNG DISEASE

While the true prevalence of interstitial (diffuse) lung disease in the pediatric population is not definitely known, estimates range from 0.13 cases/100,000 children younger than 17 years to 16.2 cases/100,000 children younger than 15 years.[3,5] However, these estimates are based on data from several years ago and, therefore, likely substantially underestimate the true prevalence in light of the recently developed classification system, increased use of lung biopsy, and increased recognition of interstitial lung disease in the pediatric population. Some studies have shown that infants and young children are disproportionately affected, with estimates of 31% to 68% of cases affecting patients less than 2 years.[5]

CHALLENGES RELATED TO PEDIATRIC INTERSTITIAL LUNG DISEASE

There are a few major challenges to the early and accurate diagnosis of chILD. First, the decreased prevalence of chILD in the pediatric population, as compared with adult interstitial lung disease, makes chILD less familiar to clinicians and radiologists. Additionally, pediatric interstitial lung disease is characterized by often subtle, nonspecific, and highly variable clinical manifestations with a lack of pathognomonic clinical or laboratory diagnostic criteria. Pathologic characterization presents another challenge, as many lung biopsies show nonspecific findings or features that overlap among more than one category of disease classification. Furthermore, there are persistent uncertainties regarding the natural history, prognostic indicators, and specific host factors in the pathogenesis of interstitial lung disease in infants and children.

IMAGING TECHNIQUES

Currently, 2 major imaging modalities for evaluating pediatric interstitial lung disease are chest radiography (CXR) and computed tomography (CT) with recent advances in magnetic resonance imaging (MRI), which are discussed in the following section.

Chest Radiography

Due to its relatively low radiation dose and cost, wide availability, and ease of performance, chest radiography is typically the preferred initial (ie, screening) imaging modality in infants and children with suspected ILD. Although it lacks specificity and sensitivity for the definitive diagnosis of chILD, chest radiography remains useful for initial screening and follow-up of previously characterized disease, as most infants and children with ILD often have abnormalities on chest radiographs (Fig. 1).[1,5] However, these abnormalities are usually nonspecific and further characterization with CT is often necessary for complete assessment.[3,5,6]

Computed Tomography

CT, usually performed as high-resolution CT (HRCT) without intravenous contrast, has been the gold standard imaging modality for the evaluation of chILD due to its superior anatomic detail and use of multiplanar reformats and 3D reconstructions.[4] The major role of CT is to confirm the presence of ILD, characterize its extent and distribution, identify features specific to certain disorders, and suggest an optimal biopsy site (Fig. 2A).[2,5] There are a variety of CT imaging manifestations of chILD, including nodules, ground-glass opacities (GGO), consolidations, air trapping, cysts, septal thickening, linear and reticular markings, and traction bronchiectasis.[2] Technologic advances in recent years allow volumetric high-resolution CT of the entire chest to be performed in a fraction of a second, decreasing the need for sedation to minimize respiratory motion in infants

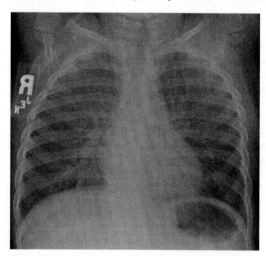

Fig. 1. Congenital surfactant deficiency (ABCA3 mutation) in a 28-month-old male. Chest radiograph shows bilateral diffuse interstitial thickening, ground-glass opacification, and multiple tiny cysts.

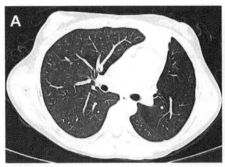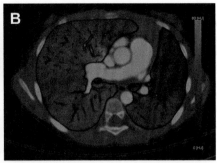

Fig. 2. Congenital lung hypoplasia in a 9-year-old female who presented with shortness of breath. (*A*) Axial lung window CT image shows an asymmetrically small left lung with attenuated vessels and airways. (*B*) Axial iodine perfusion CT image demonstrates decreased blood flow (darker) reflecting relative hypoperfusion to the hypoplastic left lung.

and young children.[2,4] However, if sedation and anesthesia with controlled breathing are required for adequate CT evaluation, lung recruitment maneuvers should be performed to prevent rapid accumulation of dependent atelectasis which can obscure underlying pathology.[4] The recent development of dual-energy computed tomography (DECT), which can also provide vital information on lung perfusion with the postprocessed iodine map, has also opened the door for evaluating both anatomic (ie, structural) and functional (ie, perfusion) abnormalities associated with chILD in the pediatric population (**Fig. 2**B).

Magnetic Resonance Imaging

Although MRI is often favored in children due to its lack of ionizing radiation, its use in the evaluation of chILD is limited due to respiratory motion artifact and inferior spatial resolution compared with CT. While there is an overall paucity of information on the efficacy of MRI for detecting abnormalities of pediatric ILD, a recent study by Sodhi and colleagues demonstrated that in comparison to HRCT, 3T MRI can also detect consolidation, parenchymal bands, and fissural thickening well in children with ILD.[7] However, the detection of other distinguishing diagnostic features, such as septal thickening, GGO, nodules, and cysts, was low by MRI compared with CT.[5,7] Therefore, the clinical utility of MRI remains limited in the initial evaluation of chILD; however, MRI may be useful for follow-up evaluation in infants and children with already known and at least moderate degree of chILD (**Fig. 3**).

NEW PEDIATRIC INTERSTITIAL LUNG DISEASE CLASSIFICATION

As the substantial clinicopathologic differences between adult and pediatric ILD became increasingly understood, particularly the large subset of genetic and heritable disorders in pediatric ILD, it has become clear that the adult ILD classification system is not applicable to chILD. In addition, substantial confusion surrounding the description and classification of pediatric ILD in prior classification systems has led to the development of a new classification system, which takes into account the combination of clinical setting, imaging findings, and pathologic correlation in the diagnosis of chILD.

The new classification system pertaining to children less than 2 years was developed in 2007 by clinicians, radiologists, and pathologists in the Children's Interstitial Lung Disease Research Cooperative of North America (chILDRN) based on a retrospective review of 186 lung biopsies, with corresponding clinical information and images, from children younger than 2 years.[8] Based on this classification system, infants with ILD are

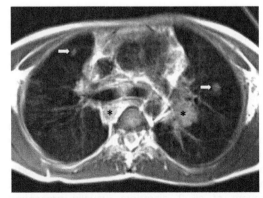

Fig. 3. Combined immunodeficiency in a 13-year-old male. Axial PD BLADE sequence MR image shows interstitial thickening and small pulmonary nodules (*arrows*) in both lungs. Also noted is mediastinal and hilar lymphadenopathy (*asterisks*).

placed in one of the following 4 categories: (1) diffuse developmental disorders, (2) alveolar growth abnormalities, (3) surfactant dysfunction disorders or (4) specific conditions of unknown or poorly understood etiology (**Table 1**).

Although this new system was widely accepted and eventually recommended for routine use by the 2013 American Thoracic Society (ATS) Clinical Guidelines, it only classified children less than age 2.[9] Therefore, chILDRN published an extended classification in 2015 based on a retrospective review of 191 lung biopsies in patients with diffuse lung disease between ages 2 and 18 years, which categorized patients by immunocompetent or immunocompromised status.[10] Immunocompetent patients were further subdivided into those with primary lung disease, lung disease related to systemic disease, or sequelae and ongoing disorders of infancy.[10]

SPECTRUM OF DISORDERS

Key clinical and imaging features of infantile interstitial lung disease are summarized in **Table 1**.

Disorders of Infancy

Diffuse developmental disorders
Acinar dysplasia/congenital alveolar dysplasia/alveolar capillary dysplasia with misalignment of pulmonary veins The diffuse developmental disorders of acinar dysplasia, congenital alveolar dysplasia (CAD), and alveolar capillary dysplasia with misalignment of pulmonary veins (ACDMPV) represent a category of diseases showing growth deficiency with variable degrees of alveolar capillary underdevelopment and associated pulmonary hypertension (**Fig. 4**). Although the precise incidence is not known, these 3 disorders are rare and only account for a small percentage of chILD, with female and male infants relatively equally affected.[11] Although the etiology is currently not entirely understood, multiple identified genetic mutations in affected infants offer strong evidence for a genetic component, with variants in the TBX4 gene implicated in acinar dysplasia and variants in the FOXF1 gene implicated in a percentage of ACDMPV cases.[12,13]

Diffuse developmental disorders most often occur in term infants, presenting with respiratory distress, rapidly progressive severe hypoxemia, and often pulmonary hypertension (PHT) shortly after birth. Acinar dysplasia is the most rare and severe of all 3 disorders, usually presenting earliest within hours after birth, with the shortest survival.[1] CXR findings are nonspecific and typically involve hypoinflation and diffuse hazy opacification (**Fig. 5**).[14] Increased pulmonary blood flow

and size of the main pulmonary artery may also be seen in infants with associated PHT. Due to the rarity and short survival of these disorders, CT findings are unknown. As current management is purely supportive, including advanced ventilation strategies, extracorporeal membrane oxygenation, and medical treatment of PHT, fatality rate remains nearly 100% within the first 2 months of life without transplant, with rare reports of a milder course with longer survival.[6]

Growth abnormalities
Trisomy 21 Disorders of alveolar growth are the most common form of ILD in infants and occur as a result of a superimposed condition or an event causing abnormal development of the lungs.[1] Trisomy 21 (Down syndrome) is one of the alveolar growth disorders with an associated, although not specific, imaging finding of small subpleural cysts (**Fig. 6**). Reported prevalence of subpleural cysts in children with Down syndrome ranges from 20% to 36%, with cysts measuring 0.1 to 2 cm and most commonly located along the lung periphery and pulmonary fissures with anteromedial predominance on CT.[2,15] The cysts are generally too small to see on chest radiographs (see **Fig. 6A**). Although the etiology and clinical relevance are not well understood, it is important to be aware of this finding so as to not confuse it with other pathology (**Fig. 7**). It has been postulated that the cysts may be a result of pulmonary hypoplasia, which is a known characteristic of Down syndrome.[15]

Surfactant dysfunction disorders and related abnormalities
The purpose of surfactant, comprised of 90% phospholipids and 10% proteins, is to reduce surface tension along the air–fluid interface to prevent alveolar collapse.[11] Each gene implicated in the surfactant dysfunction disorders has a critical role in the production of mature surfactant, and the epidemiologic, clinical, and radiological features of the 3 most common disorders, SFTPB, SFTPC, and ABCA3 genetic mutations, are discussed in this review.

The imaging findings of the surfactant dysfunction disorders include diffuse hazy or granular parenchymal opacities on CXR, and GGO with variable interlobular septal thickening and possible cyst formation on HRCT (**Fig. 8**).[1,16] SFTPC and ABCA3 genetic mutations may present later in life with enlarging cystic lung changes along with underlying lung parenchymal architectural distortion (**Figs. 9 and 10**). Pectus excavatum is also associated with these disorders, thought to be

Table 1
Key clinical and imaging features of infantile interstitial lung disease

Types of ILD	Key Clinical Features	Key Imaging Features
Diffuse Developmental Disorders		
Acinar dysplasia	Term infants, present at birth, female predominance, severe hypoxemia, high mortality	Diffuse opacities, hypoinflation
CAD	Term infants, present at birth, severe hypoxemia, high mortality	Diffuse opacities, hypoinflation, increased pulmonary blood flow/size of main PA if + PHT
ACDMPV	Term infants, present soon after birth, associated with other congenital abnormalities, severe hypoxemia, high mortality	Diffuse opacities, hypoinflation, increased pulmonary blood flow/size of main PA if + PHT
Growth abnormalities	Most common ILD, preterm and term infants, associated with underlying causes of growth abnormalities, variable clinical presentations, moderate mortality	Variable imaging findings, chromosomal abnormalities (eg, Trisomy 21) associated with small peripheral cysts
Surfactant Dysfunction Mutations and Related Disorders		
Mutation in *SFTPB* (surfactant protein-B gene)	Term infants, present at birth, autosomal recessive, severe hypoxemia, high mortality without transplant	Diffuse hazy or granular opacities on CXR, GGO with variable interlobular septal thickening on HRCT
Mutation in *SFTPC* (surfactant protein-C gene)	Term infants, present at birth, autosomal dominant, severe hypoxemia, moderate early mortality	Diffuse hazy or granular opacities on CXR, GGO with variable interlobular septal thickening on HRCT
Mutation in *ABCA3* (gene involved in surfactant transport)	Term infants, postnatal period, autosomal recessive, persistent tachypnea and hypoxemia, moderate early mortality	Diffuse hazy or granular opacities on CXR, GGO with variable interlobular septal thickening on HRCT
Specific Conditions of Undefined Etiology		
NEHI	Term infants, initially well, presents by 3 mo with persistent tachypnea, retractions, crackles, and hypoxemia, not responsive to steroids, no reported mortality	Hyperinflation with variable increased perihilar opacities on CXR, geographic GGO, and air-trapping with central predominance, especially in the lingula and right middle lobe on HRCT
PIG	Preterm and term infants, presents at birth, often associated with other conditions that affect lung growth, severe tachypnea and hypoxemia, pulsed steroids used in more severe cases, mortality related to associated disorders	Hyperinflation and diffusely increased interstitial markings on CXR, diffuse segmental or subsegmental GGO, predominantly subpleural interlobular septal thickening, and reticular changes on HRCT

Abbreviations: ABCA3, ATP binding cassette subfamily A member 3; ACDMPV, alveolar capillary dysplasia with misalignment of pulmonary veins; CAD, congenital alveolar dysplasia; CXR, chest radiographs; GGO, ground-glass opacities; NEHI, neuroendocrine cell hyperplasia of infancy; PHT, pulmonary hypertension; PIG, pulmonary interstitial glycogenosis; Sp-B, surfactant protein-B; Sp-C, surfactant protein-C.

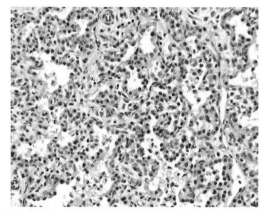

Fig. 4. Alveolar capillary dysplasia with misalignment of pulmonary veins in a 5-day-old female with respiratory failure and pulmonary hypertension. Lung biopsy shows alveolar septa with excess mesenchyme and deficient capillaries (hematoxylin and eosin; original magnification, 400x).

due to abnormal chest wall development in the setting of chronic restrictive lung disease.[5]

While certain clinical and imaging features can suggest a diagnosis of surfactant dysfunction disorder, the definitive diagnosis is made by genetic testing and/or lung biopsy (**Fig. 11**).[16] Specific treatment and prognosis are dependent on the

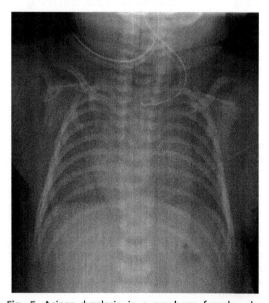

Fig. 5. Acinar dysplasia in a newborn female, also with a history of esophageal atresia, who presented with respiratory distress and progressively worsening hypoxemia. Frontal chest radiograph shows decreased lung volumes with diffuse hazy opacifications of both lungs. Also incidentally noted is an enteric tube tip located in the upper esophageal pouch (in this patient with esophageal atresia).

clinical severity and underlying mutation, but overall treatment remains largely supportive.

Surfactant protein-B genetic mutation Surfactant protein-B deficiency is associated with at least 40 different mutations in the SFTPB gene. It is inherited in an autosomal recessive pattern and most often presents immediately after birth with rapidly progressive respiratory failure and death within the first 3 to 6 months of life.[11,16] Exogenous surfactant has not proven effective, and treatment is supportive until death unless lung transplant is pursued. However, there have been some encouraging results regarding viral-mediated gene therapy for long-term expression of Sp-B in mice.[16]

Surfactant protein-C genetic mutation Surfactant protein-C deficiency is one of the more common surfactant dysfunction disorders, accounting for approximately 17% of childhood ILD, and is associated with more than 60 different mutations in the gene. SpC deficiency is inherited in an autosomal dominant pattern.[5,11] Presentation is variable and can occur at any age, usually with persistent tachypnea and hypoxemia if in the postnatal period and sometimes preceded by RSV bronchiolitis. It may also remain asymptomatic until childhood or adulthood. Treatment in the neonatal period often involves aggressive chronic ventilation, and there may be a possible response to hydroxychloroquine in older children, although recent data showed that hydroxychloroquine may exacerbate symptoms.[17]

ABCA3 genetic mutation The ABCA3 gene is a large and complex gene with more than 200 reported mutations, making it the most common known cause of surfactant deficiency and likely accounting for its highly variable clinical, radiological and pathologic phenotype.[11] It is inherited in an autosomal dominant pattern and often presents similarly to SpC deficiency with mild or absent history of neonatal lung disease. Late-presenting disease may remain stable for many years.[18] Anecdotal responses to pulsed methylprednisolone, azithromycin, and hydroxychloroquine have been reported.[11] Transplantation is an option, although it is associated with substantial morbidity and mortality.[19]

Other gene mutation

Filamin A genetic mutation The FLNA gene encodes the actin-binding filamin A, which is involved in maintaining cell shape and motility. Mutations in this gene can cause abnormal neural migration (eg, gray matter heterotopia), disorders of skeletal development, vascular abnormalities, and disordered alveolar growth.[5] Onset of

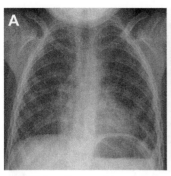
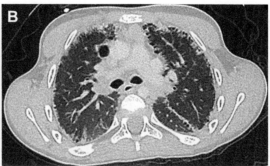

Fig. 6. Trisomy 21 in a 7-year-old male who presented with shortness of breath. (*A*) Frontal chest radiograph shows mild subsegmental atelectasis in both lungs and a suggestion of biapical pleural thickening, mildly irregular, especially on the right. No definite pulmonary cysts are seen. (*B*) Axial lung window CT image demonstrates multiple subcentimeter subpleural cysts located along the lung periphery and pulmonary fissures.

respiratory symptoms usually occurs in the neonatal period or in the first few months of life, and females are primarily affected due to an X-linked pattern of inheritance that is often lethal to males in utero. HRCT findings include predominantly upper and middle lobe hyperinflation and hyperlucency, which can resemble congenital lobar emphysema, as well as coarse septal thickening, lower lobe atelectasis, and pruning of the pulmonary vasculature (**Fig. 12**).[5] Clinical outcomes are variable and include death, making early aggressive supportive treatment important.[20]

Specific conditions of unknown/poorly understood etiology

Two chILD with specific conditions of unknown/poorly understood etiology are neuroendocrine cell hyperplasia of infancy (NEHI) and pulmonary interstitial glycogenosis (PIG).

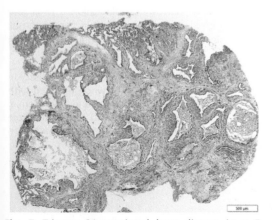

Fig. 7. Trisomy 21-associated lung disease in a 5-month-old male born prematurely. Lung biopsy shows cysts that are small and predominantly subpleural (hematoxylin and eosin).

Neuroendocrine cell hyperplasia of infancy Initially known as persistent tachypnea of infancy, NEHI is one of the most common causes of ILD in infants and is characterized by increased neuroendocrine cells in the distal airways, with otherwise normal or nearly normal lung histology. The etiology and pathophysiology are unknown, although it has been theorized that the increased neuroendocrine cells may cause bronchoconstriction and air-trapping, or may simply indicate immaturity of the lung.[21] Affected infants are predominantly male and often present with tachypnea, crackles and hypoxemia in the first few months of life after an initial period of wellbeing.[11,21]

CXR findings range from normal to nonspecific hyperinflation (**Fig. 13**A). However, HRCT findings are quite sensitive and specific, and can potentially obviate the need for biopsy if other causes of infant ILD have been excluded. A mosaic pattern of geographic centrally distributed GGO involving the right middle lobe and lingula has been shown to be 78% sensitive and 100% specific (**Fig. 13**B).[21] Because of this specificity, diagnostic biopsy is rarely pursued unless there are atypical clinical or radiologic features (**Fig. 14**).

Although there is no reported mortality, substantial morbidity in the first few years of life is usually present, including frequent respiratory exacerbations. Steroids are typically ineffective due to the absence of underlying inflammation. Infants with NEHI often require supportive treatment with supplemental oxygen, with the majority able to be weaned by age 2.[21]

Pulmonary interstitial glycogenosis Previously encompassed within the term infantile cellular interstitial pneumonitis, PIG is characterized by the presence of primitive glycogen-containing cells within the lung interstitium, thought to reflect either early disruption of lung development or a

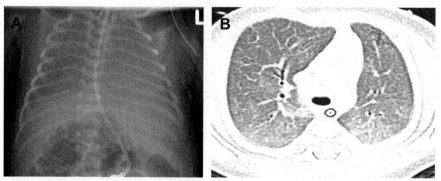

Fig. 8. Surfactant protein-B deficiency in a 13-day-old male who presented with progressive respiratory failure. (*A*) Frontal chest radiograph shows decreased lung volume with diffuse hazy and granular parenchymal opacities in both lungs. Also noted are partially visualized endotracheal and nasogastric tubes. (*B*) Axial lung window CT image demonstrates diffuse ground-glass opacities and septal thickening throughout both lungs.

response to lung injury (**Fig. 15**).[22] Often associated with other pulmonary disorders and congenital heart disease, PIG can affect preterm or term infants and typically presents with tachypnea and hypoxemia shortly after birth. It rarely presents or persists beyond 6 to 12 months, although a recent case report by Liptzin and colleagues reports a diagnosis of PIG at 14 months.[23] Unfortunately, there are no specific biomarkers or radiological features of PIG that would obviate the need for lung biopsy.

CXR often demonstrates bilateral hyperinflation and diffuse interstitial markings. HRCT findings include diffuse or segmental GGO, interlobular septal thickening, predominantly subpleural reticular changes, and occasional cystic changes.[24] Prognosis is variable and thought to be dependent on the underlying associated condition rather than PIG itself, although there have been reported fatalities in patients without another known diagnosis.[22]

Treatment is often supportive with supplemental oxygen, although pulsed dose steroids are often recommended for severe cases.[24,25]

Disorders of the Normal Host

There is a variety of chILD which occurs in the normal host. The 5 most common of these disorders encountered in clinical practice are infectious/postinfectious bronchiolitis obliterans (BO), hypersensitivity pneumonia, aspiration pneumonia, eosinophilic pneumonia, and idiopathic pulmonary hemosiderosis.

Infectious/postinfectious bronchiolitis obliterans

Viral and bacterial infections are a common underlying cause of diffuse lung disease in an immunocompetent host, with viruses accounting for 50% of pneumonia in children less than 5 years old.[1] Postinfectious bronchiolitis obliterans (PIBO) is a chronic sequela of various respiratory viruses, most commonly adenovirus, characterized by severe lower respiratory tract obstruction due to chronic inflammation and eventual fibrosis resulting in airway narrowing/obliteration.[2] It is the most common cause of irreversible chronic small airway disease in children and usually presents

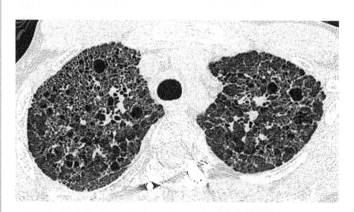

Fig. 9. Surfactant protein-C deficiency in a 2-year-old female who presented with shortness of breath and hypoxemia. Axial lung window CT shows multiple lung cysts, of variable size, in addition to extensive interlobular septal thickening throughout both lungs.

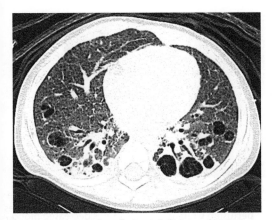

Fig. 10. Congenital surfactant deficiency (ABCA3 mutation) in a 13-month-old female who presented with respiratory distress and hypoxemia. Axial lung window CT shows bilateral lung cysts, septal thickening, and ground-glass opacities.

with prolonged recovery after a respiratory infection, followed by wheezing, shortness of breath, and fixed airway obstruction on PFTs.[1]

CXR findings can range from normal in mild disease to hyperinflation, atelectasis, and bronchial wall thickening in moderate to severe disease. Characteristic CT findings can preclude the need for biopsy and include a mosaic pattern of attenuation, air trapping, bronchiectasis, and bronchial wall thickening.[1] Expiratory CT imaging can improve the detection of the underlying mosaic pattern of attenuation and air trapping, which may not be conspicuous on inspiratory CT imaging (Fig. 16).

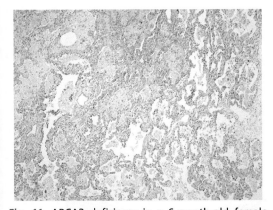

Fig. 11. ABCA3 deficiency in a 6-month-old female who developed respiratory distress within hours of birth. Lung biopsy shows intraalveolar proteinaceous material, type 2 pneumocyte hyperplasia, and thick alveolar septa (hematoxylin and eosin, original magnification, 100x).

Treatment involves a combination of inhaled and systemic corticosteroids, azithromycin, and immunoglobulin depending on severity, with clinical and radiological improvement occurring in most of the patients after treatment.[26]

Hypersensitivity pneumonia

Previously known as extrinsic allergic alveolitis, hypersensitivity pneumonia is an immune-mediated response to inhaled organic antigens, resulting in lymphocytic inflammation of the lungs, sometimes accompanied by small and poorly formed granulomas. It typically presents in later childhood or adolescence, with avian and fungal antigens being the most common triggers.[4,27] It can present acutely within 4 to 12 hours of exposure with flu-like symptoms, such as fever, chills, cough, dyspnea, and malaise. Presentation in the subacute or chronic phase is more insidious, often with exercise intolerance, cough, and weight loss. The diagnosis is made by a combination of clinical history, characteristic HRCT findings, and precipitin assay to identify a trigger antigen[27]; biopsy can also be helpful.

CXR may demonstrate diffuse micronodular interstitial prominence with opacities involving the middle and lower lung zones.[1] Classic HRCT findings in the acute phase include centrilobular ground-glass nodules, air-trapping, and sparing of the upper lung zones, whereas the chronic fibrotic phase demonstrates subpleural reticular markings, architectural distortion, and eventually honeycombing (Fig. 17).[2] Imaging findings can persist for several weeks despite a good clinical response on treatment.

Given the potential irreversible progression to fibrosis, early diagnosis and treatment with removal of the inciting exposure and systemic steroids is essential.[2,27]

Aspiration pneumonia

Aspiration pneumonia is typically a polymicrobial infection resulting from a variety of causes in children, including swallowing disorders, H-type tracheoesophageal fistula, and esophageal stricture or obstruction (Fig. 18). Aspiration pneumonia presents acutely with fever and hypoxemia, and recurrent aspiration can result in chronic lung disease in children.

CXR and HRCT findings can vary based on the timing and amount of aspiration, but typically include alveolar consolidations in the dependent aspects of the lungs, occasionally with abscess formation, and bronchiectasis in more advanced cases (Fig. 19).[1] Mucus and aspirated material accumulated within the large airways can also be observed on CT (see Fig. 19A).

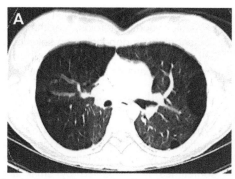
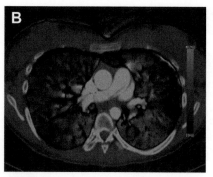

Fig. 12. Filamin A genetic mutation in a 16-year-old female who presented with respiratory distress. (*A*) Axial lung window CT image shows bilateral hyperinflation with pruning of the pulmonary vasculature and peripheral regions of relative hyperlucency in both lungs. (*B*) Axial iodine perfusion CT image demonstrates decreased blood flow (ie, darker) reflecting relative hypoperfusion in the peripheral portions of both lungs, corresponding to the areas with pruning of the pulmonary vasculature seen in Figure 12A.

Treatment involves intravenous or oral antibiotics with both aerobic and anaerobic coverage, and a recent study by Streck and colleagues demonstrated that a shorter course of antibiotics (7 days or less) in hospitalized pediatric patients did not result in increased treatment failure compared with a longer course.[28]

Eosinophilic pneumonia

Eosinophilic pneumonia is one of a diverse group of eosinophilic lung diseases, which are characterized by peripheral or tissue eosinophilia and are divided into 3 main categories. Acute and chronic eosinophilic pneumonia fall under the category of eosinophilic lung disease of unknown cause. Eosinophilic pneumonia is more common in adolescents than young children and the acute clinical syndrome is characterized by fever, hypoxemia, bronchoalveolar lavage with more than 25%

eosinophils, and prompt and complete response to steroids.[1] The chronic form has a more insidious clinical presentation and is more often associated with peripheral eosinophilia and increased serum IgE.[29] Main underlying causes include infection (particularly fungal and parasitic), drug reaction, primary eosinophilic disorders, and idiopathic conditions.

CXR findings include bilateral reticular opacities, sometimes with patchy consolidations and pleural effusions. HRCT features of acute eosinophilic pneumonia include bilateral patchy GGO and consolidations, with smooth interlobular septal thickening and occasionally pleural effusions (**Fig. 20**).[29] More organized coarse parenchymal opacities may be seen in chronic eosinophilic pneumonia (**Fig. 21**). Due to similarities between the more common entities of pulmonary edema

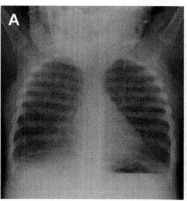
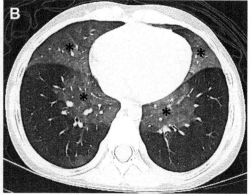

Fig. 13. Neuroendocrine cell hyperplasia of infancy (NEHI) in a 6-month-old male who presented with tachypnea, crackles, and hypoxemia. (*A*) Frontal chest radiograph shows hyperinflation and mild paramediastinal hazy opacities in both lungs. (*B*) Axial lung window CT image demonstrates ground-glass opacities in the right middle lobe, lingula, and medial aspects of bilateral lower lobes, in a symmetric bilateral paramediastinal distribution (*asterisks*).

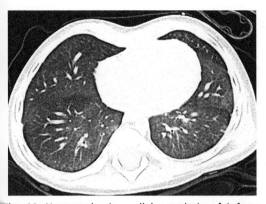

Fig. 14. Neuroendocrine cell hyperplasia of infancy (NEHI) in an 8-month-old male who presented with tachypnea and hypoxemia. Axial lung window CT image shows diffuse ground-glass opacities in both lungs without a specific pattern. Although the patient's clinical symptoms suggested possible NEHI, the patient eventually underwent lung biopsy because CT did not show characteristic imaging findings of NEHI. Lung biopsy pathology confirmed the diagnosis of NEHI.

and atypical bacterial or viral pneumonia, delayed diagnosis and rapid clinical deterioration can occur. However, outcomes are very favorable in the setting of prompt diagnosis and initiation of steroids.

Idiopathic pulmonary hemosiderosis

Initially termed *brown lung induration* by Virchow in 1864, idiopathic pulmonary hemosiderosis is a rare lung disease that can affect both children and adults. Although the etiology and

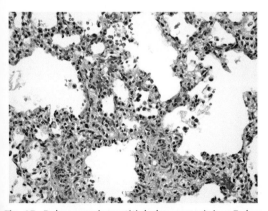

Fig. 15. Pulmonary interstitial glycogenosis in a 5-day-old female with heterotaxy and complex cyanotic congenital heart disease. Lung biopsy shows alveolar septa widened by small interstitial cells with vacuolated cytoplasm (hematoxylin and eosin; original magnification, 400x); pulmonary hypertensive remodeling was also present.

pathophysiology are unknown, there is some evidence to suggest an immunologic cause.[30] The clinical presentation involves recurrent episodes of hemoptysis, iron deficiency anemia, and diffuse lung opacities on CXR, often with a relapsing and remitting course. Less commonly, the excessive iron deposition and secondary oxidative damage can lead to fibrosis and end-stage lung disease.[30] In conjunction with the imaging findings, bronchoscopy can help suggest the diagnosis by confirming diffuse alveolar hemorrhage and ruling out infection. Although biopsy shows intra-alveolar hemosiderin-laden macrophages, it is important to correlate with the clinical findings to rule out bleeding from an airway or other upper aerodigestive source (**Fig. 22**).[30]

CXR often demonstrates diffuse alveolar opacities with a central and lower lobe predominance during the acute hemorrhage, which evolves into a more interstitial pattern after 72 hours. HRCT demonstrates GGO and consolidation in the same distribution, which can progress to a crazy-paving pattern in the subacute phase (**Fig. 23**).[30] Corticosteroids and other immunosuppressive therapies are used for treatment, and 86% of patients now survive beyond 5 years after diagnosis due to advances in diagnosis and treatment.[1]

Disorders Related to Systemic Disease Processes

Immune-mediated disorders

Granulomatosis with polyangiitis Previously known as Wegener's granulomatosis, granulomatosis with polyangiitis (GPA) is a rare multisystemic granulomatous small-vessel vasculitis that most often affects the upper and lower respiratory tract and kidneys (**Fig. 24**). Although more commonly seen in adults, GPA is the most common necrotizing systemic vasculitis in the pediatric population and is thought to be due to autoimmune-mediated endothelial injury and inflammation resulting in vasculitis and parenchymal disease.[1] Affected patients with GPA present with fever, malaise, arthralgias, chronic rhinitis and occasionally hemoptysis, dyspnea and pleuritic chest pain in those with pulmonary involvement. Elevated ESR and positive rheumatoid factor are nonspecific features; however, c-ANCA positivity is 80% to 100% specific.[31]

CXR findings are variable but include nodules, patchy or diffuse opacities, transient infiltrates, and hilar adenopathy.[31] HRCT often demonstrates multiple pulmonary nodules, which tend to cavitate when greater than 2 cm, and ground-glass opacity and/or consolidations due to pulmonary hemorrhage (**Fig. 25**).

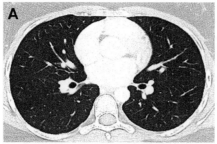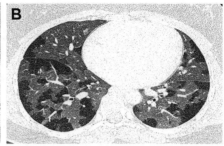

Fig. 16. Postinfectious bronchiolitis obliterans in a 6-year-old female who presented with progressively worsening wheezing and shortness of breath after severe viral pneumonia. Pulmonary function testing showed a fixed airway obstructive pattern. (A) Axial lung window CT image obtained at end-inspiration shows normally inflated lungs without definite abnormality. (B) Axial lung window CT image obtained at end-expiration demonstrates mosaic attenuation with moderate multifocal lobular air trapping throughout both lungs.

The disease is fatal if untreated, and treatment usually involves induction with cyclophosphamide and corticosteroids or rituximab, followed by maintenance treatment with azathioprine.[31]

Lymphoproliferative disease Pulmonary lymphoproliferative disorders comprise a spectrum of reactive and neoplastic disorders, characterized by abnormal proliferation or infiltration of lymphoid cells in the lung parenchyma and most commonly affecting children with immune deficiency or autoimmune disease (Fig. 26). Clarified what the reactive (non-neoplastic) disorders are (nodular lymphoid hyperplasia and lymphoid interstitial pneumonia) range from discrete nodular masses in nodular lymphoid hyperplasia to diffuse interstitial involvement, GGO, nodules, cysts, and

peribronchovascular thickening in lymphoid interstitial pneumonia (Fig. 27A).[32] Concomitant mediastinal lymphadenopathy can also be seen (Fig. 27B). The malignant disorders, the most common of which is MALT lymphoma, are characterized by consolidations, larger nodules, and pleural effusions.[32] Treatment varies by individual disorder.

Nonimmune-mediated disorders

Langerhans cell histiocytosis Also known as eosinophilic granuloma, Langerhans cell histiocytosis (LCH) is a rare multisystem disorder characterized by clonal proliferation of Langerhans cells of bone marrow origin. Childhood LCH can present with cough and dyspnea any time from age 2 weeks to 16 years.[4] The etiology of LCH may have a genetic component, given reports of

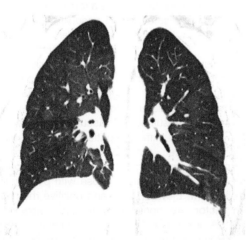

Fig. 17. Hypersensitivity pneumonia in a 15-year-old male due to exposure to bird droppings while cleaning his grandparent's barn. The patient presented with cough, dyspnea, and fever. Coronal lung window CT image shows diffuse and patchy ground-glass opacities in both lungs. The patient's symptoms resolved after treatment with corticosteroids.

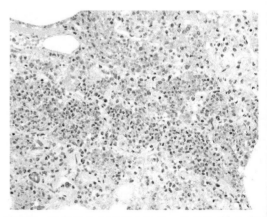

Fig. 18. Aspiration pneumonia in a 2-year-old under palliative care for progressive atypical teratoid rhabdoid tumor involving the brain and leptomeninges. Autopsy shows acute exudative pneumonia with a bronchopneumonia pattern (hematoxylin and eosin; original magnification, 400x). Postmortem culture of lung tissue grew polymicrobial species.

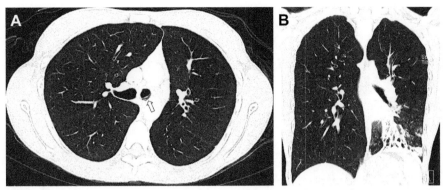

Fig. 19. Aspiration pneumonia in an 11-year-old female with swallowing disorder who presented with cough and left chest pain. (*A*) Axial lung window CT image shows aspirated debris and mucus (*arrow*) in the dependent portion of the left main stem bronchus. (*B*) Coronal lung window CT image demonstrates aspirated debris and mucus (*arrow*) in the left main stem bronchus and bronchiectasis, consolidation, and scarring with volume loss in the left lower lobe from aspiration.

familial cases and a large percentage of cases associated with a *BRAF* mutation.[1,4]

CXR findings of LCH range from indistinct nodular interstitial opacities to fibrotic architectural distortion and honeycombing in advanced disease. The most common HRCT findings are 1 to 10 mm centrilobular and peribronchial nodules, followed by thick or thin-walled cysts and alveolar consolidations, all of which can involve the lung bases in children, unlike adult pulmonary LCH which typically spares the lung bases (**Fig. 28**).[33] Although prognosis is overall favorable, up to 10% of those with lung involvement will have severe lung LCH, predisposing to pneumothorax secondary to cystic lung lesions.[34]

Treatment involves chemotherapeutic agents and prednisolone, as well as BRAF inhibitors for those with a BRAF mutation for cases without eventual and spontaneous resolution.

Sarcoidosis Childhood sarcoidosis is a rare multisystem granulomatous disorder of unknown etiology and variable presentation depending on which organ systems are involved. When there is pulmonary involvement, children can present with cough, dyspnea, fever, and occasionally hemoptysis in advanced cases.

Imaging findings vary based on disease stage, and pulmonary sarcoidosis has been classified into four stages: (1) isolated lymphadenopathy, (2) lymphadenopathy and pulmonary disease, (3) isolated pulmonary disease, and (4) pulmonary fibrosis.[1] Whereas small peribronchial nodules, interstitial thickening, and areas of GGO and consolidation are common findings in stages 2 to 3, fibrotic changes, such as architectural distortion, honeycombing, and traction bronchiectasis,

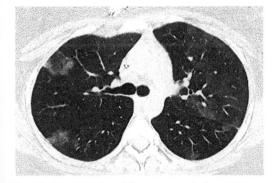

Fig. 20. Acute eosinophilic pneumonia in a 15-year-old female who presented with respiratory distress and fever. Axial lung window CT image shows bilateral patchy ground-glass opacities, in a predominantly peripheral distribution. The patient's symptoms resolved with steroid treatment.

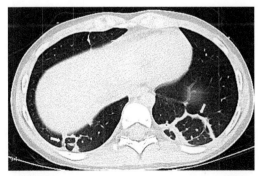

Fig. 21. Chronic eosinophilic pneumonia in a 16-year-old female who presented with progressively worsening shortness of breath. Axial lung window CT image shows nonsegmental areas of airspace consolidation (*arrows*) with peripheral predominance.

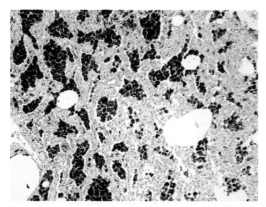

Fig. 22. Idiopathic hemosiderosis in a 3-year-old who underwent chest x-ray showing bilateral pulmonary infiltrates after profound anemia failed to respond to iron replacement therapy. Lung biopsy shows alveolar spaces filled with iron-laden (blue-staining) macrophages (iron stain; original magnification, 200x).

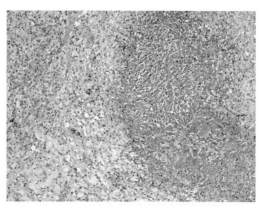

Fig. 24. Granulomatosis with polyangiitis in a 17-year-old female presenting with cough, chest pain, fevers, and night sweats. Lung biopsy shows granulomatous inflammation and palisading basophilic necrosis (hematoxylin and eosin; original magnification, 400x).

predominate in stage 4. A recent study by Gorkem and colleagues found that contrast-enhanced thoracic MRI is comparable to chest CT in the detection of stages 1, 2 and 4 pulmonary sarcoidosis, potentially allowing for decreased radiation exposure in the diagnosis and follow-up.[35] Pathologic examination shows epithelioid granulomas in a perilymphatic distribution; in the pediatric population, major considerations in the histologic differential diagnosis include infection or inborn error of immunity.

Disorders of the Immunocompromised Host

Pneumocystis jirovecii pneumonia
In immunocompromised children, opportunistic infection accounts for almost half of diffuse lung disease diagnoses, the majority of which are fungal and include *Pneumocystis jirovecii* pneumonia (PJP) (Fig. 29). Imaging features include extensive bilateral and fairly symmetric GGO, usually with a central predominance, sometimes with interlobular septal thickening and a crazy-paving pattern in more advanced cases (Fig. 30). Pulmonary cysts are also seen in a third of cases and can predispose to pneumothorax.[36] First-line treatment is with trimethoprim-sulfamethoxazole.

Posttransplant lymphoproliferative disorder
Posttransplant lymphoproliferative disorder (PTLD) is a serious complication of solid organ or bone marrow transplant and most often occurs as a result of immunosuppression and EBV infection (Fig. 31). Most cases occur within the first year after transplant, and risk of PTLD depends on the type of transplant and degree of

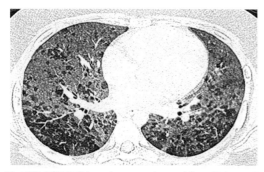

Fig. 23. Idiopathic pulmonary hemosiderosis in a 13-year-old male who presented with hemoptysis, epistaxis, and iron deficiency anemia. Axial lung window CT image shows ground-glass opacities in a "crazy-paving" pattern in the bilateral lower lung zones.

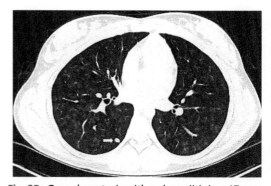

Fig. 25. Granulomatosis with polyangiitis in a 17-year-old female who presented with fever, chest pain and hemoptysis. Diffuse centrilobular ground-glass nodular opacities are seen throughout both lungs likely due to underlying pulmonary hemorrhage. Also noted is a pulmonary nodule (*arrow*).

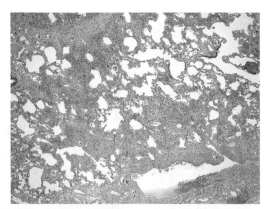

Fig. 26. Interstitial lymphoid hyperplasia in a 13-year-old boy with mixed connective tissue disease who developed pneumothorax in the setting of rash, Raynaud's phenomenon, and patulous aperistaltic esophagus. Lung tissue removed at blebectomy showed a lymphocytic infiltrate expanding alveolar septa and cuffing bronchovascular tissue (hematoxylin and eosin; original magnification, 100x).

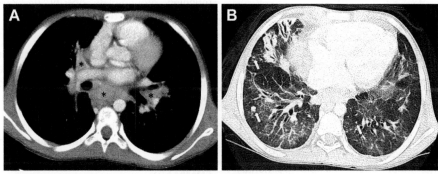

Fig. 27. Lymphoproliferative disease in a 13-year-old female with common variable immunodeficiency who presented with chest pain and shortness of breath. (*A*) Axial contrast-enhanced CT image shows mediastinal and hilar lymphadenopathy (*asterisk*). (*B*) Axial lung window CT image demonstrates diffuse interstitial thickening, ground-glass opacities, and nodules (*arrow*).

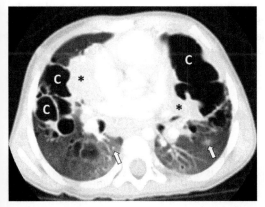

Fig. 28. Langerhans cell histiocytosis in a 2-year-old female who presented with progressively worsening cough and shortness of breath. Axial lung window CT image shows both pulmonary cysts (C), consolidations (*asterisk*), and nodules (*arrows*).

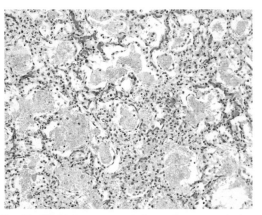

Fig. 29. Florid *Pneumocystis jirovecii* pneumonia in a 5-month-old female with hemophagocytic syndrome treated with corticosteroids and other immunomodulatory agents. Autopsy showed airspaces filled with a proteinaceous exudate (hematoxylin and eosin stain; original magnification, 600x), in which round organisms, often showing a "crushed ping-pong ball" configuration, were demonstrated on Grocott's methenamine silver stain (not shown).

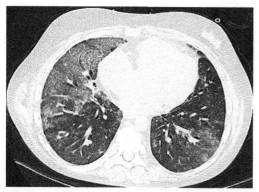

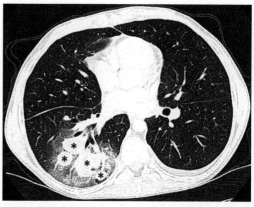

Fig. 30. *Pneumocystis jirovecii* pneumonia in a 12-year-old girl immunocompromised from chemotherapy who presented with cough and chest pain. Axial lung window CT image shows extensive bilateral ground-glass opacities with interlobular septal thickening and a "crazy-paving" pattern.

Fig. 32. Posttransplant lymphoproliferative disorder in a 17-year-old male status post lung transplant due to cystic fibrosis. Axial lung window CT image shows multiple large pulmonary nodules (*asterisk*) with surrounding ground-glass opacity (ie, ground-glass "halo" sign) in the right lower lobe.

immunosuppression. Incidence is highest following small intestine transplants, followed by lung transplants, and less commonly liver, heart, and kidney transplants in pediatric patients with solid organ transplant.[37] B cell lymphoproliferation in the setting of immunosuppression usually occurs at extranodal sites, including the lung.

Intrathoracic imaging findings include mediastinal lymphadenopathy, consolidations, pleural effusions, and most often multiple pulmonary nodules with a basal or peripheral predominance, which usually range from 1 to 4 cm and can demonstrate central necrosis or surrounding halo

(Fig. 32).[1] In lung transplant recipients, pulmonary involvement is 4x more common than mediastinal involvement. Due to its nonspecific imaging findings, biopsy is often needed for the diagnosis and staging of PTLD. Early-stage disease is treated with immune modulation, whereas advanced disease is treated as lymphoma.

SUMMARY

Pediatric ILD encompasses a wide range of diffuse lung diseases, which are constantly becoming better understood and now organized into a structured classification system based on their clinical, radiologic, and pathologic features. Given the critical role of imaging in early diagnosis and treatment, it is important for radiologists to be familiar with characteristic imaging findings and up-to-date advances in imaging which, in turn, can lead to early and accurate diagnosis as well as optimal care of patients with chILD.

CLINICS CARE POINTS

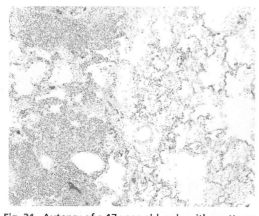

Fig. 31. Autopsy of a 17-year-old male with posttransplant lymphoproliferative disorder after lung transplant shows extensive nodular collections of monomorphic lymphoid cells in the lung (hematoxylin and eosin; original magnification, 100x). Antemortem biopsy of liver (not shown) had demonstrated the neoplastic cells to be of B cell lineage and positive for Epstein–Barr virus.

- A new structured classification system for chILD is now available, which categorizes infant ILD by etiology and childhood ILD by disorders of the immunocompetent and immunocompromised host.

- The two most commonly used imaging modalities for evaluating chILD are CXR and CT.

- The role of imaging in the diagnosis of ILD is to confirm its presence, characterize its extent

- and distribution, narrow the differential diagnosis, and suggest an optimal biopsy site.
- Due to substantial morbidity and mortality associated with chILD, it is essential for radiologists to be familiar with this spectrum of disorders and associated imaging characteristics to aid in prompt diagnosis and initiation of appropriate treatment.

DISCLOSURE

The authors have nothing to disclose.

REFERENCES

1. Cleveland RH, Lee EY. Pediatric Interstitial (Diffuse) Lung Disease. In: Lee EY, editor. Imaging in pediatric Pulmonology. 2nd edition. Cham (Switzerland): Springer Nature Switzerland AG; 2020. p. 145–96.
2. Liang TI, Lee EY. Interstitial Lung Diseases in Children, Adolescents, and Young Adults: Different from Infants and Older Adults. Radiol Clin North Am 2020;58(3):487–502.
3. Thacker PG, Vargas SO, Fishman MP, et al. Current Update on Interstitial Lung Disease of Infancy: New Classification System, Diagnostic Evaluation, Imaging Algorithms, Imaging Findings, and Prognosis. Radiol Clin North Am 2016;54(6):1065–76.
4. Semple T, Winant AJ, Lee EY. Childhood Interstitial Lung Disease: Imaging Guidelines and Recommendations. Radiol Clin North Am 2022;60(1):83–111.
5. Liang T, Vargas SO, Lee EY. Childhood Interstitial (Diffuse) Lung Disease: Pattern Recognition Approach to Diagnosis in Infants [published online ahead of print, 2019 Mar 5]. AJR Am J Roentgenol 2019;1–10. https://doi.org/10.2214/AJR.18.20696.
6. Lee EY. Interstitial lung disease in infants: new classification system, imaging technique, clinical presentation and imaging findings. Pediatr Radiol 2013;43(1):3, 129.
7. Sodhi KS, Sharma M, Lee EY, et al. Diagnostic Utility of 3T Lung MRI in Children with Interstitial Lung Disease: A Prospective Pilot Study. Acad Radiol 2018; 25(3):380–6.
8. Deutsch GH, Young LR, Deterding RR, et al. Diffuse lung disease in young children: application of a novel classification scheme. Am J Respir Crit Care Med 2007;176(11):1120–8.
9. Kurland G, Deterding RR, Hagood JS, et al. An official American Thoracic Society clinical practice guideline: classification, evaluation, and management of childhood interstitial lung disease in infancy. Am J Respir Crit Care Med 2013;188(3):376–94.
10. Fan LL, Dishop MK, Galambos C, et al. Diffuse Lung Disease in Biopsied Children 2 to 18 Years of Age.

Application of the chILD Classification Scheme. Ann Am Thorac Soc 2015;12(10):1498–505.
11. Bush A, Gilbert C, Gregory J, et al. Interstitial lung disease in infancy. Early Hum Dev 2020;150:105186.
12. Szafranski P, Coban-Akdemir ZH, Rupps R, et al. Phenotypic expansion of TBX4 mutations to include acinar dysplasia of the lungs. Am J Med Genet A 2016;170(9):2440–4.
13. Stankiewicz P, Sen P, Bhatt SS, et al. Genomic and genic deletions of the FOX gene cluster on 16q24.1 and inactivating mutations of FOXF1 cause alveolar capillary dysplasia and other malformations. Am J Hum Genet 2009;84(6):780–91 [published correction appears in Am J Hum Genet. 2009 Oct;85(4):537. multiple author names added].
14. Hugosson CO, Salama HM, Al-Dayel F, et al. Primary alveolar capillary dysplasia (acinar dysplasia) and surfactant protein B deficiency: a clinical, radiological and pathological study. Pediatr Radiol 2005; 35(3):311–6.
15. Biko DM, Schwartz M, Anupindi SA, et al. Subpleural lung cysts in Down syndrome: prevalence and association with coexisting diagnoses. Pediatr Radiol 2008;38(3):280–4.
16. Singh J, Jaffe A, Schultz A, et al. Surfactant protein disorders in childhood interstitial lung disease. Eur J Pediatr 2021;180(9):2711–21.
17. Alysandratos KD, Russo SJ, Petcherski A, et al. Patient-specific iPSCs carrying an SFTPC mutation reveal the intrinsic alveolar epithelial dysfunction at the inception of interstitial lung disease. Cell Rep 2021;36(9):109636.
18. Cho JG, Thakkar D, Buchanan P, et al. *ABCA3* deficiency from birth to adulthood presenting as paediatric interstitial lung disease. Respir Case Rep 2020; 8(7):e00633.
19. Eldridge WB, Zhang Q, Faro A, et al. Outcomes of Lung Transplantation for Infants and Children with Genetic Disorders of Surfactant Metabolism. J Pediatr 2017;184:157–64.e2.
20. Shelmerdine SC, Semple T, Wallis C, et al. Filamin A (FLNA) mutation-A newcomer to the childhood interstitial lung disease (ChILD) classification. Pediatr Pulmonol 2017;52(10):1306–15.
21. Balinotti JE, Maffey A, Colom A, et al. Clinical, functional, and computed tomography findings in a cohort of patients with neuroendocrine cell hyperplasia of infancy. Pediatr Pulmonol 2021;56(6):1681–6.
22. Galambos C, Wartchow E, Weinman JP, et al. Pulmonary interstitial glycogenosis cells express mesenchymal stem cell markers. Eur Respir J 2020;56(4): 2000853.
23. Liptzin DR, Udoko MN, Pinder M, et al. Pulmonary interstitial glycogenosis after the first year. Pediatr Pulmonol 2021;56(9):3056–8.
24. Liptzin DR, Baker CD, Darst JR, et al. Pulmonary interstitial glycogenosis: Diagnostic evaluation and

clinical course. Pediatr Pulmonol 2018;53(12): 1651–8.

25. Yonker LM, Kinane TB. Diagnostic and clinical course of pulmonary interstitial glycogenosis: The tip of the iceberg. Pediatr Pulmonol 2018;53(12): 1659–61.

26. Yazan H, Khalif F, Shadfaan LA, et al. Post-infectious bronchiolitis obliterans in children: Clinical and radiological evaluation and long-term results. Heart Lung 2021;50(5):660–6.

27. Wawszczak M, Bielecka T, Szczukocki M. Hypersensitivity pneumonitis in children. Ann Agric Environ Med 2021;28(2):214–9.

28. Streck HL, Goldman JL, Lee BR, et al. Evaluation of the Treatment of Aspiration Pneumonia in Hospitalized Children [published online ahead of print, 2021 Dec 13]. J Pediatr Infect Dis Soc 2021. https://doi.org/10.1093/jpids/piab122. piab122.

29. Hochhegger B, Zanon M, Altmayer S, et al. COVID-19 mimics on chest CT: a pictorial review and radiologic guide. Br J Radiol 2021;94(1118):20200703.

30. Saha BK, Milman NT. Idiopathic pulmonary hemosiderosis: a review of the treatments used during the past 30 years and future directions. Clin Rheumatol 2021;40(7):2547–57.

31. Cuceoglu MK, Ozen S. Pulmonary Manifestations of Systemic Vasculitis in Children. Pediatr Clin North Am 2021;68(1):167–76.

32. Hare SS, Souza CA, Bain G, et al. The radiological spectrum of pulmonary lymphoproliferative disease. Br J Radiol 2012;85(1015):848–64.

33. Della Valle V, Donadieu J, Sileo C, et al. Chest computed tomography findings for a cohort of children with pulmonary Langerhans cell histiocytosis. Pediatr Blood Cancer 2020;67(10):e28496.

34. Le Louet S, Barkaoui MA, Miron J, et al. Childhood Langerhans cell histiocytosis with severe lung involvement: a nationwide cohort study. Orphanet J Rare Dis 2020;15(1):241.

35. Gorkem SB, Köse S, Lee EY, et al. Thoracic MRI evaluation of sarcoidosis in children. Pediatr Pulmonol 2017;52(4):494–9.

36. Kanne JP, Yandow DR, Meyer CA. Pneumocystis jiroveci pneumonia: high-resolution CT findings in patients with and without HIV infection. AJR Am J Roentgenol 2012;198(6):W555–61.

37. Shin YM. Posttransplantation lymphoproliferative disorder involving liver after renal transplantation. Korean J Hepatol 2011;17(2):165–9.

MR Imaging for the Evaluation of Diffuse Lung Disease: Where Are We?

Bryan O'Sullivan-Murphy, MD, PhD, Bastiaan Driehuys, PhD, Joseph Mammarappallil, MD, PhD*

KEYWORDS

- Hyperpolarized [129]Xenon MR imaging ● MR imaging ● Diffuse lung disease ● Pulmonary imaging
- Long-COVID ● ILD ● Cystic fibrosis ● COPD

KEY POINTS

- Hyperpolarized [129]Xe-MR lung imaging permits evaluation of pulmonary ventilation, microstructure, and gaseous exchange.
- MR lung imaging has demonstrated utility in evaluation of 1) obstructive lung diseases including COPD and asthma, 2) diffuse lung diseases including pulmonary fibrosis, cystic fibrosis, and 'long COVID', and 3) pulmonary vascular imaging.

INTRODUCTION

Diffuse lung disease represents an umbrella term comprising a collection of lung disorders. Clinical assessment of patients requires thorough medical and social history and physical examinations, coupled with laboratory tests, pulmonary function tests (PFTs), and radiologic imaging. Often, a multidisciplinary team involving pulmonology, radiology, and pathology are needed to discern the diagnosis and treatment plan. From the radiologic viewpoint, chest radiography and computed tomography (CT) are the general imaging workhorses in diffuse lung diseases. Chest radiography is useful for initial work-up and can identify acute exacerbation and detect macroscopic parenchymal changes associated with progression of lung disease, although it is generally poor at identifying subtle changes.[1] High-resolution CT (HRCT) is far superior in determining the extent and progression of diffuse lung diseases given the noninvasive, rapid technique and intricate high-resolution images of the airway, pulmonary parenchyma, and bronchovascular anatomy.[2] For interstitial lung diseases (ILDs) in particular,

HRCT is the key diagnostic approach in defining the specific diagnosis.[3] MR imaging, however, which is often considered the pinnacle of radiologic imaging because of its superior tissue characteristic distinction, has conventionally not been an ideal choice in pulmonary imaging given the dearth of protons in lung parenchyma, magnetic field inhomogeneities, and physiologic motion of the lungs and heart.[4] Advancements in pulmonary MR imaging technology and protocols including those using ultrashort echo times have improved lung tissue definition.[5] Furthermore, pulmonary MR imaging using inhaled hyperpolarized (HP-MR imaging) gases can offer further detail of structural changes and regions of diseased lung, while also determining functional dynamics of impaired gas exchange and vascular flow in the lung.[6] Considering that diffuse lung diseases affect the airways and pulmonary parenchyma including the alveolar-capillary interface in the vascular bed, HP-MR imaging may represent a unique imaging approach in understanding the cause of these diseases, detection of early changes of progression, or response to treatment. The following review presents the current state of imaging of

Department of Radiology, Duke University Medical Center, PO Box 3808, 2301 Erwin Road, Durham, NC 27710, USA
* Corresponding author. m
E-mail address: joseph.mammarappallil@duke.edu

Radiol Clin N Am 60 (2022) 1021–1032
https://doi.org/10.1016/j.rcl.2022.06.007
0033-8389/22/© 2022 Elsevier Inc. All rights reserved.

various diffuse lung diseases by HP-MR imaging and highlights the superior morphologic and functional information gained from this modality.

HYPERPOLARIZED 129XE-MR IMAGING OF THE LUNGS

The lungs consist of multidimensional complex anatomic domains with soft tissue, vascular, and gas compartments domains, with respiratory and cardiac motion complicating imaging approaches. Pulmonary MR imaging is not in widespread clinical use because of several inherent issues, although recent advances with motion gating and ultrashort echo time MR imaging sequences have improved the spatial resolution and tissue definition of the lung.[5] Given the improved visualization of lung anatomy, it is plausible that MR imaging may become an imaging tool in diffuse lung diseases, possibly interlaced between HRCT examinations, with the goal to decrease ionizing radiation in these patients.

Intravascular contrast in CT and MR imaging improves visualization of soft tissues and vascular structures. However, given that inhaled air comprises a significant volume of the lung, the novel approach of using exogenously inhaled gas as a contrast media, with specifically tuned MR imaging protocols to identify the inhaled gas atoms, would further enhance the information that is currently achievable through conventional MR imaging. Historically, helium 3 (^{3}He) was used as the inhaled gas in HP-MR imaging, although decreased supply chains and increasing costs of ^{3}He gas limited adoption into pulmonary imaging.[7] Imaging with xenon 129 (^{129}Xe) gas has increased because of its availability, affordability, and excellent safety profile.[8] Imaging the dynamic flow of inhaled gas and transfer into the bloodstream could provide detailed information about pulmonary ventilation and gas exchange and position pulmonary MR imaging as an integral component in evaluating and monitoring diffuse lung diseases.

An important aspect of this approach is the ability to image the inhaled gas within the lungs; to overcome their inherent signal deficit caused by their low density, the magnetization of gas atoms is enhanced 100,000-fold via a process termed hyperpolarization. The physical principles pertaining to hyperpolarization of gases have been previously outlined[8]; basically, the increase in nuclear spin polarization is accomplished via the processes of optical pumping and spin exchange. Optical pumping involves the use of a circularly polarized laser light to align the valence electron of a heavy alkali metal, such as rubidium, after which spin

exchange occurs when polarized electron spins of rubidium collide with the nuclei of the adjacent ^{3}He or ^{129}Xe, transferring the alignment of electrons to the noble gas.[8,9]

MR imaging using HP gas offers several distinct advantages in determining pulmonary anatomy and function. HP-^{129}Xe-MR imaging is a fast, well-tolerated study that has enabled a multitude of structural and functional pulmonary characteristics, including ventilation and diffusion imaging.[10] The imaged distribution of inhaled gas permits the detection of focal MR imaging voids representing ventilation defects, termed the ventilation defect percent (VDP).[11] Using diffusion-weighted imaging, the apparent diffusion coefficient is used to measure airspace enlargement, such as that found in emphysema and cystic regions in fibrotic lung disease.[12,13] The solubility and wide chemical shift range of HP-^{129}Xe gas permits the detection of the gas as it partitions across the alveolar (gas) to membrane (interstitium and plasma) to red blood cell (RBC) phases (**Fig. 1**), and is used to characterize pulmonary gas flow mechanics, similar to that of inhaled oxygen.[14–16] Gaseous and dissolved xenon generates a set of three detectable MR imaging spectral peaks at distinct frequencies corresponding to gaseous xenon in the airspaces (0 ppm), xenon dissolved in the barrier membrane tissues (198 ppm), and xenon associated with hemoglobin in the RBC (218 ppm) (see **Fig. 1**).

CHRONIC OBSTRUCTIVE PULMONARY DISEASE IMAGING

Chronic obstructive pulmonary disease (COPD) is a common respiratory condition characterized by airflow limitation and a leading cause of morbidity and mortality throughout the world.[17] Clinically, pulmonologists depend on PFTs, to provide whole-lung measures of pulmonary function, including a measurement of the conductance of gas transfer, termed the diffusing capacity for carbon monoxide (DLCO). However, PFTs are insensitive for the detection of minor changes heralding disease progression or defining responses to novel COPD therapies. Thus, it is apparent that management of this disease would benefit from earlier identification and functional imaging of disease progression.

Although chest radiography is useful in detection of emphysema, HRCT is the imaging modality of choice in COPD and used to quantify the distribution and degree of disease with accuracy and reproducibility, with visual characterization and severity of emphysema on HRCT correlating with mortality.[18] More recent developments with

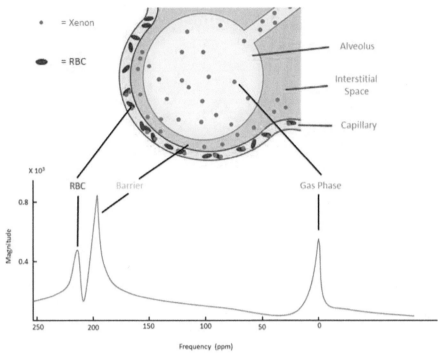

Fig. 1. Spectrum of ^{129}Xe exhibits three distinct resonance peaks in the lung that correspond to specific locations: 0 ppm in the "gas phase," 198 ppm in the membrane phase (interstitial tissues and plasma), and 217 ppm in the RBC-bound phase.

artificial intelligence have led to the emergence of quantitative CT analysis as a powerful tool to augment visual assessment of COPD and other diffuse lung diseases.[19] MR imaging using HP ^{3}He or ^{129}Xe has shown promise as a complementary tool to HRCT in the detection of regional ventilation defects in patients with COPD.[10,20,21] A recent study by Qing and colleagues[22] used a multi-pronged approach with chest CT, perfusion MR imaging, and ventilation and gas uptake by HP-^{129}Xe-MR imaging to demonstrate the unique potential for HP- ^{129}Xe-MR imaging in identifying alterations in lung physiology. To determine the utility of HP-^{129}Xe MR imaging in monitoring response to therapy for COPD, Mummy and colleagues[23] examined the changes in xenon gas transfer following the administration of long-acting β-agonist/long-acting muscarinic-antagonist bronchodilators (Fig. 2), showing improved ventilation in patients with COPD with preserved barrier uptake and DLCO, although the uncovered ventilated regions demonstrated underlying RBC transfer defects. Overall, HP-^{129}Xe-MR imaging provides insights into lung injury and physiology that can detect COPD at an earlier phase, determine functional decline before that found by conventional PFTs, and distinguish response to therapy, positioning HP-^{129}Xe-MR imaging as a prime tool in COPD imaging.

PULMONARY VASCULAR IMAGING

Pulmonary arterial hypertension is a disease of the pulmonary vasculature classified into five groups based on cause and mechanism.[24] Echocardiography is used for initial assessment for suspected pulmonary hypertension, with chest radiography, CT, ventilation/perfusion scans, and cardiac MR imaging as ancillary imaging techniques.[25] Chest CT angiography, in particular, is useful in identifying causes and sequelae of pulmonary hypertension.[26] A possible alternative approach is to directly and noninvasively image the vascular abnormalities in the lung with the goal of defining regions of decreased microvasculature function using HP-MR imaging. An initial study by Dahhan and colleagues[27] using HP-^{129}Xe-MR imaging in two patients with suspected pulmonary vascular disease demonstrated normal ventilation patterns but markedly reduced gas transfer, suggesting the utility of this novel imaging technique in the diagnosis of pulmonary vascular disease and possibly monitoring response to therapy. Although still at the experimental phase, cardiogenic oscillations of the dissolved HP-^{129}Xe signal in the RBC phase can be detected.[28,29] Teasing apart the details of these RBC oscillations revealed lower amplitude and greater lower percentage in patients with pulmonary arterial hypertension when

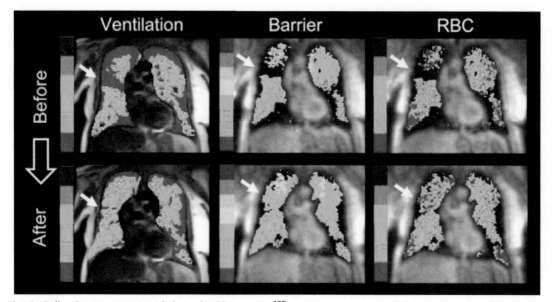

Fig. 2. Following treatment with bronchodilators, HP-^{129}Xe-MR imaging revealed improvement of ventilation and barrier xenon gas uptake in patients with COPD. Example of a subject where a region of improved ventilation following therapy (*arrows*) revealed areas of normal barrier uptake but poor RBC transfer. (*From* Mummy DG, Coleman EM, Wang Z, Bier EA, Lu J, Driehuys B, Huang YC. Regional Gas Exchange Measured by ^{129} Xe Magnetic Resonance Imaging Before and After Combination Bronchodilators Treatment in Chronic Obstructive Pulmonary Disease. J Magn Reson Imaging. 2021 Sep;54(3):964-974.)

compared with healthy control patients.[30] Advancements in this research by Wang and colleagues[31] showed that various cardiopulmonary diseases generated distinct xenon MR imaging signatures (**Fig. 3**). Taken together, HP-^{129}Xe-MR imaging has the potential to be an additional tool in pulmonary vascular imaging as a noninvasive, nonionizing approach to assess lung structure and disease, in addition to providing information regarding gas exchange and regional pulmonary microvasculature function.

ASTHMA

Asthma is a common chronic airway inflammatory disease, with the classic reporting signs and symptoms of wheezing, dyspnea, chest tightness, and cough that vary in intensity and duration.[32] Globally, approximately 5% of the adult population is affected, resulting in significant health care–associated costs and economic burden. Asthma diagnosis and management is routinely performed using PFTs. However, similar to COPD, PFTs are used to determine the global lung function, but are insensitive to small airway perturbations.[33] Earlier diagnosis of asthma, evaluation of potential exacerbations, and response to treatment would be beneficial for improving patient outcomes.

The role of imaging in asthma is not to diagnose the disease, but primarily focused on identifying possible complications, such as allergic bronchopulmonary aspergillosis, or to suggest an alternative diagnosis.[34] HRCT is useful in defining anatomic abnormalities, such as bronchial wall thickening, air-trapping, and bronchiectasis.[34] Recent imaging approaches, including via HP-MR imaging, have been geared to understanding the complexities of regional lung ventilation and gas exchange in patients with asthma. A comprehensive review by Kooner and colleagues[35] highlights the history and potential clinical use of HP-MR imaging in asthma management. Fundamentally, HP-MR imaging is used to identify regional ventilation defects in patients with asthma, and these have been shown to correlate with disease severity and are exacerbated following bronchoprovocation.[36,37] Mummy and colleagues[38,39] used HP-^{3}He-MR imaging to demonstrate VDP in patients with asthma that are strongly associated with future exacerbations, suggesting this as a promising asthma biomarker. HP-^{129}Xe-MR imaging recapitulates the ventilation defects seen in patients with asthma, with a moderate to strong correlation with PFTs, although HP-^{129}Xe-MR imaging is believed to be more sensitive to airflow in the entire bronchial tree.[40] Comparing HP-^{3}He with HP-^{129}Xe MR imaging in patients with asthma, the latter was superior in defining more ventilation deficits.[6] HP-MR imaging has been trialed as a method to assess therapy in

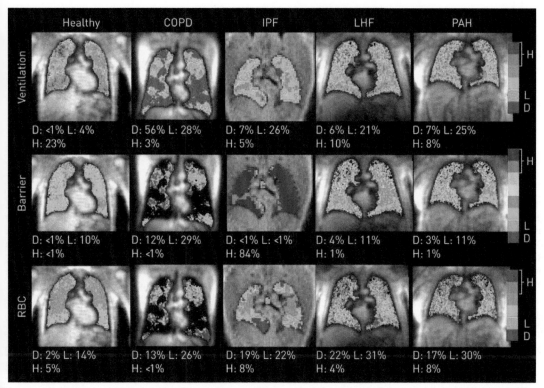

Fig. 3. Ventilation, normalized barrier uptake, and RBC transfer maps of representative subjects from each cohort. IPF, idiopathic pulmonary fibrosis; LHF, left heart failure; PAH, pulmonary arterial hypertension. The color bins represent signal intensity, with *red* for the lowest, *blue/purple* for the highest, and *green* representing voxels in the healthy reference range. Each map is quantified by the percentage of defect (D), low (L), and high (H), calculated as the voxel fraction of the lowest, second lowest, and the highest two bins for each map, respectively. The voxels with ventilation defect were excluded from the analysis of barrier uptake and RBC transfer maps. Reproduced with permission of the © ERS 2022: Wang Z, Bier EA, Swaminathan A, Parikh K, Nouls J, He M, Mammarappallil JG, Luo S, Driehuys B, Rajagopal S. Diverse cardiopulmonary diseases are associated with distinct xenon magnetic resonance imaging signatures. European Respiratory Journal 201954: 1900831; DOI: 10.1183/13993003.00831-2019.

asthma: following bronchodilator treatment in asthma, Svenningsen and colleagues[7] demonstrated discrete improvements in ventilation deficits identified by HP-MR, supporting this modality as a means of assessing response to therapy (**Fig. 4**). In a promising single study of patients with severe asthma, the response to the monoclonal antibody dupilumab was evaluated with HP-MR imaging, whereupon ventilation heterogeneity was normalized, despite PFT showing some airflow limitation.[41] Thus, it seems that HP-MR imaging has the potential to be used clinically to identify small airway changes in asthma, prognosticate the potential for exacerbations, and drive the clinical development of novel therapies.

INTERSTITIAL LUNG DISEASE

The term ILD includes a large group of complex parenchymal lung diseases that cause various patterns of inflammation and fibrosis throughout the alveolar, interstitial, and vascular compartments of the lung.[42] Among the ILD subtypes, idiopathic pulmonary fibrosis (IPF) is the most common and confers a poor prognosis with less than 5-year survival after diagnosis.[3,43] Although there is no cure for IPF, survival time is prolonged with earlier diagnosis and management. Newer antifibrotic medications, nintedanib and pirfenidone, have been shown to slow progression of disease and decrease acute exacerbations, with decreased all-cause mortality.[44] Prompt diagnosis of IPF is paramount to ensure appropriate care and earlier initiation of antifibrotic therapy.

Imaging is essential in IPF diagnosis, with a usual interstitial pneumonia pattern on HRCT being diagnostic of IPF.[3] PFTs are limited in IPF because they tend to be insensitive to early fibrotic changes and are complicated by comorbidities. HP-[129]Xe-MR imaging is a promising tool for definition of early markers of IPF and clarifying disease progression in IPF, and has been comprehensively reviewed.[45]

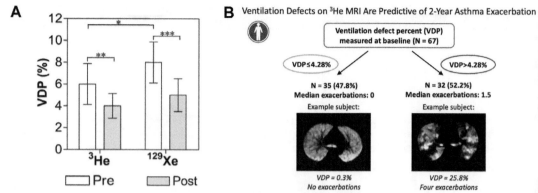

Fig. 4. (*A*) Bronchodilator response using HP-³He- and HP-¹²⁹Xe-MR imaging (*$*p \leq 0.01$, **$p \leq 0.001$, ***$p \leq 0.0001$). (*B*) The ventilation defect percent (VDP) derived from hyperpolarized gas lung MR imaging is predictive of 2-year asthma exacerbation. (*From* [*A*] Svenningsen S, Kirby M, Starr D, Leary D, Wheatley A, Maksym GN, McCormack DG, Parraga G. Hyperpolarized (3) He and (129) Xe MRI: differences in asthma before bronchodilation. J Magn Reson Imaging. 2013 Dec;38(6):1521-30; and [*B*] Mummy DG, Carey KJ, Evans MD, Denlinger LC, Schiebler ML, Sorkness RL, Jarjour NN, Fain SB. Ventilation defects on hyperpolarized helium-3 MRI in asthma are predictive of 2-year exacerbation frequency. J Allergy Clin Immunol. 2020 Oct;146(4):831-839.e6.)

Initial studies evaluating IPF in whole-lung spectroscopy demonstrated a decreased RBC/membrane ratio of xenon gas in patients with IPF compared with healthy volunteers, correlating with DLCO values.[46] From there, HP-¹²⁹Xe-MR imaging in IPF has further defined the dynamics of xenon gas transfer across the blood/gas interface, with Stewart and colleagues[47,48] showing the increased septal thickness in lungs of patients with IPF and systemic sclerosis compared with healthy volunteers. Further developments in MR imaging approaches to distinguish the gas phase, barrier phase, and RBC-bound HP-¹²⁹Xe gas allowed Kaushik and colleagues[46] to demonstrate regions of impaired gas exchange in patients with IPF that correlated with fibrosis on HRCT in a peripheral and basilar pattern.

Extrapolating the data acquired by MR imaging at the voxel level allowed the development of three-dimensional quantitative color maps of lung function with ventilation, barrier xenon uptake, and RBC transfer histograms generated.[49–51] Extension of these research endeavors led Wang and colleagues[49] to discover that, in addition to regions of decreased RBC transfer, there was increased barrier uptake of xenon in patients with IPF, suggesting regions of decreased diffusivity related to fibrosis. Recent studies have shown the value of HP-¹²⁹Xe-MR imaging in detecting disease progression in patients with IPF as manifested through decreasing RBC/barrier ratio before these findings were evident on standard PFTs (**Fig. 5**).[51,52]

HP-¹²⁹Xe MR imaging is not exclusive to evaluating IPF, with a recent study from Mummy and colleagues[53] showing increased barrier uptake, decreased RBC transfer, and overall reduced RBC/barrier ratio in patients with nonspecific interstitial pneumonia. Furthermore, Eaden and colleagues[54] used HP-¹²⁹Xe-MR imaging to differentiate the airway microstructure between fibrotic and inflammatory ILDs with observed differences on diffusion-weighted imaging. In addition, their study revealed declining gas exchange in fibrotic ILD compared with patients with inflammatory ILD based on xenon RBC/barrier ratio, suggesting that HP-¹²⁹Xe-MR imaging could be used to assess the progression of fibrotic ILD.[54]

Although HRCT is an essential tool in defining ILD, HP-¹²⁹Xe-MR imaging provides an exciting nonionizing technique that can be added to the arsenal of ILD imaging tools to establish the severity of the disease, monitor progression, and determine response to treatment.

CYSTIC FIBROSIS

Cystic fibrosis (CF) is a fatal autosomal-recessive disorder highly prevalent in populations of Northern European descent. In the lungs, the dysfunctional Cystic Fibrosis Transmembrane conductance Regulator (*CFTR*) protein causes chronic stasis of viscous mucus secretions in the airways, resulting in airway obstruction and inflammation, culminating in progressive morphologic changes. Clinically, CF manifests as a persistent productive cough, with hyperinflated lungs, obstructive airway pathology, and recurrent infections.

HRCT is the gold standard in CF imaging with dedicated protocols including inspiratory and expiratory phases that aid in the delineation of bronchiectasis and degree of air-trapping. Studies over the past two decades evaluating pulmonary MR

A

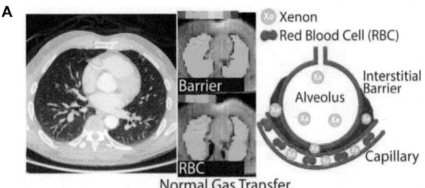

Normal Gas Transfer

B

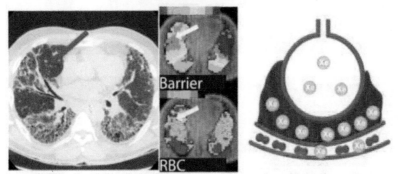

Diffusion Block - High Barrier, Impaired RBC Transfer

C

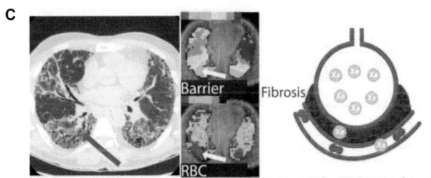

End Stage Fibrosis - Low/Normal Barrier, Little RBC Transfer

D

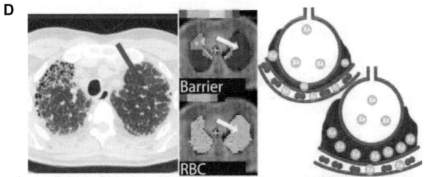

Active Disease - High Barrier, Preserved RBC Transfer

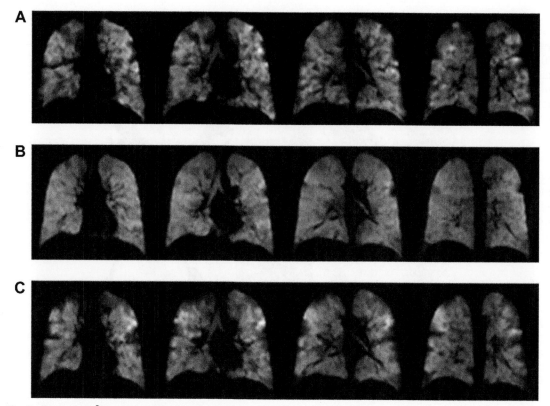

Fig. 6. Coronal HP-³He-MR imaging images of patient 002 in *A*. Typical images are shown (expanded image sets of the same case are given). Following inhalation of the hyperpolarized gas, well-ventilated lung regions appear *bright white*, and poorly ventilated regions (termed "ventilation defects") appear *dark gray/black*. (*A*) Baseline (Day 15): ppFEV₁: 62.2; TVD_H: 51.7%; TVD_C: 48.4%. (*B*) End of 4 weeks of ivacaftor treatment (Day 43): ppFEV₁: 83.0; TVD_H: 27.1%; TVD_C: 17.4%. (*C*) End of 2 weeks of placebo washout (Day 57): ppFEV₁: 71.6; TVD_H: 57.4%; TVD_C: 40.9%. (ppFEV₁ = percent predicted offorced expiratory volume in 1 second; TVD_H = total ventilation defect human reader; TVD_C = total ventilation defect computer algorithm). (*From* Altes TA, Johnson M, Fidler M, Botfield M, Tustison NJ, Leiva-Salinas C, de Lange EE, Froh D, Mugler JP 3rd. Use of hyperpolarized helium-3 MRI to assess response to ivacaftor treatment in patients with cystic fibrosis. J Cyst Fibros. 2017 Mar;16(2):267-274.)

imaging have shown that MR imaging provides similar structural changes related to CF comparable with CT images.[55] In addition, HP-¹²⁹Xe-MR imaging has been suggested as a complementary imaging tool in assessing complicated asthma cases.[56]

Initial studies by several groups using HP-³He-MR imaging showed the underlying ventilation heterogeneity in patients with CF that were concordant with structural changes seen on CT imaging and stronger than spirometry.[57,58] Thomen and colleagues[59] used HP-¹²⁹Xe-MR imaging to show marked ventilation defects in patients with CF with normal spirometry, positing that HP-¹²⁹Xe-MR imaging may be used to detect

Fig. 5. Proposed models of gas transfer for various barrier uptake (*red* = low, *plum/orchid* = high) and RBC transfer patterns (*red* = low, *blue* = high). In a healthy lung (*A*), gaseous ¹²⁹Xe efficiently diffuses from the alveolus, across a thin barrier to RBCs, resulting in signal intensities in the normal range for both compartments. In IPF, however, interstitial fibrosis thickens the barrier tissue, which increases xenon uptake. In some regions of barrier enhancement (*B, arrows*), diffusion across it is slowed, causing RBC transfer to decrease. As the disease progresses (*C, arrows*), scarring becomes so severe that ¹²⁹Xe no longer diffuses into or through the barrier. Therefore barrier uptake returns to the normal or low range, whereas RBC transfer is dramatically reduced. Most interesting are regions depicting the coexistence of increased barrier uptake with preserved RBC transfer (*D, arrows*). This may represent regions of disease activity that could be responsive to therapy. (*From* Wang JM, Robertson SH, Wang Z, He M, Virgincar RS, Schrank GM, Smigla RM, O'Riordan TG, Sundy J, Ebner L, Rackley CR, McAdams P, Driehuys B. Using hyperpolarized 129Xe MRI to quantify regional gas transfer in idiopathic pulmonary fibrosis. Thorax. 2018 Jan;73(1):21-28.)

mild pulmonary changes in CF. HP-MR imaging has also been used to demonstrate the effectiveness of bronchodilator therapy.[60] Gene-specific mucolytic therapies, such as ivacaftor and Trikafta, are exciting prospects in CF therapy. Altes and colleagues[61] used HP-³He-MR imaging to identify short- and long-term improvements in ventilation following treatment with ivacaftor (Fig. 6).

Overall, imaging with HP-MR imaging has been shown to be a reproducible means of obtaining noninvasive, nonionizing, high-resolution regional lung functional data, outperforming spirometry in detecting early changes of CF lung disease and being effective in monitoring response to novel CF therapies.

COVID-19

In late 2019, a novel coronavirus, severe acute respiratory syndrome coronavirus 2 (SARS-CoV-2 or COVID-19), emerged leading to a worldwide pandemic public health emergency.[62] Symptoms of COVID-19 infection range in severity although predominantly affect the lungs. Imaging with chest radiographs and CT increased for detection of pneumonia and complications.[63] MR imaging of the lungs depicted peripheral consolidations similar to those noted on chest CT.[64] As the pandemic progressed, there were escalating medical accounts of "recovered" COVID-19 patients exhibiting persistent symptoms, such as fatigue and breathlessness, described medically as "long-COVID."[65] Despite the persistence of symptoms in patients with long-COVID, PFTs showed abnormal pulmonary diffusion in 27% of patients and minimal subpleural changes noted on CT.[66] To further explore pulmonary function post-COVID-19, Li and colleagues[67] used HP-¹²⁹Xe-MR imaging to demonstrate higher VDP in discharged COVID-19 patients compared with healthy control subjects. Their research proposed that interstitial thickening and subpleural fibrosis in the lungs of post-COVID-19 patients, similar to that seen with SARS viral infection, contributed to impaired gas exchange.[68] A recent study by Grist and colleagues[69] used HP-¹²⁹Xe-MR imaging to show abnormalities in the lungs of some COVID-19 patients many months after discharge from the hospital. HP-¹²⁹Xe-MR imaging demonstrated a significant difference in the RBC to tissue/plasma ratio between post-COVID-19 patients and healthy control subjects, localizing the regions of the lungs where gas exchange was impaired in post-COVID patients.[69] Given the unprecedented impact of the COVID-19 pandemic and symptoms of long COVID, continued research with HP-¹²⁹Xe-MR imaging is underway and may become essential in identifying those patients at risk of prolonged symptoms and provide a way of assessing potential therapies.

SUMMARY

MR imaging using HP gases, and in particular ¹²⁹Xe, represents a unique and sensitive technique to advance the structural definition and functional characteristics of the lung, providing quantitative physiologic information. HP-MR imaging has the potential to ascertain lung abnormalities earlier than PFTs and has the ability to prognosticate exacerbations in ILD, COPD, and CF, allowing earlier intervention or therapy to mitigate further damage. Ventilation imaging with HP-¹²⁹Xe is highly sensitive to changes associated with therapy and could strengthen the outcome of clinical trials of novel therapeutic agents. In addition, the absence of ionizing radiation with HP-MR imaging allows safer chronic monitoring of disease progression and therapy. Currently, HP-¹²⁹Xe-MR imaging is approved for clinical use in the United Kingdom, with the modality under Food and Drug Administration review for clinical approval in the United States, possibly in late 2022. Ultimately, the complementary use of HP-MR imaging alongside HRCT may be the optimal approach to evaluate structural-functional relationships and monitor progression and therapeutic responses.

CLINICS CARE POINTS

- Hyperpolarized gas MR imaging of the lungs is a novel approach to define lung parenchyma and functional characteristics of the lung, with the potential for advancing ILD diagnosis and management.

DISCLOSURE

B. O'Sullivan-Murphy disclosed no relevant relationships. B. Driehuys' activities related to the present article: disclosed no relevant relationships. Activities not related to the present article: is founder of and a board member for Polarean Imaging; has patents planned, pending, or issued; receives royalties from a xenon gas-exchange MR imaging patent; and holds stock/stock options in Polarean Imaging. Other relationships: has intellectual property licensed and issued and also receives royalties for intellectual property. J. Mammarappallil disclosed no relevant relationships.

REFERENCES

1. Behr J. Approach to the diagnosis of interstitial lung disease. Clin Chest Med 2012;33(1):1–10.

2. Mayo JR. CT evaluation of diffuse infiltrative lung disease: dose considerations and optimal technique. J Thorac Imaging 2009;24(4):252–9.

3. Raghu G, Remy-Jardin M, Myers JL, et al. Diagnosis of idiopathic pulmonary fibrosis. An official ATS/ERS/JRS/ALAT Clinical Practice Guideline. Am J Respir Crit Care Med 2018;198(5):e44–68.

4. Weatherley ND, Eaden JA, Stewart NJ, et al. Experimental and quantitative imaging techniques in interstitial lung disease. Thorax 2019;74(6):611–9.

5. Johnson KM, Fain SB, Schiebler ML, et al. Optimized 3D ultrashort echo time pulmonary MRI. Magn Reson Med 2013;70(5):1241–50.

6. Marshall H, Stewart NJ, Chan HF, et al. In vivo methods and applications of xenon-129 magnetic resonance. Prog Nucl Magn Reson Spectrosc 2021;122:42–62.

7. Svenningsen S, Kirby M, Starr D, et al. Hyperpolarized (3) He and (129) Xe MRI: differences in asthma before bronchodilation. J Magn Reson Imaging 2013;38(6):1521–30.

8. Roos JE, McAdams HP, Kaushik SS, et al. Hyperpolarized gas MR imaging: technique and applications. Magn Reson Imaging Clin N Am 2015;23(2):217–29.

9. Norquay G, Collier GJ, Rao M, et al. {129}Xe-Rb spin-exchange optical pumping with high photon efficiency. Phys Rev Lett 2018;121(15):153201.

10. Driehuys B, Martinez-Jimenez S, Cleveland ZI, et al. Chronic obstructive pulmonary disease: safety and tolerability of hyperpolarized 129Xe MR imaging in healthy volunteers and patients. Radiology 2012;262(1):279–89.

11. Kirby M, Svenningsen S, Owrangi A, et al. Hyperpolarized 3He and 129Xe MR imaging in healthy volunteers and patients with chronic obstructive pulmonary disease. Radiology 2012;265(2):600–10.

12. Ouriadov A, Farag A, Kirby M, et al. Lung morphometry using hyperpolarized (129) Xe apparent diffusion coefficient anisotropy in chronic obstructive pulmonary disease. Magn Reson Med 2013;70(6):1699–706.

13. Chan HF, Stewart NJ, Norquay G, et al. 3D diffusion-weighted 129 Xe MRI for whole lung morphometry. Magn Reson Med 2018;79(6):2986–95.

14. Qing K, Ruppert K, Jiang Y, et al. Regional mapping of gas uptake by blood and tissue in the human lung using hyperpolarized xenon-129 MRI. J Magn Reson Imaging 2014;39(2):346–59.

15. Kaushik SS, Robertson SH, Freeman MS, et al. Single-breath clinical imaging of hyperpolarized (129) Xe in the airspaces, barrier, and red blood cells using an interleaved 3D radial 1-point Dixon acquisition. Magn Reson Med 2016;75(4):1434–43.

16. Wang Z, Rankine L, Bier EA, et al. Using hyperpolarized 129Xe gas-exchange MRI to model the regional airspace, membrane, and capillary contributions to diffusing capacity. J Appl Physiol (1985) 2021;130(5):1398–409.

17. Global Strategy for Prevention, Diagnosis and Management of COPD: 2021 Report (PDF). Global Initiative for Chronic Obstructive Lung Disease. 25 November 2020. https://goldcopd.org/wp-content/uploads/2020/11/GOLD-REPORT-2021-v1.1-25Nov20_WMV.pdf Accessed 01/01/2022.

18. Lynch DA, Moore CM, Wilson C, et al. CT-based visual classification of emphysema: association with mortality in the COPDGene Study. Radiology 2018;288(3):859–66.

19. Chen A, Karwoski RA, Gierada DS, et al. Quantitative CT analysis of diffuse lung disease. Radiographics 2020;40(1):28–43.

20. van Beek EJ, Dahmen AM, Stavngaard T, et al. Hyperpolarised 3He MRI versus HRCT in COPD and normal volunteers: PHIL trial. Eur Respir J 2009;34(6):1311–21.

21. Virgincar RS, Cleveland ZI, Kaushik SS, et al. Quantitative analysis of hyperpolarized 129Xe ventilation imaging in healthy volunteers and subjects with chronic obstructive pulmonary disease. NMR Biomed 2013;26(4):424–35.

22. Qing K, Tustison NJ, Mugler JP 3rd, et al. Probing changes in lung physiology in COPD using CT, perfusion MRI, and hyperpolarized Xenon-129 MRI. Acad Radiol 2019;26(3):326–34.

23. Mummy DG, Coleman EM, Wang Z, et al. Regional gas exchange measured by 129 Xe magnetic resonance imaging before and after combination bronchodilators treatment in chronic obstructive pulmonary disease. J Magn Reson Imaging 2021;54(3):964–74.

24. Simonneau G, Montani D, Celermajer DS, et al. Haemodynamic definitions and updated clinical classification of pulmonary hypertension. Eur Respir J 2019;53(1):1801913.

25. Ascha M, Renapurkar RD, Tonelli AR. A review of imaging modalities in pulmonary hypertension. Ann Thorac Med 2017;12(2):61–73.

26. Remy-Jardin M, Ryerson CJ, Schiebler ML, et al. Imaging of pulmonary hypertension in adults: a position paper from the Fleischner Society. Radiology 2021;298(3):531–49.

27. Dahhan T, Kaushik SS, He M, et al. Abnormalities in hyperpolarized (129)Xe magnetic resonance imaging and spectroscopy in two patients with pulmonary vascular disease. Pulm Circ 2016;6(1):126–31.

28. Bier EA, Robertson SH, Schrank GM, et al. A protocol for quantifying cardiogenic oscillations in dynamic 129 Xe gas exchange spectroscopy:

the effects of idiopathic pulmonary fibrosis. NMR Biomed 2019;32(1):e4029.

29. Ruppert K, Altes TA, Mata JF, et al. Detecting pulmonary capillary blood pulsations using hyperpolarized xenon-129 chemical shift saturation recovery (CSSR) MR spectroscopy. Magn Reson Med 2016; 75(4):1771–80.

30. Niedbalski PJ, Bier EA, Wang Z, et al. Mapping cardiopulmonary dynamics within the microvasculature of the lungs using dissolved 129Xe MRI. J Appl Physiol (1985) 2020;129(2):218–29.

31. Wang Z, Bier EA, Swaminathan A, et al. Diverse cardiopulmonary diseases are associated with distinct xenon magnetic resonance imaging signatures. Eur Respir J 2019;54(6):1900831.

32. Dharmage SC, Perret JL, Custovic A. Epidemiology of asthma in children and adults. Front Pediatr 2019; 7:246.

33. Gallucci M, Carbonara P, Pacilli AMG, et al. Use of symptoms scores, spirometry, and other pulmonary function testing for asthma monitoring. Front Pediatr 2019;7:54.

34. Richards JC, Lynch D, Koelsch T, et al. Imaging of asthma. Immunol Allergy Clin North Am 2016; 36(3):529–45.

35. Kooner HK, McIntosh MJ, Desaigoudar V, et al. Pulmonary functional MRI: detecting the structure-function pathologies that drive asthma symptoms and quality of life. Respirology 2022;27(2):114–33.

36. de Lange EE, Altes TA, Patrie JT, et al. Evaluation of asthma with hyperpolarized helium-3 MRI: correlation with clinical severity and spirometry. Chest 2006;130:1055–62.

37. Samee S, Altes T, Powers P, et al. Imaging the lungs in asthmatic patients by using hyperpolarized helium-3 magnetic resonance: assessment of response to methacholine and exercise challenge. J Allergy Clin Immunol 2003;111(6):1205–11.

38. Mummy DG, Kruger SJ, Zha W, et al. Ventilation defect percent in helium-3 magnetic resonance imaging as a biomarker of severe outcomes in asthma. J Allergy Clin Immunol 2018;141(3): 1140–1.e4.

39. Mummy DG, Carey KJ, Evans MD, et al. Ventilation defects on hyperpolarized helium-3 MRI in asthma are predictive of 2-year exacerbation frequency. J Allergy Clin Immunol 2020;146(4):831–9.e6.

40. Ebner L, He M, Virgincar RS, et al. Hyperpolarized 129Xenon magnetic resonance imaging to quantify regional ventilation differences in mild to moderate asthma: a prospective comparison between semiautomated ventilation defect percentage calculation and pulmonary function tests. Invest Radiol 2017; 52(2):120–7.

41. Svenningsen S, Haider EA, Eddy RL, et al. Normalisation of MRI ventilation heterogeneity in severe asthma by dupilumab. Thorax 2019;74(11):1087–8.

42. Wallis A, Spinks K. The diagnosis and management of interstitial lung diseases. BMJ 2015;350:h2072.

43. Nicholson AG, Colby TV, du Bois RM, et al. The prognostic significance of the histologic pattern of interstitial pneumonia in patients presenting with the clinical entity of cryptogenic fibrosing alveolitis. Am J Respir Crit Care Med 2000;162(6):2213–7.

44. Petnak T, Lertjitbanjong P, Thongprayoon C, et al. Impact of antifibrotic therapy on mortality and acute exacerbation in idiopathic pulmonary fibrosis: a systematic review and meta-analysis. Chest 2021; 160(5):1751–63.

45. Mammarappallil JG, Rankine L, Wild JM, et al. New developments in imaging idiopathic pulmonary fibrosis with hyperpolarized xenon magnetic resonance imaging. J Thorac Imaging 2019;34(2):136–50.

46. Kaushik SS, Freeman MS, Yoon SW, et al. Measuring diffusion limitation with a perfusion-limited gas: hyperpolarized 129Xe gas-transfer spectroscopy in patients with idiopathic pulmonary fibrosis. J Appl Physiol (1985) 2014;117(6):577–85.

47. Stewart NJ, Leung G, Norquay G, et al. Experimental validation of the hyperpolarized 129 Xe chemical shift saturation recovery technique in healthy volunteers and subjects with interstitial lung disease. Magn Reson Med 2015;74(1):196–207.

48. Stewart NJ, Horn FC, Norquay G, et al. Reproducibility of quantitative indices of lung function and microstructure from 129 Xe chemical shift saturation recovery (CSSR) MR spectroscopy. Magn Reson Med 2017;77(6):2107–13.

49. Wang Z, Robertson SH, Wang J, et al. Quantitative analysis of hyperpolarized 129 Xe gas transfer MRI. Med Phys 2017;44(6):2415–28.

50. He M, Driehuys B, Que LG, et al. Using hyperpolarized 129Xe MRI to quantify the pulmonary ventilation distribution. Acad Radiol 2016;23(12):1521–31.

51. Weatherly N, Stewart N, Norquay G, et al. Hyperpolarized 129Xe MR spectroscopy detects short-term changes in lung gas exchange efficiency in idiopathic pulmonary fibrosis. Proc Intl Soc Mag Reson Med 2018;26:0966.

52. Wang JM, Robertson SH, Wang Z, et al. Using hyperpolarized 129Xe MRI to quantify regional gas transfer in idiopathic pulmonary fibrosis. Thorax 2018;73(1):21–8.

53. Mummy DG, Bier EA, Wang Z, et al. Hyperpolarized 129Xe MRI and spectroscopy of gas-exchange abnormalities in nonspecific interstitial pneumonia. Radiology 2021;301(1):211–20.

54. Eaden J, Collier G, Norquay G, et al. S75 Hyperpolarised 129-xenon MRI in differentiating between fibrotic and inflammatory interstitial lung disease and assessing longitudinal change. Thorax 2021; 76:A46–7.

55. Roach DJ, Crémillieux Y, Fleck RJ, et al. Ultrashort echo-time magnetic resonance imaging is a

sensitive method for the evaluation of early cystic fibrosis lung disease. Ann Am Thorac Soc 2016; 13(11):1923–31.

56. Mussell GT, Marshall H, Smith LJ, et al. Xenon ventilation MRI in difficult asthma: initial experience in a clinical setting. ERJ Open Res 2021;7(3):00785–2020.

57. McMahon CJ, Dodd JD, Hill C, et al. Hyperpolarized 3helium magnetic resonance ventilation imaging of the lung in cystic fibrosis: comparison with high resolution CT and spirometry. Eur Radiol 2006;16(11): 2483–90.

58. Donnelly LF, MacFall JR, McAdams HP, et al. Cystic fibrosis: combined hyperpolarized 3He-enhanced and conventional proton MR imaging in the lung: -preliminary observations. Radiology 1999;212(3):885–9.

59. Thomen RP, Walkup LL, Roach DJ, et al. Hyperpolarized 129Xe for investigation of mild cystic fibrosis lung disease in pediatric patients. J Cyst Fibros 2017;16(2):275–82.

60. Mentore K, Froh DK, de Lange EE, et al. Hyperpolarized HHe 3 MRI of the lung in cystic fibrosis: assessment at baseline and after bronchodilator and airway clearance treatment. Acad Radiol 2005; 12(11):1423–9.

61. Altes TA, Johnson M, Fidler M, et al. Use of hyperpolarized helium-3 MRI to assess response to ivacaftor treatment in patients with cystic fibrosis. J Cyst Fibros 2017;16(2):267–74.

62. Coronaviridae Study Group of the International Committee on Taxonomy of Viruses. The species severe acute respiratory syndrome-related coronavirus: classifying 2019-nCoV and naming it SARS-CoV-2. Nat Microbiol 2020;5(4):536–44.

63. Yoon SH, Lee KH, Kim JY, et al. Chest radiographic and CT findings of the 2019nNovel Coronavirus disease (COVID-19): analysis of nine patients treated in Korea. Korean J Radiol 2020;21(4):494–500.

64. Ates OF, Taydas O, Dheir H. Thorax magnetic resonance imaging findings in patients with coronavirus disease (COVID-19). Acad Radiol 2020;27(10): 1373–8.

65. Doykov I, Hällqvist J, Gilmour KC, et al. The long tail of Covid-19': the detection of a prolonged inflammatory response after a SARS-CoV-2 infection in asymptomatic and mildly affected patients. F1000Res 2020;9:1349.

66. Han X, Fan Y, Alwalid O, et al. Six-month follow-up chest CT findings after severe COVID-19 pneumonia. Radiology 2021;299(1):E177–86.

67. Li H, Zhao X, Wang Y, et al. Damaged lung gas exchange function of discharged COVID-19 patients detected by hyperpolarized 129Xe MRI. Sci Adv 2021;7(1):eabc8180.

68. Hon KL, Leung CW, Cheng WT, et al. Clinical presentations and outcome of severe acute respiratory syndrome in children. Lancet 2003;361(9370): 1701–3.

69. Grist JT, Chen M, Collier GJ, et al. Hyperpolarized 129Xe MRI abnormalities in dyspneic patients 3 months after COVID-19 pneumonia: preliminary results. Radiology 2021;301(1):E353–60.

Artificial Intelligence in the Imaging of Diffuse Lung Disease

Jessica Chan, MD[a], William F. Auffermann, MD, PhD[b],*

KEYWORDS

- Artificial intelligence • Interstitial lung disease • Computed tomography • Deep learning
- Convolutional neural networks

KEY POINTS

- Diffuse lung diseases are a heterogeneous group of disorders which can be difficult to differentiate by imaging using traditional methods of evaluation.
- The overlap between various disorders results in difficulty when medical professionals attempt to interpret images.
- Artificial intelligence offers new tools for the evaluation and quantification of imaging of patients with diffuse lung disease.

INTRODUCTION

Health-care providers use imaging to characterize, quantify, and monitor diseases. There have been many changes in the way in which radiologists interact with images during the past several decades. Radiologists have transitioned from viewing medical images on film to a more interactive evaluation on computerized radiology workstations. Yet to date, our use of computers to quantitatively evaluate medical images has been limited. Radiologists may make size and Hounsfield unit measurements on computer but further quantitative evaluation of radiology images is generally not currently the norm. In addition, when quantitative evaluation of radiology images does occur, this has historically has been done by designing specific algorithms to explicitly evaluate for certain predefined patterns in the images. This approach is problematic for diseases with less well-defined imaging appearances. This is especially true for diffuse lung disease, which includes many abnormalities of the lungs,[1] notably interstitial lung diseases (ILD).

Radiologic evaluation of interstitial lung disease is challenging given relatively nonspecific image findings and the overlap of findings for different disorders. In addition, human evaluation of computed tomography (CT) and magnetic resonance images are limited by interobserver variability. For example, a study examined 43 radiologists rating the presence of honeycombing on 80 CT images. The agreement of radiologists with the reference standard as measured by Cohen's kappa coefficient ranged from 0.40 to 0.58, corresponding to an overall moderate agreement.[2] More quantifiable and automated methods for characterization of interstitial lung disease would be helpful.

There has been recent interest in quantitative methods for the evaluation of chest CTs. These quantitative methods may use measures such as threshold-based measures,[3] first-order statistics including kurtosis and skew,[4] texture analysis,[5] and more complex image features.[6] Although such

Disclosures: None.
a Department of Radiology and Imaging Sciences, University of Utah Health, 30 North 1900 East, Room # 1A71, Salt Lake City, UT 84132, USA; b Interim Section Chief of Cardiothoracic Imaging, Department of Radiology and Imaging Sciences, University of Utah School of Medicine, University of Utah Health, 30 North 1900 East, Room # 1A71, Salt Lake City, UT 84132, USA
* Corresponding author.
E-mail address: william.auffermann@hsc.utah.edu

Radiol Clin N Am 60 (2022) 1033–1040
https://doi.org/10.1016/j.rcl.2022.06.014
0033-8389/22/© 2022 Elsevier Inc. All rights reserved.

radiologic.theclinics.com

quantitative methods are very useful, they suffer from the disadvantage that they often require predefined image features for the analysis. That is, the computer algorithm needs to be told what features to look for. As a consequence, one will find what they are looking for but not find what they are not looking for. This limitation may be more severe than it initially appears. Computers are capable of analyzing multidimensional data sets where the number of variables is well beyond the capacity for humans to understand. Consequently, using human-derived features will restrict a computer to operate in a limited problem space, and not take full advantage of its ability to work with large sets of variables and complex image features.

It would be helpful to have a class of computer algorithms that are able to define their own features for analysis, based on the characteristics of the data. Newer artificial intelligence (AI) algorithms are able do this with improving accuracy. The goals of this article are to provide a brief review of AI, their use for analysis of ILD, recent advances in the field, and challenging areas where further research is needed.

ARTIFICIAL INTELLIGENCE OVERVIEW

AI has been defined as "The capacity of computers or other machines to exhibit or simulate intelligent behavior."[7] AI basically refers to computer algorithms that are able to perform tasks that historically only a human could perform. Older variants of AI algorithms depended on human beings to hard code the AI's rules of operation and did not learn from the data on their own. Such algorithms had limited success in their application to complex medical data. Later iterations of AI algorithms called machine learning algorithms were able to learn on their own but only from subsets of the data and not from the full data set. For older machine learning algorithms, humans needed to specify features of interest in the data for subsequent AI analysis. An example of such an algorithm may be an AI algorithm attempting to estimate the probability of malignancy in a nodule based on the nodule size, contour, and attenuation. Even though these algorithms were able to learn, they could only learn based on the predefined features they were provided.[8]

Newer AI algorithms are able to learn directly from the data. In medical imaging, the more popular methods involve deep learning (DL) and convolutional neural networks (CNNs). DL has been defined as "Machine learning based on artificial neural networks in which multiple layers of processing are used to extract progressively higher level features from data."[9] Such algorithms often have multiple

levels of processing, allowing for improved feature extraction and characterization.[10]

CNNs are modeled on the nervous system. There are multiple data and computational units (neurons) and the flow from one neuron to another is mediated by data transfer links (axons). An AI algorithm is run several times for a training dataset and the importance of data associated with each axon is adjusted to minimize the error of algorithm output (such as disease classification). Once an algorithm is trained, it may be tested on an independent dataset to estimate the accuracy of classification. DL algorithms utilizing CNNs have become an important class of AI algorithms in medical image processing.[10]

DETECTION

Interstitial lung disease is a broad category of diseases with diverse etiologies presenting in patients of divergent demographics. The imaging appearance of these different ILDs can both overlap and be strikingly different such as chronic hypersensitivity pneumonitis, idiopathic pulmonary fibrosis (IPF), and pulmonary sarcoidosis. Detection of some ILDs are not challenging for the radiologist, such as chronic obstructive pulmonary disease (COPD). Many ILDs, especially early in their disease course, can be difficult to detect from other non-ILD pulmonary pathologic conditions, such as infection, or subpleural subsegmental atelectasis. These imaging characteristics of ILD make the development of algorithms that can identify ILD without contextual clinical information a challenging task. Some AI algorithms have been developed to answer narrower clinical questions related to the detection of ILD, such as "Are there interstitial lung abnormalities (ILAs) on this CT chest examination of a patient with risk factors for ILAs?" Other commercially available DL tools have been developed to detect, segment, and characterize lung texture. Interestingly, some of the most salient imaging features of ILD identified by DL models are not detectable to the human imager. These discussion points are elaborated on below.

ILAs-nondependent lung abnormalities, such as reticular abnormalities, traction bronchiectasis, or ground glass opacities, involving 5% or greater of the lung are an emerging area of research with promising clinical significance.[11] ILAs are more common in older patients and smokers and are associated with poor clinical outcomes and increased mortality, even in the absence of ILD.[12] Furthermore, ILAs can be a precursor to the development of IPF or acute interstitial pneumonia (AIP).[11] Using DL algorithms to detect ILAs on CT is a hot topic of research. A recent study explored the use of an ensemble of 7 deep CNNs with 2-dimensional (2D), 2.5 dimensional, and 3-dimensional (3D) architectures, to detect ILAs on chest CT examinations from the COPDGene study.[13] The authors tailored features of the algorithm to detect ILAs, such as the use of relatively small kernels in the convolutional layers to prevent the inclusion of nonlocalized texture patterns because ILAs involve only a small part of the lung.[13] The algorithm was able to detect the presence of ILAs with a sensitivity of 91% and a specificity of 98%. ILAs are a rich area for future AI research, particularly in determining which ILAs are predictive of poor clinical outcome or the development of IPF or AIP.

Computer-Aided Lung Informatics for Pathology Evaluation and Rating (CALIPER) is a versatile commercially available DL tool that can detect, segment, and characterize parenchymal texture patterns. CALIPER uses both supervised and unsupervised DL approaches and was developed with pathologic correlates from the Lung Tissue Research Consortium.[14,15] Although the tool was developed at the Mayo Clinic, it is now licensed as Lung Texture Analysis (Imbio, Minneapolis, Minnesota, USA). The software divides the lung into 15 × 15 × 15 voxel VOIs, for which histogram-based analysis is performed, and a DL approach is used to characterize each volume of interest (VOI) as: normal, ground glass, low attenuation, honeycombing, or reticular.[6] This process is repeated until the entire lung is segmented and characterized. CALIPER has been used in numerous research studies exploring quantitative analysis of ILD.

One of the novel advantages of DL over feature engineering or radiomics is the model's freedom to identify imaging biomarkers not detectable by the human eye, which may offer better assessment of ILDs. One such model derived feature "vessel related structures" quantitation of pulmonary vasculature and perivascular fibrosis. This feature has been shown to correlate well with pulmonary function test (PFT) variables, differentiate usual interstitial pneumonia (UIP) CT pattern in IPF from UIP CT pattern in connective tissue disease, and is an independent marker of prognosis for various forms of ILD.[16–19] Ultimately, however, the greatest clinical value of DL applications in ILD imaging may not be detection, but instead characterization, prognosis, and accurate assessment of the extent of disease, for these applications guide treatment management.

CHARACTERIZATION

Characterization of ILD is an area fraught with difficulty. One reason is that it is difficult to confidently establish a diagnosis using current technology and criteria. There can be substantial disagreement about the ILD diagnosis among radiologists. A recent study showed that for CT examinations with findings of ILD, 41% of CTs read by nonacademic radiologists did not report a specific diagnosis, whereas second-opinion reports did not provide a specific diagnoses in 7%.[20] In addition, the clinical-consensus diagnosis was concordant with the academic radiologist diagnosis in 85% of cases but concordant with the initial interpretation in only 44% of cases.[20] There is also often discordance between the radiological read, pathology read, and multidisciplinary discussion (MDD) consensus. For example, a recent study showed that for 41.9% of patients with a diagnosis before MDD, the MDD changed the diagnosis; for 79.5% of patients without a diagnosis before MDD, MDD provided a diagnosis when the referring physician did not.[21]

These examples of discordant diagnoses show the need for improved interpretation. Not all radiology groups have chest-trained radiologists. Such groups may be ill equipped to provide subspecialized interpretations. In such instances, AI may be particularly useful. AI algorithms have been applied to CT datasets for the characterization of ILD with increasing success. Earlier work in application of AI to classification of ILD used a machine learning approach, requiring manual feature selection before attempted classification. One example is a study that examined using Fourier analysis, modeling the lung using sinusoidal waves, to characterize interstitial lung disease.[22] Subsequent attempts to move away from human-selected features included using support vector machines.[23] More recently, CNNs and DL have been used for the classification of interstitial lung disease. AI has been used to classify the types of interstitial abnormalities present. A recent article examined using CNNs and DL methods to classify regions of lung as having ground-glass opacity, consolidation, reticular opacity, emphysema, and honeycombing; with up to 95% accuracy.[24]

AI has also been used to provide an overall classification of the type of interstitial lung disease present on a CT. An article by Christe and colleagues[25] reported that their CNN algorithms were able to correctly specify the type of interstitial lung disease with an accuracy of 81%. Another article by Shaish and colleagues[26] used a CNN to identify CT scans with UIP and probable UIP pattern lung disease with a sensitivity and specificity of 74% and 58%, respectively.

QUANTIFICATION/SEGMENTATION

The task of segmenting normal or abnormal anatomy within medical images is a common application of DL. Similarly, CNNs have had great success in segmenting abnormal lung parenchyma in the setting of diffuse or interstitial lung disease. Accurate segmentation is the foundation for characterization of the type of abnormal lung parenchyma and broader classification of the CT-pattern of ILD. Furthermore, accurate segmentation is critical to reproducibly determining the extent of disease and following disease progression on serial CT chest examinations.

DL models have outperformed other quantitative methods of segmenting the lung in ILD. For example, researchers compared a stacked 2D U-Net DL model to a density threshold-based method, using a manually annotated dataset of CT chest images from 617 patients with organizing pneumonia, nonspecific interstitial pneumonia, and UIP CT-patterns of ILD.[27] The segmentation performance of the DL model was statistically significantly better than that of the threshold-based method, and was in excellent agreement with the gold standard, yielding a Dice similarly coefficient greater than 98%. The lung texture abnormalities of ILD, such reticular opacities, ground glass opacities, and honeycombing, are readily apparent on axial CT chest images and do not typically require visualization with coronal or sagittal reformats. As such, it is unsurprising that 2D models have generally performed as well as 3D models in segmenting ILD because interslice content plays little role in identifying areas of lung texture abnormality in ILD. For example, a recent study, validated on an external dataset, compared 2D and 3D U-Net model segmentation of normal lung parenchyma from abnormal lung parenchyma, on CT chest examinations of patients with ILD, emphysema, and lung cancer among other pulmonary diseases.[28] The researchers found excellent model performance exceeding 98% for both the 2D and 3D models, without statistical significance between the models' performance.

Quantitative segmentation of the abnormal portions of the lung allows for precise determination of extent of disease. Imaging extent of disease is an important clinical marker in ILD because a patient's symptoms and even PFTs can be affected by non-ILD pathologic conditions such as a superimposed infection or development of pulmonary hypertension. In systemic sclerosis, for example, studies have found that imaging extent of disease is an independent predictor of outcome and mortality.[29,30] A recent study, used a DL model, specifically AlexNet, to segment and quantify the extent of ILD on CT chest images of patients with systemic sclerosis, trained on an annotated dataset.[31] The model's approach was to identify areas of

lung abnormality, not to characterize the abnormality as ground glass or reticular opacities. The model was able to segment the lung equally well to a radiologist; furthermore, the quantitative extent of disease showed good correlation with PFT parameters.

Imaging findings of disease progression is an important consideration in the treatment management of ILDs, especially with the development of effective and expensive antifibrotic medications. As fibrotic-type ILDs progress, more areas of the lung may be affected but also the volume of the affected areas of the lung decrease. This presents a challenge to DL models that only follow the total volume of abnormal lung parenchyma on serial CT chest examinations. One recent study overcame this challenge by the use of elastic registration combined with a DL model on CT chest examinations of patients with systemic sclerosis to provide a more accurate longitudinal assessment of extent of ILD.[32] This model was able to predict a morphologic progression of disease with an accuracy of 80%. Another study found that changes in abnormal lung pattern, as determined by CALIPER on serial CT chest examinations of patients with systemic sclerosis, was not accurate in predicting disease progression but total lung volume did predict progression.[33] Another research group also found that serial total lung volumes as determined by a U-net based DL model (CT Pulmo Auto Results, IntelliSpace Portal ISP11.1, Philips Healthcare) was an accurate imaging biomarker of disease progression in patients of various forms of ILD.[34] Furthermore, the researchers found that an annual total lung volume loss of 7.9% or greater was associated with a higher risk of major adverse event, and that patients with IPF had on average a volume loss of 156 mL per year, whereas those with non-IPF ILD had only a loss of 51 mL. Overall, following total lung volumes, as determined by a DL model, or a more sophisticated approach by combining elastic-regression techniques with a DL model, are currently the most accurate methods of determining imaging disease progression on serial CT chest examinations.

ARTIFICIAL INTELLIGENCE USE CASE

What follows in this section is an example of how current AI technology may be used to facilitate the image evaluation and care of a patient with ILD.

A CT chest to evaluate for ILD is ordered by a pulmonologist for a 70-year-old man with shortness of breath for the past 6 months. A recent chest radiograph (CXR) showed findings suspicious for ILD. The CT chest without contrast is performed per protocol, including image reconstruction kernels and slice thickness, specified by a commercially available software package, which identifies, segments, and characterizes ILD. The software uses a CNN algorithm trained on a large multi-institutional database consisting of thousands of CT chest examinations manually segmented and labeled with an expert consensus derived ILD CT pattern. The completed examination is sent to a server where the algorithm is run, and a summary image of the results is sent back to the institution's Picture Archiving and Communication System within an hour. The summary image shows the distribution of abnormal lung parenchyma and provides a differential diagnosis and probability of these diagnoses.

A radiologist opens the CT chest examination and identifies features on the inspiratory and expiratory views that lead to a differential diagnosis of UIP CT pattern, chronic hypersensitivity pneumonitis, and nonspecific interstitial pneumonia CT pattern. The summary image identifies similar areas of lung parenchymal abnormality, and yields a differential diagnosis favoring UIP CT pattern. After receiving the radiologist's report, the pulmonologist and patient discuss the results, along with recent PFT results. Antifibrotic medications are prescribed. Every 6 months, the pulmonologist has a follow-up visit with the patient and repeat PFTs and a CT chest are performed. The patient's PFT values and CT chest examination findings remain stable for 4 years. However, in the fifth year of treatment, the extent of abnormal lung parenchyma, as determined by the commercially available software, decreases. As the radiologist reviews the images and reads the report, it is determined that there has been volume loss in the areas of abnormal lung, compatible with disease progression. PFT values however remain unchanged and there is no change in treatment. On the subsequently obtain CT chest examination, there are been further volume loss and key PFT values have just begun to decrease. The patient is then referred for enrollment in a clinical trial of an experimental medicine for treating IPF, during which repeat CT chest examinations are obtained and key quantitative findings from the summary image are followed to analyze treatment efficacy.

Challenges to the Use of Artificial Intelligence for Diffuse Lung Disease (DLD)

The number of artificial intelligence algorithms available

AI algorithms have been become more advanced and efficient. There is a proliferation of new algorithms capable of performing an ever-increasing number of tasks. PubMed was searched for the term "artificial intelligence" on 1/02/2022, and the resulting number of search results by year is shown in **Fig. 1**. Based on this search, the number of AI publications between 2000 and the end of 2021 increased from 1,248 to 25,994, a near 20-fold increase. The number of AI algorithms in existence has probably undergone a similar increase in number. This dramatic increase in AI algorithms is beneficial in that there are more AI algorithms for a multitude of clinical questions and purposes. However, it may be difficult for a health-care organization to decide which is the best AI algorithms for a given task. In order to select the best algorithm, it is helpful to understand how the algorithm is designed and have a standardized method for testing algorithms.

Proprietary algorithms

A subset of AI algorithms has their computer code publicly available on code repositories such as GitHub (https://github.com/). However, many AI algorithms are proprietary. One may be able to use the compiled program to process a dataset but not have access to the computer code in which the algorithm was written. Consequently, the user does not have direct knowledge regarding the way in which the data is processed. This can lead to difficulties in comparing algorithms and understanding which algorithm is the best for a particular application. In addition, software algorithms may undergo frequent upgrades that may alter performance. Therefore, even if there is data available for AI product A-version-1 and B-version-1, we may not know how product A-version-2 compares to B-version-1. The challenge of dealing with multiple variations of different proprietary algorithms may be addressed by adequate testing on standardized data sets.

Lack of a standardized method for validation

Earlier study in the use of AI to characterize ILD was applied to smaller nonpublic datasets. Consequently, it was difficult to compare these results across different studies. There is an increasing effort to use larger publicly available datasets for AI validation for numerous application. There are several radiologic image repositories that include CheXpert, a database with 224,316 chest radiographs of 65,240 patients at the time this article was written.[35] However, most of these databases are not specific to interstitial lung disease. Recently, new publicly accessible datasets for interstitial lung disease have become available. One such database is the University Hospitals of Geneva (HUG) ILD dataset.[36] The HUG ILD dataset includes CTs from 128 patients with 13

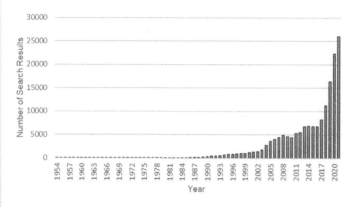

Fig. 1. AI publications per year based on PubMed Search.

different types of histologically confirmed ILD. At the time this article was written, this data has been used by several AI researchers and their article has been cited at least 22 times. Another publicly available database is the National Institutes of Health Lung Tissue Research Consortium Database.[37] Some consider it advisable that AI algorithms undergo testing on such publicly available datasets before clinical implementation, the results can be more readily compared.

Artificial intelligence generalization

A significant concern for AI in is the generalizability of an AI algorithm, trained on one dataset, then applied to other independent datasets. Generalization issues are a concern for AI as a whole,[38] and tends to be a greater issue for smaller datasets, as may be seen in the case of radiology studies where data sets are smaller. Consider that some AI research outside the medical domain may have image databases containing millions of images. For example, the ImageNet Large Scale Visual Recognition Challenge 2017 database contains over one million images (https://image-net.org/challenges/LSVRC/2017/). Now consider interstitial lung disease and the HUG database, one of the few public ILD databases, contains only 128 CT studies.[36] Lack of generalizability results in AI algorithms that may perform well on the datasets they are trained and initially tested on but perform poorly when applied to new data from different sources. This is more problematic for small datasets as is seen in radiology and medicine. The development of new, large, and heterogeneous datasets will likely contribute positively to the development of AI algorithms and improved generalization.

LEARNING MORE ABOUT ARTIFICIAL INTELLIGENCE

This article provides a brief overview of AI and its relation to radiology. There are several helpful review articles regarding AI and the applications of AI in radiology in general.[39–41] Radiologists interested in learning about how to become in more involved with AI in radiology may find the article by Richardson and colleagues[42] helpful. For a more comprehensive in-depth review of AI algorithms, the book by Goodfellow and colleagues may be helpful.[43]

SUMMARY

The practice of medicine has evolved rapidly during the past several years. The application of computer and AI technologies has changed the way medicine is practiced, particularly in radiology. AI is taking an increasingly important role in the evaluation of medical images. To date, AI algorithms have been used to help radiologists do their jobs, not take those jobs away. Given the complexity of medical image interpretation, computers will likely provide an important increasingly important role but will probably not supplant humans entirely.

CLINICS CARE POINTS

- The application of computer and AI technologies have changed the way medicine is practiced, particularly in radiology.
- AI is taking an increasingly important role in evaluation of medical images.
- Given the complexity of medical image interpretation, computers will likely provide an important increasingly important role, but will probably not supplant humans entirely.

REFERENCES

1. Hansell DM. Classification of diffuse lung diseases: why and how. Radiology 2013;268(3):628–40.
2. Watadani T, Sakai F, Johkoh T, et al. Interobserver variability in the CT assessment of honeycombing in the lungs. Radiology 2013;266(3):936–44.

3. Crossley D, Renton M, Khan M, et al. CT densitometry in emphysema: a systematic review of its clinical utility. Int J Chron Obstruct Pulmon Dis 2018; 13:547–63.

4. Kim GB, Jung KH, Lee Y, et al. Comparison of shallow and deep learning methods on classifying the regional pattern of diffuse lung disease. J Digit Imaging 2018;31:415–24.

5. Mahon RN, Hugo GD, Weiss E. Repeatability of texture features derived from magnetic resonance and computed tomography imaging and use in predictive models for non-small cell lung cancer outcome. Phys Med Biol 2018;31:415–24.

6. Chen A, Karwoski RA, Gierada DS, et al. Quantitative CT analysis of diffuse lung disease. Radiographics 2020;40(1):28–43.

7. Dictionary OE. Artificial intelligence, n. In: Oxford English dictionary. Oxford University Press Online Dictionary; 2017. Accessed 27 July 2022.

8. Suzuki K. Overview of deep learning in medical imaging. Radiological Phys Technol 2017;10(3): 257–73.

9. Oxford-English-Dictionary. deep learning n. In. Oxford English Dictionary 2022. Online Dictionary. Available at: www.oed.com. Accessed January 4,2022.

10. LeCun Y, Bengio Y, Hinton G. Deep learning. Nature 2015;521:436.

11. Hata A, Schiebler ML, Lynch DA, et al. Interstitial lung abnormalities: state of the art. Radiology 2021;301(1):19–34.

12. Putman RK, Hatabu H, Araki T, et al. Association between interstitial lung abnormalities and all-cause mortality. JAMA 2016;315(7):672–81.

13. Bermejo-Peláez D, Ash SY, Washko GR, et al. Classification of interstitial lung abnormality patterns with an ensemble of deep convolutional neural networks. Scientific Rep 2020;10(1):338.

14. Bartholmai BJ, Raghunath S, Karwoski RA, et al. Quantitative computed tomography imaging of interstitial lung diseases. J Thorac Imaging 2013;28(5): 298–307.

15. Jankharia BG, Angirish BA. Computer-Aided quantitative analysis in interstitial lung diseases - A pictorial review using CALIPER. Lung India 2021;38(2): 161–7.

16. Chung JH, Adegunsoye A, Cannon B, et al. Differentiation of Idiopathic pulmonary fibrosis from connective tissue disease-related interstitial lung disease using quantitative imaging. J Clin Med 2021; 10(12):2663.

17. Chung JH, Adegunsoye A, Oldham JM, et al. Vessel-related structures predict UIP pathology in those with a non-IPF pattern on CT. Eur Radiol 2021;31(10):7295–302.

18. Jacob J, Bartholmai BJ, Rajagopalan S, et al. Predicting outcomes in idiopathic pulmonary fibrosis using automated computed tomographic analysis. Am J Respir Crit Care Med 2018;198(6):767–76.

19. Jacob J, Bartholmai BJ, Rajagopalan S, et al. Mortality prediction in idiopathic pulmonary fibrosis: evaluation of computer-based CT analysis with conventional severity measures. Eur Respir J 2017; 49(1):1601011.

20. Filev PD, Little BP, Duong PT. Second-opinion reads in interstitial lung disease imaging: added value of subspecialty interpretation. J Am Coll Radiol 2020; 17(6):786–90.

21. De Sadeleer LJ, Meert C, Yserbyt J, et al. Diagnostic ability of a dynamic multidisciplinary discussion in interstitial lung diseases: a retrospective observational study of 938 cases. Chest 2018;153(6): 1416–23.

22. Monnier-Cholley L, MacMahon H, Katsuragawa S, et al. Computerized analysis of interstitial infiltrates on chest radiographs: a new scheme based on geometric pattern features and Fourier analysis. Acad Radiol 1995;2(6):455–62.

23. Xu Y, van Beek EJ, Hwanjo Y, et al. Computer-aided classification of interstitial lung diseases via MDCT: 3D adaptive multiple feature method (3D AMFM). Acad Radiol 2006;13(8):969–78.

24. Kim GB, Jung K-H, Lee Y, et al. Comparison of shallow and deep learning methods on classifying the regional pattern of diffuse lung disease. J Digit Imaging 2018;31(4):415–24.

25. Christe A, Peters AA, Drakopoulos D, et al. Computer-aided diagnosis of pulmonary fibrosis using deep learning and CT images. Invest Radiol 2019; 54(10):627–32.

26. Shaish H, Ahmed FS, Lederer D, et al. Deep learning of computed tomography virtual wedge resection for prediction of histologic usual interstitial pneumonitis. Ann Am Thorac Soc 2020;18(1):51–9.

27. Park B, Park H, Lee SM, et al. Lung segmentation on HRCT and volumetric CT for diffuse interstitial lung disease using deep convolutional neural networks. J Digit Imaging 2019;32(6):1019–26.

28. Yoo SJ, Yoon SH, Lee JH, et al. Automated lung segmentation on chest computed tomography images with extensive lung parenchymal abnormalities using a deep neural network. Korean J Radiol 2021; 22(3):476–88.

29. Goh NS, Desai SR, Veeraraghavan S, et al. Interstitial lung disease in systemic sclerosis: a simple staging system. Am J Respir Crit Care Med 2008; 177(11):1248–54.

30. Moore OA, Goh N, Corte T, et al. Extent of disease on high-resolution computed tomography lung is a predictor of decline and mortality in systemic sclerosis-related interstitial lung disease. Rheumatology (Oxford) 2013;52(1):155–60.

31. Chassagnon G, Vakalopoulou M, Régent A, et al. Deep learning-based approach for automated

assessment of interstitial lung disease in systemic sclerosis on CT images. Radiol Artif Intell 2020; 2(4):e190006.

32. Chassagnon G, Vakalopoulou M, Régent A, et al. Elastic Registration-driven Deep Learning for Longitudinal Assessment of Systemic Sclerosis Interstitial Lung Disease at CT. Radiology 2021;298(1):189–98.

33. Occhipinti M, Bosello S, Sisti LG, et al. Quantitative and semi-quantitative computed tomography analysis of interstitial lung disease associated with systemic sclerosis: a longitudinal evaluation of pulmonary parenchyma and vessels. PLoS One 2019;14(3):e0213444.

34. Si-Mohamed SA, Nasser M, Colevray M, et al. Automatic quantitative computed tomography measurement of longitudinal lung volume loss in interstitial lung diseases. Eur Radiol 2018;31:415–24.

35. Irvin J, Rajpurkar P, Ko M, et al. CheXpert: a large chest radiograph dataset with uncertainty labels and expert comparison. Proceedings of the AAAI Conference on Artificial Intelligence. 2019;33(01): 590-597. Honolulu, Hawaii USA — January 27– February 1, 2019.

36. Depeursinge A, Vargas A, Platon A, et al. Building a reference multimedia database for interstitial lung diseases. Comput Med Imaging Graph 2012;36(3): 227–38.

37. NIH. Lung tissue research Consortium. National Institutes of Health; 2022. Available at: https://www.nhlbi.nih.gov/science/lung-tissue-research-consortium-ltrc. Accessed 1/02/2022.

38. Barbiero P, Squillero G, Tonda A. Modeling generalization in machine learning: a methodological and computational study. arXiv 2018;31:415–24.

39. McBee MP, Awan OA, Colucci AT, et al. Deep learning in radiology. Acad Radiol 2018;31:415–24.

40. Chartrand G, Cheng PM, Vorontsov E, et al. Deep learning: a primer for radiologists. RadioGraphics 2017;37(7):2113–31.

41. Erickson BJ, Korfiatis P, Akkus Z, et al. Machine learning for medical imaging. Radiographics 2017; 37(2):505–15.

42. Richardson ML, Adams SJ, Agarwal A, et al. Review of artificial intelligence training tools and courses for radiologists. Acad Radiol 2021;28(9):1238–52.

43. Goodfellow I, Bengio Y, Courville A. Deep learning. Cambridge (MA): The MIT Press; 2016.

UNITED STATES POSTAL SERVICE ®

Statement of Ownership, Management, and Circulation
(All Periodicals Publications Except Requester Publications)

1. Publication Title	2. Publication Number	3. Filing Date
RADIOLOGIC CLINICS OF NORTH AMERICA	596 – 510	9/18/2022

4. Issue Frequency	5. Number of Issues Published Annually	6. Annual Subscription Price
JAN, MAR, MAY, JUL, SEP, NOV	6	$529.00

7. Complete Mailing Address of Known Office of Publication (Not printer) (Street, city, county, state, and ZIP+4®)

ELSEVIER INC.
230 Park Avenue, Suite 800
New York, NY 10169

Contact Person
Malathi Samayan
Telephone (Include area code)
91-44-4299-4507

8. Complete Mailing Address of Headquarters or General Business Office of Publisher (Not printer)

ELSEVIER INC.
230 Park Avenue, Suite 800
New York, NY 10169

9. Full Names and Complete Mailing Addresses of Publisher, Editor, and Managing Editor (Do not leave blank)

Publisher (Name and complete mailing address)

DOLORES MELONI, ELSEVIER INC.
1600 JOHN F KENNEDY BLVD. SUITE 1800
PHILADELPHIA, PA 19103-2899

Editor (Name and complete mailing address)

JOHN VASSALLO, ELSEVIER INC.
1600 JOHN F KENNEDY BLVD. SUITE 1800
PHILADELPHIA, PA 19103-2899

Managing Editor (Name and complete mailing address)

PATRICK MANLEY, ELSEVIER INC.
1600 JOHN F KENNEDY BLVD. SUITE 1800
PHILADELPHIA, PA 19103-2899

10. Owner (Do not leave blank. If the publication is owned by a corporation, give the name and address of the corporation immediately followed by the names and addresses of all stockholders owning or holding 1 percent or more of the total amount of stock. If not owned by a corporation, give the names and addresses of the individual owners. If owned by a partnership or other unincorporated firm, give its name and address as well as those of each individual owner. If the publication is published by a nonprofit organization, give its name and address.)

Full Name	Complete Mailing Address
WHOLLY OWNED SUBSIDIARY OF REED/ELSEVIER, US HOLDINGS	1600 JOHN F KENNEDY BLVD. SUITE 1800 PHILADELPHIA, PA 19103-2899

11. Known Bondholders, Mortgagees, and Other Security Holders Owning or Holding 1 Percent or More of Total Amount of Bonds, Mortgages, or Other Securities. If none, check box ► ☐ None

Full Name	Complete Mailing Address
N/A	

12. Tax Status (For completion by nonprofit organizations authorized to mail at nonprofit rates) (Check one)
The purpose, function, and nonprofit status of this organization and the exempt status for federal income tax purposes:
☒ Has Not Changed During Preceding 12 Months
☐ Has Changed During Preceding 12 Months (Publisher must submit explanation of change with this statement)

PS Form **3526**, July 2014 [Page 1 of 4 (see instructions page 4)] PSN: 7530-01-000-9931 PRIVACY NOTICE: See our privacy policy on www.usps.com.

13. Publication Title	14. Issue Date for Circulation Data Below
RADIOLOGIC CLINICS OF NORTH AMERICA	JULY 2022

15. Extent and Nature of Circulation			Average No. Copies Each Issue During Preceding 12 Months	No. Copies of Single Issue Published Nearest to Filing Date
a. Total Number of Copies (Net press run)			847	766
b. Paid Circulation (By Mail and Outside the Mail)	(1)	Mailed Outside-County Paid Subscriptions Stated on PS Form 3541 (Include paid distribution above nominal rate, advertiser's proof copies, and exchange copies)	592	548
	(2)	Mailed In-County Paid Subscriptions Stated on PS Form 3541 (Include paid distribution above nominal rate, advertiser's proof copies, and exchange copies)	0	0
	(3)	Paid Distribution Outside the Mails Including Sales Through Dealers and Carriers, Street Vendors, Counter Sales, and Other Paid Distribution Outside USPS®	198	179
	(4)	Paid Distribution by Other Classes of Mail Through the USPS (e.g., First-Class Mail®)	0	0
c. Total Paid Distribution (Sum of 15b (1), (2), (3), and (4))		►	790	727
d. Free or Nominal Rate Distribution (By Mail and Outside the Mail)	(1)	Free or Nominal Rate Outside-County Copies included on PS Form 3541	40	25
	(2)	Free or Nominal Rate In-County Copies Included on PS Form 3541	0	0
	(3)	Free or Nominal Rate Copies Mailed at Other Classes Through the USPS (e.g., First-Class Mail)	0	0
	(4)	Free or Nominal Rate Distribution Outside the Mail (Carriers or other means)	0	0
e. Total Free or Nominal Rate Distribution (Sum of 15d (1), (2), (3) and (4))		►	40	25
f. Total Distribution (Sum of 15c and 15e)		►	830	752
g. Copies not Distributed (See Instructions to Publishers #4 (page #3))		►	17	14
h. Total (Sum of 15f and g)		►	847	766
i. Percent Paid (15c divided by 15f times 100)		►	95.18%	96.67%

* If you are claiming electronic copies, go to line 16 on page 3. If you are not claiming electronic copies, skip to line 17 on page 3.

PS Form **3526**, July 2014 (Page 2 of 4)

16. Electronic Copy Circulation		Average No. Copies Each Issue During Preceding 12 Months	No. Copies of Single Issue Published Nearest to Filing Date
a. Paid Electronic Copies	►		
b. Total Paid Print Copies (Line 15c) + Paid Electronic Copies (Line 16a)	►		
c. Total Print Distribution (Line 15f) + Paid Electronic Copies (Line 16a)	►		
d. Percent Paid (Both Print & Electronic Copies) (16b divided by 16c × 100)	►		

☒ I certify that 50% of all my distributed copies (electronic and print) are paid above a nominal price.

17. Publication of Statement of Ownership

☒ If the publication is a general publication, publication of this statement is required. Will be printed ☐ Publication not required.

in the NOVEMBER 2022 issue of this publication.

18. Signature and Title of Editor, Publisher, Business Manager, or Owner	Date
Malathi Samayan - Distribution Controller *Malathi Samayan*	9/18/2022

I certify that all information furnished on this form is true and complete. I understand that anyone who furnishes false or misleading information on this form or who omits material or information requested on the form may be subject to criminal sanctions (including fines and imprisonment) and/or civil sanctions (including civil penalties).

PS Form **3526**, July 2014 (Page 3 of 4) PRIVACY NOTICE: See our privacy policy on www.usps.com.

Moving?

Make sure your subscription moves with you!

To notify us of your new address, find your **Clinics Account Number** (located on your mailing label above your name), and contact customer service at:

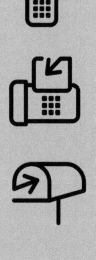

Email: journalscustomerservice-usa@elsevier.com

800-654-2452 (subscribers in the U.S. & Canada)
314-447-8871 (subscribers outside of the U.S. & Canada)

Fax number: 314-447-8029

Elsevier Health Sciences Division
Subscription Customer Service
3251 Riverport Lane
Maryland Heights, MO 63043

ELSEVIER

Printed and bound by CPI Group (UK) Ltd, Croydon, CR0 4YY

08/05/2025

01864723-0020